Obstetric Decision-Making and Simulation

Obstetric Decision-Making and Simulation

Edited by

Kirsty MacLennan
Manchester University Hospitals NHS Trust

Catherine Robinson
Manchester University Hospitals NHS Trust

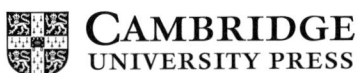
CAMBRIDGE
UNIVERSITY PRESS

CAMBRIDGE
UNIVERSITY PRESS

University Printing House, Cambridge CB2 8BS, United Kingdom

One Liberty Plaza, 20th Floor, New York, NY 10006, USA

477 Williamstown Road, Port Melbourne, VIC 3207, Australia

314–321, 3rd Floor, Plot 3, Splendor Forum, Jasola District Centre, New Delhi – 110025, India

79 Anson Road, #06-04/06, Singapore 079906

Cambridge University Press is part of the University of Cambridge.

It furthers the University's mission by disseminating knowledge in the pursuit of education, learning, and research at the highest international levels of excellence.

www.cambridge.org
Information on this title: www.cambridge.org/9781108296779
DOI: 10.1017/9781108296793

© Cambridge University Press 2019

First published 2019

Printed in the United Kingdom by TJ International Ltd. Padstow Cornwall

A catalogue record for this publication is available from the British Library.

Cambridge University Press has no responsibility for the persistence or accuracy of URLs for external or third-party internet websites referred to in this publication and does not guarantee that any content on such websites is, or will remain, accurate or appropriate.

Every effort has been made in preparing this book to provide accurate and up-to-date information that is in accord with accepted standards and practice at the time of publication. Although case histories are drawn from actual cases, every effort has been made to disguise the identities of the individuals involved. Nevertheless, the authors, editors, and publishers can make no warranties that the information contained herein is totally free from error, not least because clinical standards are constantly changing through research and regulation. The authors, editors, and publishers therefore disclaim all liability for direct or consequential damages resulting from the use of material contained in this book. Readers are strongly advised to pay careful attention to information provided by the manufacturer of any drugs or equipment that they plan to use.

Contents

Contributors

Omar Asghar
Cardiologist
Manchester Heart Centre
Manchester, UK

Charlotte Ash
Anaesthetist
Health Education North West
Speciality trainee, UK

Dougal Atkinson
Intensivist
Manchester University NHS Foundation Trust
Manchester, UK

Kailash Bhatia
Anaesthetist
Manchester University NHS Foundation Trust
Manchester, UK

Sophie Bishop
Anaesthetist
Manchester University NHS Foundation Trust
Manchester, UK

Samantha Bonner
Obstetrician
St Mary's Hospital,
Manchester, UK

Annemarie Brown
Emergency Medicine
Royal Liverpool and Broadgreen University
Hospitals Trust Liverpool, UK

John Butler
Emergency Medicine and Intensivist
Manchester University NHS Foundation
Trust Manchester, UK

Craig Carroll
Neuroanaesthetist
Salford Royal Foundation Trust
Salford, UK

Laura Coleman
Anaesthetist
Manchester University NHS Foundation Trust
Manchester, UK

Samantha Cox
Obstetrician
St Mary's Hospital
Manchester, UK

Susan Davies
Anaesthetist
Manchester University NHS Foundation
Trust Manchester, UK

Shuayb Elkhalifa
Immunologist
Manchester University NHS Foundation Trust
Manchester, UK

Joanne Gillham
Obstetrician
St Mary's Hospital
Manchester, UK

Katie Gott
Anaesthetist
Health Education North West
Speciality trainee, UK

James Hanison
Intensivist
Manchester University Hospitals Foundation Trust
Manchester, UK

Mark Hellaby
Simulation Education Network Manager
NHS Health Education England

Daniel Holsgrove
Neurosurgeon
Salford Royal Foundation Trust
Salford, UK

Lorna Howie
Anaesthetist
Manchester University NHS Foundation Trust
Manchester, UK

Jonathan Hurst
Neonatologist
Liverpool Women's Hospital
Liverpool, UK

Simon Hyde
Gynaecological Oncologist
Mercy Hospital for Women
Melbourne, Ausralia

Shahid Karim
Cardiologist
Manchester Heart Centre
Manchester, UK

Sophie Kimber-Craig
Anaesthetist
Royal Bolton Hospital
Bolton, UK

Stuart Knowles
Anaesthetist
Health Education North West
Speciality trainee, UK

Pavan Kochhar
Anaesthetist
Manchester University NHS Foundation Trust
Manchester, UK

Kenneth Ma
Gynaecologist
St Mary's Hospital
Manchester, UK

Kirsty MacLennan
Anaesthetist
Manchester University NHS Foundation Trust
Manchester, UK

Kim Macleod
Obstetrician
St Mary's Hospital
Manchester, UK

Anita Macnab
Cardiologist
Manchester University NHS Foundation Trust
Manchester, UK

Al May
Anaesthetist
Scottish Centre for Simulation
Glasgow, UK

Michael McGinlay
Anaesthetist
Health Education North West
Speciality trainee, UK

Richard McGuire
Anaesthetist
Health Education North West
Speciality trainee, UK

Michelle MacKintosh
Gynaecologist
St Mary's Hospital
Manchester, UK

Simon Mercer
Trauma Anaesthetist
Aintree University Hospital NHS Foundation Trust
Liverpool, UK

Yara Mohammed
Obstetrician
St Mary's Hospital
Manchester, UK

Kristen Moloney
Fellow in Gynaecologic Oncology
University of Melbourne Victoria, Australia

Suna Monaghan
Anaesthetist
Manchester University NHS Foundation Trust
Manchester, UK

Mark Murphy
Clinical Skills and Simulation
Training Manager
Royal Liverpool and Broadgreen
University Hospitals Trust
Liverpool, UK

Jenny Myers
Obstetrician
St Mary's Hospital
Manchester, UK

Debra Nestel
Professor of Simulation Education in Healthcare
Monash University for Health & Clinical Education,
Monash University
Professor of Surgical Education
Deparment of Surgery
University of Melbourne
Victoria, Australia

Owen O'Sullivan
Anaesthetist
UL Hospitals
Limerick, Ireland

Shane O'Sullivan
Anaesthetist
UL Hospitals
Limerick, Ireland

Andrew Parkes
Anaesthetist and Anaesthetic Allergy Expert
Manchester University NHS Foundation Trust
Manchester, UK

Ian Parkinson
Anaesthetist
Royal Lancaster Infirmary
Lancaster, UK

Samiksha Patel
Obstetrician
St Mary's Hospital Manchester, UK

Shimma Rehman
Obstetrician
St Mary's Hospital
Manchester, UK

Jonathan Schofield
Diabetologist
Manchester University NHS Foundation Trust
Manchester, UK

Emma Shawkat
Obstetrician
St Mary's Hospital
Manchester, UK

Cliff Shelton
Anaesthetist
Health Education North West
Speciality trainee, UK

David Simcox
Haematologist
Royal Liverpool University Hospital
Liverpool, UK

Louise Simcox
Obstetrician
St Mary's Hospital
Manchester, UK

Andrew F. Smith
Anaesthetist
Royal Lancaster Infirmary and Lancaster University
Lancaster, UK

Sharon Smith
Anaesthetist
Manchester University NHS Foundation Trust
Manchester, UK

Sarah Vause
Obstetrician
St Mary's Hospital
Manchester, UK

Melissa Whitworth
Obstetrician
St Mary's Hospital
Manchester, UK

Kathryn Wood
Anaesthetist
Sheffield Children's Hospital
Sheffield, UK

Stephanie Worton
Obstetrician
St Mary's Hospital
Manchester, UK

Foreword

Simulation is now firmly established within medical education at undergraduate and postgraduate levels. Increasingly multiprofessional team-based, simulation is being undertaken to improve the performance of the clinical workforce and thus clinical outcomes, in a variety of emergency situations. The maternity unit is an area with an abundance of emergency situations amenable to, and that would benefit from, team-based simulation training. The pros and cons of high- versus low-fidelity simulation are often debated, with each having its own relative merits. There is one message that is consistent – undertaking simulation training is better than none at all. Even for low-fidelity simulation barriers still exist; devising a 'good' scenario, who should be involved, what kit is required and what key elements of clinical practice need to be demonstrated in the scenario? For individual units and clinicians addressing even these simple aspects requires a significant amount of work. This publication, serving as a brilliant 'simulation recipe book' removes many of the practical barriers that can prevent the development of local simulation training. The clinical scenarios are all presented in a standardized format to ensure easy navigation.

Crucially the book also contains a powerful section about the role of Human Factors, providing an invaluable context to the simulation scenarios. Raising awareness and promoting Human Factors principles and practices in healthcare and embedding an understanding of Human Factors into clinical training are major commitments of the Human Factors in Healthcare Concordat. This was published in 2013 by the National Quality Board and signed by multiple stakeholders including the CQC and the GMC.

I congratulate all the contributors on putting together what I'm sure will become the 'go to' book on simulation in the maternity unit.

Dr Nuala Lucas
Consultant Anaesthetist, Northwick Park Hospital, UK

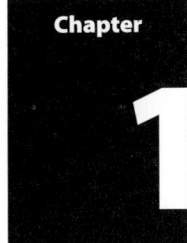

Setting the Scene for Simulation-Based Education

Debra Nestel, Kristen Moloney and Simon Hyde

I still can't believe that we did that difficult epidural scenario right before it happened for real. We knew exactly what to do. So very proud of our teamwork. [Delivery suite team participant in simulation]

Practising speculum insertion on the pelvic model built my confidence before doing my first Pap smear. Although it was different on my patient, I'd rehearsed the manoeuvres and knew how to handle the speculum. [Medical student]

We tried out the functionality of our new delivery suite before it was fully fitted out by simulating a whole day of clinical practice. Probably saved a lot of money but even more importantly uncovered some flaws in our processes from patient and staff perspectives. [Hospital manager]

Introduction

Whether healthcare simulation is providing an opportunity to develop teamwork skills, build individuals' confidence and psychomotor skills, or testing processes in a new facility, its impact can be profound. Simulation practice and research has matured sufficiently such that we need no longer focus on proving that it works, but on how to use it optimally and efficiently. The question is: how can we use simulation to support students and clinicians in developing safer practices and to design safer healthcare systems? The first chapter of an edited book is written with the intent of setting the scene. It is both a privilege and a responsibility to offer the foundations for the contributions from other authors. This book focuses on the use of simulation as an educational method and contributes to the broader conversation on safer healthcare systems. We start by defining simulation and describing the current healthcare landscape with reference to drivers for simulation uptake. We then offer an overview of simulation modalities and considerations for designing and implementing simulation-based education (SBE).

Scoping the Healthcare Simulation Landscape

Simulation is

> a technique – not a technology – to replace or amplify real experiences with guided experiences that evoke or replicate substantial aspects of the real world in a fully interactive manner. (Gaba, 2007)

Healthcare simulation is not a new concept. Quite conversely, it has historical origins. Take, for example, Madam du Coudray's fully simulation-based curriculum for midwives which was implemented in rural France in the eighteenth century (Owen, 2016). The drivers for that programme related in part to *macro-level* factors of the day. These agricultural populations were vulnerable to numerous socioeconomic stressors, among which high infant mortality made significant negative contribution. An important point here is that significant change occurred not because of *evidence* for the effectiveness of simulation but in response to large-scale social, economic and political demands. Today we are in a similar position, where our own modern macro-level factors are influencing simulation uptake. However, we are also equipped with knowledge about how simulation works, when and for whom. Empowered by this understanding, we can move towards addressing macro-level considerations, with simulation as an evidence-based and useful tool in our educational armamentarium.

What are some of these contemporary macro factors? Newspaper reports in 2017 document the apparently high numbers of infant deaths in one National Health Service (NHS) Trust in the United Kingdom (UK). Just as in eighteenth-century France, simulation could play a key role in addressing this issue. Despite recommendations from earlier investigations to improve professional practices and systems, the standards of care remain insufficient to meet societal expectations (Buchanan, 2017; Donnelly, 2017). The negative financial and reputational implications of these events to the NHS are significant. Perhaps even more so are the immeasurable emotional, psychological and social costs to the families and healthcare providers involved in adverse events. Although there can be no doubt that such expenses far outweigh the cost of targeted simulation training and systems testing, high-level political commitment is still required to effect change. In 2009, the UK's Chief Medical Officer (Sir Liam Donaldson) wrote that simulation was one of the top priorities of the health services for the next decade (Donaldson, 2009). He emphasised the utility of simulation in rehearsal for emergency situations, for the fostering of teamwork and for the development of psychomotor skills in safe settings that do not place patients at risk. He also questioned the logic of charging clinicians to undertake training to make their practice safer.

In Australia, a macro driver for significant government investment in healthcare simulation infrastructure and faculty development was the estimated shortfall of clinical placement opportunities for healthcare students. Of course, patient safety is an important consideration, but the pressing need for training the future healthcare workforce remains. So far, investment has largely been at entry-level health professions (Australian Government Department of Health, 2015), although several initiatives were funded in 2010 for specialty medical and surgical training. However, only the Training in Professional Skills (TIPS) programme at the Royal Australasian College of Surgeons (RACS) has been sustained (Bearman et al., 2011, 2012).

Other drivers for SBE are well reported (Box 1.1). We have already identified patient safety and the expanding numbers of health professional students, while other key drivers may be values-based, education-focused, or initiatives at *meso-* or *micro-*level. The shift to competency-based education, combined with growing evidence supporting SBE as an effective instructional approach, is also important (Nestel et al., 2013). Herein, we are seeing *accountability* arising from published standards for simulation practice, certification of practitioners and accreditation of programmes. Higher-educational systems in healthcare now offer short and award courses which feature prominent roles for simulation, thus facilitating quality control and improvement, as well as mitigation of the *human factors*. There is a vibrant research community with

---

Box 1.1 Drivers for Uptake of Simulation-Based Education, Adapted from Nestel et al. (2011).

Values-based drivers
- Ethical imperative of causing no harm to patients
- Recognition of importance of patients' perspectives
- Responsibility of preparing healthcare practitioners to work in a changing clinical landscape

Education-oriented drivers
- Facilitating a systematic approach to curriculum activities
- Shifting to competency-based curricula
- Assuring students/clinicians have direct/indirect exposure to certain clinical events
- Allowing for adjustment in the level of challenge offered to participants
- Identifying boundaries of competence of participants
- Providing rehearsal and assessment of technical, communication and other professional skills essential for safe clinical practice
- Enabling rehearsal of infrequently occurring events

Meso-level drivers
- Growing prominence of the patient safety movement

- Reducing length of hospital stays for patients and therefore reducing access to patients for learning
- Growing evidence of simulation as an effective educational method
- Increasing number of professional networks/societies/associations with a simulation orientation
- Establishing standards for optimal simulation practice including certification of simulation practitioners, accreditation of simulation centres or programmes

Macro-level drivers
- Working time directives/safer working hours initiatives
- Maturing national quality improvement strategies
- Growing prominence of the patient safety movement
- Increasing numbers of medical and health professional students
- Expanding national assessments for professional practice
- Billion-dollar worldwide healthcare simulation industry

new healthcare simulation-focused journals and several new textbooks such as this one. We provide a list of additional resources at the end of the chapter. It is also important to acknowledge that healthcare simulation is a billion-dollar global industry.

Healthcare simulation also has limitations and these are shared across the book. A major limitation remains the operational cost of simulation. An important area of research will be economic evaluations of SBE and other simulation applications (Maloney and Haines, 2016; Nestel et al., 2017). Further, assumptions are also often made about learning in simulation being *safe*. Although it is *patient* safe it is not necessarily safe for participants. High levels of stress, anxiety, different power relationships and the same sorts of physical risks of working in a clinical setting may all be present during SBE. Clinician safety is essential and it is incumbent on simulation practitioners to design *safe learning environments* in which all participants can develop their practice without harm.

Simulation Modalities

Simulation modalities are diverse. Most introductory books on healthcare simulation document these according to type and create a hierarchy of realism or fidelity – a highly contested notion (see later). We offer examples of core modalities and their combined use, especially in simulation scenarios. These modalities may be available in simulation centres and skills labs in higher education units and health services or may be offered *onsite* or *in situ* (Posner et al., 2017). See Chapter 5 for more information.

Simulated, or *standardised*, *participants* (SPs) refer to individuals who are paid or volunteers (patients, actors, health professionals or students) who are trained to portray specific roles within a simulation and to offer feedback to participants. As proxies for patients, SPs must be empowered to accurately represent (or simulate) them. Given that clinicians (with their own view of healthcare experiences) often train SPs, there can be challenges to the delivery of authentic *patient* perspectives (Nestel, 2015). (See example in Table 1.1.)

Task trainers enable participants to learn psychomotor skills applicable to procedures or operations. They vary in sophistication and technology from simple benchtop models (e.g. suturing, intubation) to sophisticated virtual reality models (e.g. laparoscopy; Aggarwal et al., 2007; Larsen et al., 2009) and virtual reality environments (Huber et al., 2018) (see example in Table 1.1).

Manikins are commonly used for developing team-based interprofessional care. They vary in technological sophistication and can be programmed to demonstrate physiological indicators of a patient's condition. Depending on the manikin, participants can also undertake a diverse range of clinical procedures. Examples include *SimMom* (Laerdal; enabling SBE through all phases of labour) and *Desperate Debra* (Adam Rouilly; enabling SBE in the management of impacted fetal head at caesarean section).

Screen-based simulators use different technologies to provide learners with opportunities to develop knowledge of diverse clinical skills including diagnostic decision-making, steps in operative procedures, patient-centred communication and more. They often have a tremendous advantage of being highly accessible, including at the point of care.

Hybrid simulations are those in which simulation modalities are combined. They usually involve an SP with a task trainer (e.g. urinary catheter model, rectal examination model) and enable a staged approach to the development of psychomotor and communication skills (Higham et al., 2007).

Simulation-based training packages are widely available in obstetrics. Developed in the UK, PRactical Obstetric Multi-Professional Training (PROMPT) is designed to support the development of interprofessional collaborative practice for obstetric emergencies. The package is used internationally and has demonstrated direct improvements in perinatal outcome and improvements in practitioners' knowledge, clinical skills and team-working (*PROMPT – Making Childbirth Safer, Together*, 2017). *Advanced Life Support in Obstetrics* (ALSO) and *Become a Breech Expert* (BABE) are Australian-based examples (Advanced Maternal and Reproductive Education).

Robotic surgery is emerging as a minimally invasive operative modality in gynaecology. Benefits over existing modalities include improved surgeon ergonomics, *wristed* nature of robotic instruments, and elimination of requirement for counterintuitive motion in the operative field. While we are watching this space, steady emergence of robotics must be recognised as limited by cost, access (currently available within the private health system only) and lack of robust data demonstrating global superior efficacy over techniques such as laparoscopy (Manolitsas, 2012). With increasing availability and utility of robotic surgery, simulation

Table 1.1 Considerations of tasks for simulation practitioners using the simulation phases in three examples. For each example, we have assumed that the session is either mandated, addresses a curriculum gap, meets a clinical need or is experimental. It is not possible to include all tasks but we have attempted to identify some critical ones and those that characterise simulation as an educational method.

	SP-based formative assessment for medical students explaining vaginal examination and Pap smear to a patient	Laparoscopic simulator for trainees to learn basic skills	In situ delivery suite simulation with hybrid simulator for interprofessional collaborative practice
Preparing	• Align assessment with curriculum requirement and set learning objectives • Write simulation plan for all phases noting Calgary–Cambridge[1] guide for debriefing • Choose simulators – simulated patient • Set up the environment – consultation room • Recruit SP and provide training for role portrayal and feedback • Identify rating forms • Rehearse the consultation including timings; note differences to a real encounter • Recruit and train faculty	• Set learning objectives for distributed training package that is trainee-led • Check simulator is available and working • Write simulation plan for all phases • Write guidance notes for trainees to optimise use considering different levels of experience • Ensure trainees will have access to simulators	• Set learning objectives • Develop scenario in a consultative process (with other stakeholders) • Write simulation plan for all phases noting pause and discuss feedback during the simulation and SHARP[2] after the scenario with video-assisted debriefing (VAD)[3] • Choose simulators – simulated patient and birthing suit • Recruit SP and provide training for role portrayal, using a birthing suit and debriefing process • Obtain permissions/notify all staff of the *in situ* simulation • Rehearse the whole scenario including timings; note differences to a real encounter • Recruit and train faculty
Briefing	• Inform faculty and students about the simulation • Orient students to the task, learning objectives and process for feedback • Orient students to the environment and SP including differences to a real encounter • Give observer students specific tasks • Ask for questions	• Trainees new to the simulator will need orientation to its set up, tasks, data capture for feedback • Ensure reporting process if simulator is not working	• Inform faculty and participants about the simulation • Orient participants to the task, learning objectives, pause and discuss and debriefing approaches • Discuss current strengths and areas for development of collaborative team practice • Discuss respect issues relevant to participants' performances and ideas shared in the debriefing • Orient participants to *in situ* simulation, the SP and the limitations of the birthing suit • Ask for questions
Simulating	• Implement the simulation activity as planned	• Trainees to use the simulator as requested over 6-week training package and in response to meeting end goals	• Start video-recording • Use pause and discuss approach to feedback if necessary • Ensure *in situ* simulation does not compromise safety in ongoing clinical activity
Debriefing/ offering feedback	• Give time for completion of rating forms • Use Calgary–Cambridge approach to feedback • Invite observer students to participate • Check SP has come out of role for feedback	• Use feedback generated from simulator to improve their performance	• Use SHARP for debriefing • Illustrate key points with VAD • Check SP has come out of role for feedback
Reflecting	• Ask students to complete a 500-word written reflection to be placed in portfolios • Ask students to commit to a peer discussion about the task once they have had practice in real settings	• Trainees encouraged to note progress in portfolio; to identify their improvements and areas for development to help set new goals for the next training session	• Ask participants to plan how they will use the learning from the simulation in their future practice • Faculty can use OSAD[2] to reflect on their debriefing practice
Evaluating	• Ask faculty, SP and students to complete a rating form about the effectiveness of the session • Use evaluation data to inform planning for next session	• Ask trainees to complete an evaluation form after the completion of the whole training package • Use evaluation data to inform planning for next training package	• Ask faculty, SP and participants to complete a rating form about the effectiveness of the session • Use evaluation data to inform planning for next session

[1]Kurtz, S. and Silverman, J. (1996). The Calgary–Cambridge Referenced Observation Guides: an aid to defining the curriculum and organizing the teaching in communication training programmes. *Medical Education*, 30, 83–89.

[2]Imperial College London. (2012). *The London Handbook for Debriefing: Enhancing Performance Debriefing in Clinical and Simulated Settings*. Retrieved from: https://workspace.imperial.ac.uk/ref/Public/UoA%2001%20-%20Clinical%20Medicine/Iw2222ic_debrief_book_a5.pdf

[3]Krogh, K., Bearman, M. and Nestel, D. (2015). Expert practice of video-assisted debriefing. *Clinical Simulation in Nursing*, 11, 180–187.

will play a key role in ensuring adequate operator training, maintenance of skills and patient safety.

Considerations in Designing Simulation-Based Education

McGaghie et al.'s (2010) review of the SBE literature identifies features and best practices for effective use of simulation as an educational method (see Box 1.2). Being well described both in their article and then throughout this book, it is beyond the scope of this chapter to discuss them in further detail. However, key points are that *simulation is optimal when embedded in a curriculum or broader programme of learning activities relevant to the participants*. Educational design is an overarching topic for many items in the list. The importance of setting and making explicit the *educational objectives* is emphasised. Opportunities for *repetitive practice* and *feedback* are highlighted. Selecting simulation modalities that are fit for purpose is important. Although included in the list, the notion of *fidelity* is contested, with some scholars recommending dropping the term. Hamstra et al. (2014) propose that *functional task alignment* and *learner engagement* are more useful concepts. Nestel et al. (2018) argue that the fidelity (or realism) of a simulator or a simulation depends in part on the participants' willingness to engage in the activity 'as if' it were real (Dieckmann, 2009). They offer *meaningfulness* as a more useful concept for faculty involved in educational design. Finally,

---

Box 1.2 Features and Best Practices of Simulation-Based Education.

1. Feedback
2. Deliberate practice
3. Curriculum integration
4. Outcome measurement
5. Simulation fidelity
6. Skill acquisition and maintenance
7. Mastery learning
8. Transfer to practice
9. Team training
10. High-stakes testing
11. Instructor training
12. Educational and professional context

Reproduced with permission from: McGaghie, W. C., Issenberg, S. B., Petrusa, E. R. and Scalese, R. J. (2010). A critical review of simulation-based medical education research: 2003–2009. *Medical Education*, 44(1), 50–63.

---

faculty development is considered critical; this includes acknowledgement that clinical experience is not a proxy for simulation instructor effectiveness.

There are many theories that inform SBE from behaviourist, cognitivist and constructivist traditions. Each has a specific offering and may be valuable in considering SBE design, in understanding *transfer* of learning from simulation to real clinical settings, and in appreciating the variety of participants' responses to engagement in simulation. Behaviourist theories are closely linked with the setting of learning objectives, of learning in response to a stimulus, of behaviour shaped by feedback. In SBE, the simulation activity becomes the stimulus and the briefing and debriefing (including feedback) helps to shape desired behaviour. The notions of *deliberate practice* as described by Ericsson (2015) and *mastery learning* applied extensively by McGaghie and his colleagues (McGaghie, 2015) are linked to this tradition, although they intersect with others too (Ericsson, 2015). Stimulus-response learning is insufficient in itself for sustained learning. Cognitivist theories of learning explore individuals' thinking and knowing, memory capacities and problem-solving schema (Battista and Nestel, in press). Cognitive load theory is commonly cited by simulation educators in design considerations (Reedy, 2015). Too little or too much cognitive load at any stage of the simulation activity will influence capacity to learn. Finding the optimal load is the work of the simulation practitioner. While these two traditions have the learner at their centre, they focus on the teacher *teaching*. In the *constructivist* tradition, the experiences that learners bring to the learning are valued with the acknowledgement that individuals will make meaning for themselves. *Reflective practice* is commonly described as an illustration of a constructivist approach to learning (Schon, 1983). This theory proposes that during and after an unexpected or critical event, practitioners (learners) will reflect-in-action *and* reflect-on-action. Constructivist theories also acknowledge the context in which learning occurs and its social nature. Recently, attention has shifted to a range of complexity theories and the role of non-human objects and humans influencing learning, of the influence of the broader social and political environment (Battista, 2015, 2017; Fenwick and Dahlgren, 2015). The role of theory in SBE is further discussed in a series of articles (Eppich and Cheng, 2015; Husebo et al., 2015; Nestel and Bearman, 2015; Reedy, 2015).

Important considerations for any SBE activity are outlined in Box 1.3. Although there are limitations

Box 1.3 Phases in Simulation Design.

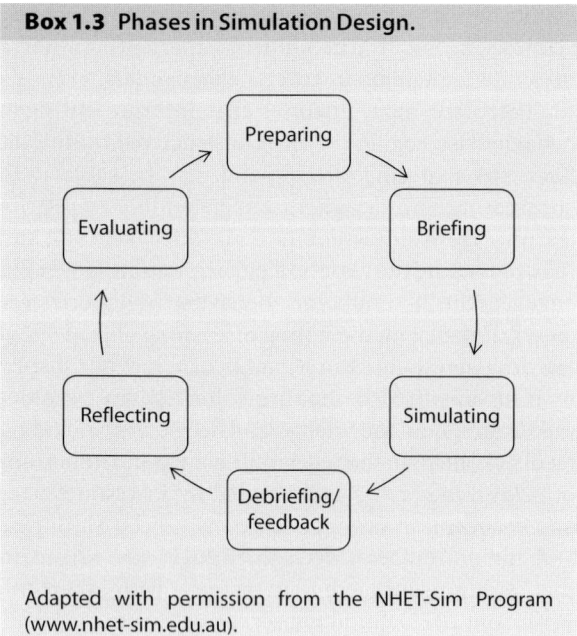

Adapted with permission from the NHET-Sim Program (www.nhet-sim.edu.au).

with oversimplifying complex processes, these defined phases help to remind the simulation practitioner of the interrelatedness of all activities. Box 1.3 illustrates these phases and Table 1.1 sets out the associated tasks for three different types of simulations.

The *preparing* phase refers to all the activities that take place before the simulation event starts, such as: identifying learners' needs; setting learning objectives; designing the scenario, sourcing simulators, medical equipment, props, etc.; booking rooms; recruiting and identifying faculty, confederates and SPs; scheduling the learners; catering, etc. The range of tasks will depend on the local simulation facility and practices.

The *briefing* phase is given relatively little attention in literature but is really important in setting up valuable learning experiences (Donnelly, 2017). The briefing for faculty includes the learning objectives, the learners' characteristics, logistics such as time frames, starting, pausing and ending the simulation activity, simulator programming, technical support, communication with the control room, audiovisual capacity, debriefing and feedback processes, reflective exercises and evaluation forms, etc. An opportunity for final questions can ensure smooth functioning. Briefing learners will include most of the above and may also include inviting learners to set their own goals relative to those prescribed and their experiences (Kneebone and Nestel, 2005).

Orientation of learners to the simulation is important. This will include explicit discussion on what is similar and what is different to reality. This is linked to what is called a *fiction contract.* Some learners find simulation stressful and it may be important to normalise the experience during the briefing. This involves acknowledgement that learners often find simulations stressful. Creating a safe learning environment involves several strategies and learner-centred attitudes from faculty. Orientation strategies include giving a clear explanation of the simulation phases and their responsibilities in each, clarity over who is observing, what will happen with audiovisual recordings, confidentiality among those involved, seeking their buy-in with respect to doing their best, the orientation or familiarisation of the simulators and setting.

During the *simulation* it is important to indicate a clear start to the simulation and observe for physical and psychological safety of those within the simulation (Donaldson, 2009). Minimal talking is often desirable to facilitate acute observation. Encouraging observers to make notes to enable specific feedback during debriefing can be valuable. If there is a pause-and-discuss option, then enact as planned. Respond to cues for finishing the scenario. Depending on the simulation modalities, during the simulation activity cues may need to be pre-programmed on to the simulators (e.g. manikin) and/or given to confederates, SPs and learners (Donaldson, 2009; Buchanan, 2017).

Once the simulation is over, observations of participants and observers can be really important in helping the facilitator to frame the opening debriefing statements. During this transition period, there can be a lot of emotion expressed that is relevant to the debriefing and feedback. Encouraging participants to regroup and spend a few minutes thinking about what has just happened can be useful, including asking them to think about what worked well and what could have been improved. If observer tools are being used, then this is a good time to complete them.

On ending the scenario, participants move to the debriefing room. As faculty, it is helpful to have the learning objectives handy to stay focused. It is easy to be sidetracked by participants' responses. Follow the processes outlined in the briefing, although flexibility is also important to ensure learner-centredness. Invite observers, confederates and SPs to participate. Use opportunities, especially for communication-based scenarios, to rehearse micro elements of the scenario. This can be a valuable way of getting observers involved.

The *debriefing and feedback* phase complements the briefing, almost as bookends to the simulation activity. Facilitators explore participants' feelings, address goals and learning objectives, seek other perspectives, summarise, affirm positive behaviours, explore unplanned issues, and seek to establish new goals (Decker et al., 2013). One goal of the debriefing is to promote reflection. However, we include this as a separate phase to highlight the importance of the locus of control for learning residing with the learner once they have left the simulation event.

Evidence of the effectiveness of debriefing has been reported (Benbow et al., 1998; Issenberg et al., 2005; Rudolph et al., 2006; Fanning and Gaba, 2007; Decker et al., 2013; Motola et al., 2013; Cheng et al., 2014). Debriefing formats vary and are usually undertaken immediately after the simulation event/warm or delayed/cold (Huber et al., 2018). Formats can be relatively unstructured to highly structured. Examples of debriefing tools include *the diamond debrief* (Laerdal, 2017) and others are provided in the London Handbook of Debriefing (Adam Rouilly, 2017). Similarly, debriefer rating tools such as the *Objective Structured Assessment of Debriefing* (Arora et al., 2012; Imperial College London, 2012; Runnacles et al., 2014) and *The Debriefing Assessment for Simulation in Healthcare* (Centre for Medical Simulation, 2011) have been developed to provide evidence-based guidelines for conducting debriefings in simulated and real clinical settings. Guidelines for video-assisted debriefing have been published (Grant et al., 2010; Grant and Marriage, 2012; Levett-Jones and Lapkin, 2013; Krogh et al., 2015), but optimal use remains unclear.

For the *reflecting* phase, learners (usually individually) are encouraged to make sense of the simulation in the light of their own experiences and those they plan. Similarly, faculty and SPs are also encouraged to reflect on all facets of their contributions. Reflecting is usually an individual activity; while debriefing is often collective and connected to the simulation activity, reflecting has a wider reach. During briefing, learners can be informed of reflecting activities and reinforced after the debriefing. Of course, there is overlap between these phases and reflecting can occur before the debriefing. There are several approaches to reflecting that have been adopted in SBE (Kolb and Fry, 1975; Schön, 1987; Husebo et al., 2015).

Learners can be directed to evidence their reflective practice following simulations by uploading and tagging digital learning resources (audio, photographs, video and podcasts, etc.) within an e-portfolio (Donnelly, 2017) or blogs, social networking sites and wikis (McGaghie, 2015). Permissions need to be considered with respect to use and storage of these images.

Evaluating refers to the success and limitations of the session in meeting its goals, rather than assessment of the individual. This phase benefits from involvement of all stakeholders although practically it is often only learners, faculty, confederates and SPs. It is well recognised in the literature and evident in simulation frameworks that evaluation is a crucial element to drive improvements in education, healthcare practice and ultimately patient care (Jeffries, 2005; Gough, 2016).

While it is essential to consider the degree to which the SBE intervention has supported learning, meaningful evaluations require more sophisticated methods. Complex learning interventions require equally complex evaluations, using qualitative and quantitative methods to draw on multiple sources and triangulating data alongside exploring multiple levels of impact can provide more meaningful evaluations (Battista and Nestel, in press).

Closing Summary

In summary, the international landscape of healthcare simulation has changed rapidly. From our opening quotations, we see that simulation has diverse applications. It responds to changes in healthcare practices (trialling new equipment or processes), addresses critical patient safety issues (reproduces sentinel or other events for learning), enables examination and development of effective interprofessional collaborative practice and supports development and assessment of clinical skills (or their components). It is an exciting time to learn how to use simulation. The remaining chapters in this book offer valuable insights to theoretical and evidence-based simulation practice.

Recommended Resources
Peer-Reviewed Journals
*Indicates open access.

Simulation in Healthcare, http://journals.lww.com/simulationinhealthcare/Pages/default.aspx: Journal of the Society for Simulation in Healthcare (SSH).

Advances in Simulation,* https://advancesinsimulation.biomedcentral.com/: Journal of the Society in Europe for Simulation Applied to Medicine (SESAM).

Clinical Simulation in Nursing, www.nursingsimulation.org/: Journal of the International Nursing

Association for Clinical Simulation and Learning (INACSL).

BMJ STEL, http://stel.bmj.com/: Journal of the Association for Simulated Practice in Healthcare (ASPiH).

Simulation and Gaming, http://journals.sagepub.com/home/sag: published in association with the International Simulation and Gaming Association (ISAGA).

Reference Books

The books cover different facets of simulation practice. Although speciality- or modality-specific, they all offer valuable insights and all have been published in the last five years.

Dudley, F. (2012). *The Simulated Patient Handbook: A Comprehensive Guide for Facilitators and Simulated Patients*. London: Radcliffe Publishing.

Grant, V., and Cheng, A. (Eds.). (2016). *Comprehensive Healthcare Simulation: Paediatrics*. Switzerland: Springer.

Levine, S., DeMaria, A., Schwartz, A. and Sim, A. (Eds.). (2013). *The Comprehensive Textbook of Healthcare Simulation*. New York, NY: Springer.

Nestel, D., and Bearman, M. (Eds.). (2016). *Simulated Patient Methodology: Theory, Evidence and Practice*. Chichester: Wiley Blackwell.

Nestel, D., Kelly, M., Jolly, B. and Watson, M. (Eds.). (2018). *Healthcare Simulation Education: Evidence, Theory and Practice*. Chichester: John Wiley & Sons.

Palaganas, J., Maxworthy, J., Epps, C. and Mancini, M. (Eds.). (2015). *Defining Excellence in Simulation Programs*. Philadelphia, PA: Wolters Kluwer.

Riley, R. (Ed.). (2016). *Manual of Simulation in Healthcare*, 2nd edition. Oxford: Oxford University Press.

Other Online Resources

Debrief2Learn provides resources on debriefing and other practices associated with healthcare simulation: http://debrief2learn.org/

PROMPT (PRactical Obstetric Multi-Professional Training) is an evidence-based multiprofessional training package for obstetric emergencies: www.promptmaternity.org/

Simulcast offers podcasts on topics of interest to simulation practitioners and guidance to other resources: http://simulationpodcast.com/

SimGhosts specialises in faculty development for simulation technologists and operations specialists: www.simghosts.org/sim/default.asp

Professional Society Websites

All listings host an annual conference and are inter-professional (except for INACSL).

Society for Simulation in Healthcare (SSH) is the largest simulation society by membership and is based in the USA: www.ssih.org/

Society in Europe for Simulation Applied to Medicine (SESAM) is based in Europe: www.sesam-web.org/

Association for Simulated Practice in Healthcare (ASPiH) is based in the UK: www.aspih.org.uk/

International Nursing Association for Clinical Simulation and Learning (INACSL) is based in the USA: www.inacsl.org/i4a/pages/index.cfm?pageid=1

International Pediatric Simulation Society (IPSS): http://ipssglobal.org/

Bibliography

Adam Rouilly. *Desperate Debra – Impacted Fetal Head Simulator* (cited November 20, 2017). Available from: www.adam-rouilly.co.uk/productdetails.aspx?pid=3566%26cid=

Advanced Maternal and Reproductive Education (cited November 27, 2017). Available from: www.amare.org.au/.

Aggarwal, R., Ward, J., Balasundaram, I., et al. (2007). Proving the effectiveness of virtual reality simulation for training in laparoscopic surgery. *Annals of Surgery*, 246(5), 771–779.

Arora, S., Ahmed, M., Paige, J., et al. (2012). Objective Structured Assessment of Debriefing (OSAD): bringing science to the art of debriefing in surgery. *Annals of Surgery*, 256(6), 982–988.

Australian Government Department of Health (2015). *Final Annual Report – Health Workforce Australia – Building Capacity* (cited July 2, 2017). Available from: www.health.gov.au/internet/publications/publishing.nsf/Content/hwa-annual-report~2-building-capacity

Battista, A. (2015). Activity theory and analyzing learning in simulations. *Simulation and Gaming*, 46(2), 187–196.

(2017). An activity theory perspective of how scenario-based simulations support learning: a descriptive analysis. *Advances in Simulation*, 2, 23.

Battista, A. and Nestel, D. (2018, forthcoming). Simulation in medical education. In T. Swanwick (Ed.), *Understanding Medical Education*. Chichester: Wiley.

Bearman, M., Anthony, A. and Nestel, D. (2011). A pilot training program in surgical communication, leadership and teamwork. *Australia and New Zealand Journal of Surgery*, 81(4), 213–215.

Bearman, M., O'Brien, R., Anthony, A., et al. (2012). Learning surgical communication, leadership and teamwork through simulation. *Journal of Surgical Education*, 69(2), 201–207.

Benbow, E. W., Harrison, I., Dornan, T. L. and O'Neill, P. A. (1998). Pathology and the OSCE: insights from pilot study. *Journal of Pathology*, 184(1), 110–114.

Buchanan, M. (2017). *Parents' anger at baby deaths NHS trust*. BBC News. Available from: www.bbc.com/news/health-39591929.

Centre for Medical Simulation (2011). *Debriefing Assessment for Simulation in Healthcare* (cited May 1, 2013). Available from: www.harvardmedsim.org/debriefing-assessment-simulation-healthcare.php.

Cheng, A., Eppich, W., Grant, V., Sherbino, J., Zendejas, B. and Cook, D. A. (2014). Debriefing for technology-enhanced simulation: a systematic review and meta-analysis. *Medical Education*, 48(7), 657–666.

Decker, S., Fey, M., Sideras, S., et al. (2013). Standards of best practice: Simulation Standard VI: The debriefing process. *Clinical Simulation in Nursing*, 9(6), S26–S29.

Dieckmann, P. (Ed.). (2009). *Using Simulations for Education, Training and Research*. Lengerich: PABST.

Donaldson, L. (2009). *150 Years of the Chief Medical Officer's Annual Report 2008*. London: Department of Health.

Donnelly, L. (2017). Avoidable deaths of at least seven babies at NHS trust where midwives 'couldn't be bothered'. *The Telegraph*.

Eppich, W. and Cheng, A. (2015). Cultural historical activity theory (CHAT) – informed debriefing for interprofessional teams. *Clinical Simulation in Nursing*, 11, 383–389.

Ericsson, K. A. (2015). Acquisition and maintenance of medical expertise: a perspective from the expert-performance approach with deliberate practice. *Academic Medicine*, 90(11), 1471–1486.

Fanning, R. M. and Gaba, D. M. (2007). The role of debriefing in simulation-based learning. *Simulation in Healthcare*, 2(2), 115–125.

Fenwick, T. and Dahlgren, M. A. (2015). Towards socio-material approaches in simulation-based education: lessons from complexity theory. *Medical Education*, 49(4), 359–367.

Gaba, D. (2007). The future vision of simulation in healthcare. *Simulation in Healthcare*, 2, 126–135.

Gough, S. (2016). *The Use of Simulation-based Education in Cardio-respiratory Physiotherapy*. Manchester: Manchester Metropolitan University.

Grant, D. J. and Marriage, S. C. (2012). Training using medical simulation. *Archives of Diseases of Childhood*, 97(3), 255–259.

Grant, J., Moss, J., Epps, C. and Watts, P. (2010). Using video-facilitated feedback to improve student performance following high-fidelity simulation. *Clinical Simulation in Nursing*, 6(5), e177–e184.

Hamstra, S. J., Brydges, R., Hatala, R., Zendejas, B. and Cook, D. A. (2014). Reconsidering fidelity in simulation-based training. *Academic Medicine*, 89(3), 387–392.

Higham, J., Nestel, D., Lupton, M. and Kneebone, R. (2007). Teaching and learning gynaecology examination with hybrid simulation. *The Clinical Teacher*, 4, 238–243.

Huber, T., Wunderling, T., Paschold, M., Lang, H., Kniest, W. and Hansen, C. (2018). Highly immersive virtual reality laparoscopy simulation: development and future aspects. *International Journal of Computer Assisted Radiology and Surgery*, 13(2), 281–290.

Husebo, S., O'Regan, S. and Nestel, D. (2015). Reflective practice and its role in simulation. *Clinical Simulation in Nursing*, 11(8), 368–375.

Imperial College London. (2012). *The London Handbook for Debriefing: Enhancing Performance Debriefing in Clinical and Simulated Settings*. London: London Deanery.

Issenberg, S. B., McGaghie, W., Petrusa, E. R., Gordon, D. L. and Scalese, R. J. (2005). Features and uses of high-fidelity medical simulations that lead to effective learning: a BEME systematic review. *Medical Teacher*, 27(1), 10–28.

Jeffries, P. (2005). A framework for designing, implementing, and evaluating simulations. *Nurse Education Perspectives*, 26(2), 97–104.

Kneebone, R. and Nestel, D. (2005). Learning clinical skills – the place of simulation and feedback. *The Clinical Teacher*, 2(2), 86–90.

Kolb, D. and Fry, R. (1975). Toward an applied theory of experiential learning. In C. Cooper (Ed.), *Theories of Group Process*. London: John Wiley.

Krogh, K., Bearman, M. and Nestel, D. (2015). Expert practice of video-assisted debriefing. *Clinical Simulation in Nursing*, 11, 180–187.

Laerdal. *SimMom*. (cited November 20, 2017). Available from: www.laerdal.com/au/SimMom.

Larsen, C. R., Sørensen, J. L. and Grantcharov, T. (2009). Effect of virtual reality training in laparoscopic surgery: a randomised controlled trial. *British Medical Journal*, 338, b1802.

Levett-Jones, T. and Lapkin, S. (2013). A systematic review of the effectiveness of simulation debriefing in health professional education. *Nurse Education Today*, 34(6), e58–e63.

Maloney, S. and Haines, T. (2016). Issues of cost–benefit and cost–effectiveness for simulation in health professions education. *Advances in Simulation*, 1, 13.

9

Manolitsas, T. (2012). Robotic surgery. *O&G Magazine*, 14(1), 25–27.

McGaghie, W. C. (2015). Mastery learning: it is time for medical education to join the 21st century. *Academic Medicine*, 90(11), 1438–1441.

McGaghie, W. C., Issenberg, S. B., Petrusa, E. R. and Scalese, R. J. (2010). A critical review of simulation-based medical education research: 2003–2009. *Medical Education*, 44(1), 50–63.

Motola, I., Devine, L. A., Chung, H. S., Sullivan, J. E. and Issenberg, S. B. (2013). Simulation in healthcare education: a best evidence practical guide. AMEE Guide No. 82. *Medical Teacher*, 35(10), e1511–e1530.

Nestel, D. (2015). Expert's corner: Standardized (simulated) patients in health professions education: a proxy for real patients? In J. Palaganas, J. C. Maxworthy, C. A. Epps and M. E. Mancini (Eds.), *Defining Excellence in Simulation Programs*, p. 394. Philadelphia, PA: Wolters Kluwer.

Nestel, D. and Bearman, M. (2015). Theory and simulation-based education: definitions, worldviews and applications. *Clinical Simulation in Nursing*, 11, 349–354.

Nestel, D., Tabak, D., Tierney, T., et al. (2011). Key challenges in simulated patient programs: an international comparative case study. *BMC Medical Education*, 11, 69.

Nestel, D., Pritchard, S., Watson, M., Andreatta, P., Bearman, M. and Morrison, T. (2013). Strategic approaches to simulation-based education: a case study from Australia. *Journal of Health Specialties*, 1(1), 4–12.

Nestel, D., Brazil, V. and Hay, M. (2017). You can't put a value on that ... Or can you? Economic evaluation in simulation-based medical education. *Medical Education*, 52, 139–147.

Nestel, D., Krogh, K. and Kolbe, K. (2018). Exploring realism in healthcare simulations. In D. Nestel, B. Jolly, M. Watson and M. Kelly (Eds.), *Healthcare Simulation Education: Evidence, Theory & Practice* (Chapter 4, pp. 23–28). Chichester: Wiley.

Owen, H. (2016). *Simulation in Healthcare Education: An Extensive History*. Switzerland: Springer.

Posner, G., Clark, M. D. and Grant, V. (2017). Simulation in the clinical setting: towards a standard lexicon. *Advances in Simulation*, 2, 15.

PROMPT – Making Childbirth Safer, Together (2017) (cited April 24, 2017). Available from: www.promptmaternity.org/.

Reedy, G. (2015). Using cognitive load theory to inform simulation design and practice. *Clinical Simulation in Nursing*, 11, 350–360.

Rudolph, J. W., Dufresne, S. R. and Raemer, D. B. (2006). There's no such thing as 'nonjudgmental' debriefing: a theory and method for debriefing with good judgment. *Simulation in Healthcare*, 1(1), 49–55.

Runnacles, J., Thomas, L., Sevdalis, N., Kneebone, R. and Arora, S. (2014). Development of a tool to improve performance debriefing and learning: the paediatric Objective Structured Assessment of Debriefing (OSAD) tool. *Postgraduate Medical Journal*, 90(1069), 613–621.

Schon, D. (1983). *The Reflective Practitioner: How Professionals Think in Action*. London: Temple Smith.

(1987). *Educating the Reflective Practitioner*. San Francisco, CA: Jossey-Bass.

Chapter

2

The Where of Simulation Training

Al May

Simulation is by no means a new phenomenon in medical education; it is an ever-developing learning modality. When agreeing the learning objectives and goals of the simulation, consideration of the locality of your session is essential to maximise the focus of the learning.

In Situ Simulation Versus the Simulation Centre

In situ simulation can be generally taken to mean simulation that is integrated into the real environment. In its broadest sense within healthcare, this could include actual clinical areas where patients are managed, and areas set aside solely for simulation but within a wider clinical area (e.g. a side room of a labour ward permanently set up for simulation). To take this further, it is clear that the *in situ* environment must be the actual clinical environment for the specific people participating in the simulation. They may be participating in the simulation as part of their normal working day while simultaneously engaged with the clinical care of real patients, or participating solely in simulation with no other responsibilities. The importance of this difference is highlighted under the heading of safety for patients. This is contrasted with simulation centre simulation, which will be isolated either physically or functionally from real clinical areas. Although an isolated simulation set up may not be referred to locally as a 'Centre', it clearly should be considered as such. In either case, the simulation modality could of course be anything from a paper-based drill walk-through in the real clinical environment to fully immersive, real-time, psychologically high-fidelity simulation.

What are the Similarities Between *In Situ* Simulation and Simulation in a Dedicated Centre?

Similarities: Aims of Simulation

With the potential exception of systems assessment (discussed below in What Are the Differences?), the simulation centre and the *in situ* environment can be used for all the same aims. You will almost certainly soon get tired of people asking you to 'come and do some simulation'. The first question you should be asking is, 'What do we need to achieve?' This needs to be followed up with a serious consideration of whether simulation (in all its many forms) is the most efficient and effective way to achieve that aim for your learner/organisation.

In terms of volume of learning for time spent, constructively aligned, planned learning through debriefing of actively driven simulation is probably the most efficient. This may make use of anything from simple table-top exercises to fully immersive real-time, real-team events. The planned learning content could be equally diverse from practising an uncommon drill in a step-by-step way, to learning how to hand over information in real time. Simulation for formative assessment is commonly used, but in reality, is only efficient for a minority of high-performing, well-trained stable teams: there is usually some planned learning that could be delivered first. Summative assessment of individuals, teams, equipment or work processes can clearly be done in both environments, but the simulation centre is usually better placed in terms of resource and research expertise to create a validated assessment tool which would stand up to scrutiny.

Once the aims are clarified and the specific objectives defined, you will select the cheapest and most efficient simulation modality to deliver what you plan, both *in situ* and in a simulation centre. You will consider everything from table-top exercise simulation, through individual task trainers, to full-body manikin immersive simulation.

Similarities: Structured Developmental Conversations and Debriefing

A developmental conversation of some form is equally important in both *in situ* and simulation centre environments. This is both to ensure the objective of the simulation is achieved, but also to maintain the psychological safety of the participants. Of prime relevance here is Ericsson's assertion that practice merely makes permanent. Development is unlikely without deliberate practice; the sandwiching of active efforts to improve through reflection, facilitated reflection or feedback, between episodes of performance (Ericsson et al., 1993).

When participants are engaging with simulation in their real clinical environment, where there may be resource pressure in terms of time or space, they still require the same amount and quality of debriefing as they would for the same objectives in the centre. If time is tight and you think you may have to cut some debriefing, you're trying to pack too much in and the simulation activity or scenario needs to be shorter.

What are the Differences Between *In Situ* Simulation and Simulation in a Dedicated Centre?

Differences: Aims of Simulation

The main potential difference in what objectives can be achieved using *in situ* simulation pertains to 'the system', or the interaction of staff, patients and system with the healthcare process. If a real-time immersive simulation can allow participants, the system and the simulation itself to act and react exactly as they do in real life, then there is a relevance to using this technique. If any of these aspects depart from reality, the data that are discovered are at best less likely to be representative and at worst dangerously misrepresentative of the system being analysed. By extension, this means that using real-time immersive simulation to test a system must have the sole objective of testing the system. Any interference in the running of the 'scenario' activity in order to create learning for participants within debriefing is highly likely to pollute and therefore invalidate the systems testing information.

So where does this leave *in situ* real-time immersive simulation for systems testing? There are various publications associating *in situ* simulation with the detection of latent safety threats (Patterson et al., 2013; Wetzel et al., 2013; Auerbach et al., 2015). This includes assessment of new facilities and systems before patients are treated, as practised by the UK army for several years (Ingram, M. Col., Clinical Director Army Medical Services Training Centre, personal communication; Kobayashi et al., 2006). However, consider how latent safety threats could be discovered in a more efficient way, or put another way, consider how many of these latent threats are truly 'hidden' if we actually look for them in the right way. Gathering key relevant staff together from the top of the organisation all the way to the clinical floor will allow you to identify a process map for the specific 'system' that requires testing. Overlaying a failure mode and effects analysis will identify the majority of 'system problems', which could be eliminated or mitigated before the manikin even gets out of the box. More importantly, this approach provides you with a structure for data collection if and when you decide to run a real-time immersive *in situ* simulation system test. In a way, you can sit around the table and conceptually drive a patient through a system within your department. Because our systems within healthcare are complex, as for any other complex system, we would expect errors or latent threats not to be independent. Therefore, running a manikin through the system in real time will only pick up one error chain; one snapshot of things that happened once and not a rich overview of how the system works and what it needs for resilience. Having considered this, you may get to the end of the table-top exercises and then decide that an *in situ* simulation is in fact warranted, but it certainly should not be your first port of call. Other methodologies for understanding your systems are available and specifically the functional resonance analysis method (FRAM, available at: http://functionalresonance.com/index.html; Hollnagel, 2012) is gaining utility within healthcare, and the reader with aspirations of improving healthcare systems is directed to further reading on this.

Taking a step back to look at the whole picture, perhaps one of the broader aims of *in situ* simulation is to promote learning in the workplace and a culture of continual support for improvement. Using simulation to make debriefing and learning an everyday occurrence can create a learning opportunity from every clinical encounter, fostering a culture that is continually striving to improve through recognising and understanding success and learning from mistakes. Linking your simulation activity to the clinical governance systems within your organisation will help stakeholders see relevance and value in what you are doing. Perhaps this is the true added value of *in situ* simulation versus the simulation centre.

Differences: Resources

The first consideration is whether the equipment you want to use is portable enough. Along with this goes a consideration of what you actually need to use to achieve the intended outcomes. As a general rule, the responsible approach is to use the cheapest, simplest and most portable equipment that will deliver the intended outcome with the optimal degree of engagement and psychological fidelity for that outcome. Most modern equipment can be moved around, but employing a trained simulation technician within your organisation will almost certainly be cheaper than the cost of ongoing repairs of badly maintained equipment.

If video capture is part of your process then ensure you have a robust organisational policy governing its use. Increasingly, video capture of real patients being treated is used for staff development through video-assisted debriefing, and modifications to policy already written for this purpose will often suffice. Retention of video must have specific consent that would usually include the purpose and likely uses of this video in the future. The big question to ask first is 'Why do I need this piece of video?' and the answer is usually that you don't. Retaining pieces of debriefing video for a limited time (e.g. 2 weeks) to allow in-house faculty development is probably the only purpose you should consider.

Differences: Time

Having tightly planned simulation activity ensures that the 'on the ground' time is minimal. This should include as much information as possible including requirements in terms of simulation, ancillary and audiovisual equipment, environmental set-up, running instructions, faculty roles, debrief notes, intended outcomes, evaluation of event and clean up procedure. In fact, if you have a library of simulation-based packages (not simply full-body manikin immersive simulations) then you will find that education can fit in to the occasional ten minutes of downtime – even over a cup of tea!

Differences: Space

When performing *in situ* simulation, you should automatically have a higher degree of environmental fidelity; the environment is actually real! This will be useful, depending on what your aims are. Having the real environment means the location and time to retrieve equipment and staff are close to reality so helping people to learn about this will be easier than in the simulation centre. A simple example could be an equipment race; simulating gathering equipment for a task without needing to run an immersive, real-time simulation. Being in the real environment will almost

certainly make achieving high psychological fidelity (the perception of reality in the participant mind) easier, which will be useful when achieving the objectives that require real behaviours, in real time, from the participants. Having said this, you would be striving for the same level of psychological fidelity to achieve these objectives in the simulation centre also.

With the *in situ* environment, you may not have the luxury of a remote area set up with audiovisual for a wider group of participants to watch the simulation and then take part in the debriefing. You may not have a separate area to debrief in while the next simulation is being set up. You may not have a separate control room from which to drive the simulation. Thankfully, you will find that these logistical differences are easy to overcome, primarily by focusing everyone on the process of learning through simulation. People soon forget about these logistical potential problems. There are also some physical things you can do if you feel it necessary. Using a fishbowl set-up whereby participant observers are placed around the edges of the simulation can be useful. The observers are briefed that they are there to watch and not interfere in any way with the simulation but to get involved in the debriefing conversation afterwards. You will find that the participants within the simulation soon forget there are people at the periphery. This is certainly preferable to involving everyone in the simulation itself because you think you should, but it in fact detracts from the reality of the situation. A laptop, webcam and long cable can simply and cheaply achieve the same.

Differences: Experience for Patients

It is obvious but vital to be aware of patients in the proximity of simulation. If a patient understands the intended outcome of the event as being aimed at improving performance and patient safety they are much more likely to be accepting of the process, when it is happening in an adjacent cubicle. In fact, more than accepting, patients are often reassured that training appears to be occurring. As a general rule, debriefing should probably not be carried out within earshot of patients. The reason for this is that through the process of debriefing participants may be moving from having displayed a performance gap towards conceptualising the underpinnings of that and considering strategies for the future, all of which is likely to be out of context and sound concerning from the outside. Letting patients know that simulation is going to be happening is essential and giving handouts and even having 'simulation training happens here' signs up can go a long way to helping patients understand what could otherwise be distressing for them. Actively seeking structured feedback from patients in the vicinity, after the event, can help you to ensure that they don't leave with any concerns or misunderstandings about what they may have seen or overheard. More importantly, feedback from patients will inform the development of your events, and could also be useful in terms of buy-in from stakeholders.

Differences: Safety for Patients

There is a potential risk to patients in terms of equipment and drugs used during *in situ* simulation. Using real drugs and equipment probably poses the lowest risk to patients as nothing artificial, simulated or expired is brought into the clinical area. This does clearly have cost and restocking implications, but will add to fidelity, if this is what is required for immersion. Using drugs and equipment specifically labelled as 'simulation' or 'simulated' will reduce but not eliminate the risk of passing in to the care of patients. This may also have a trade-off in terms of fidelity and immersion, but will almost certainly be irrelevant for most other simulation modalities. Also consider whether there is an infection risk with the things you are bringing into the clinical space; this includes your manikin or task trainer as well. Expired medication vials or equipment without 'simulation' labels carry the highest risk to patients. Nothing should be taken away from the simulation by participants (which could of course be accidental), as again there is a risk of being put in to clinical use.

What if there's an actual clinical emergency, particularly if the simulation is within the working day while participants are engaged with caring for real patients? There needs to be a senior clinical oversight with no other role than to terminate the simulation in the event of potential real patient harm. It can be useful to set criteria in advance for terminating early or cancelling the simulation. If this occurs, consider the continuing need for a delayed debriefing conversation depending on how much of the simulation occurred.

Differences: Safety for Participants

Do not underestimate the potential psychological impact of simulation (particularly with immersive simulation) on your individual participants. In contrast to the simulation centre, *all* participants will be colleagues or peers, and they may even have to go back to clinical work with each other after the event. Creation of a psychologically safe learning environment every time is as important, if not more, for *in situ* simulation, particularly when starting an organisational programme and for new members of staff. Some of this can be done before the actual event. This could include circulating information in advance about what things you are trying to achieve for the individual and the organisation. If you are using immersive, real-time simulation then specific details of the event should not be shared as this would almost certainly alter the fidelity and behaviours, but any other type of simulation could benefit from specific advance information to maximise the learning from face-to-face time. Perhaps a 'meet the manikin' session, dropping by with your simulation equipment and some refreshments, will allow people to familiarise themselves with both you and the equipment. If you are gaining written consent for participation in simulation with or without audiovisual recording then this could be the time to do that.

No matter how much work you have done in preparing people prior to the event, setting that safe learning environment must be done on the day, every time. When people believe that 'what happens here stays here', 'we'll only take the learning away' and 'anything goes … within the bounds of professionalism!' then they will act and react as they would do in real life. More importantly they will have frank and open developmental conversations, even when mistakes have been made. As time goes by in your organisation, with simulation becoming the norm rather than a novelty and with people seeing the process in action, creating a safe learning environment will become easier but no less important.

Briefing and orientation regarding the simulation activity itself become less important *in situ* compared with simulation in a dedicated centre, as people are generally in their place of work, doing their usual job, with their usual colleagues. Again, a lot of this can be reinforced at some time in advance of the event.

Motivation will profoundly affect the mindset of the participants and working with intrinsic motivators will make everything easier in the long run. Consider the differences of walking in to a mandatory event followed by a summative assessment versus one that is optional but with a reputation for being engaging, engendering deep learning with improvement of performance for all. Start small, giving people a challenging yet supportive developmental experience and word will spread.

Summary: Top Tips for *In Situ* Simulation

- *In situ* simulation can be a powerful catalyst to drive organisational change.
- *In situ* simulation is essentially the same as in-centre simulation but there will be some differences in how you get there.
- Your faculty need to be experts in simulation, just as they are in the simulation centre.
- Engaging the skills of a simulation technician will save you money.
- Do some ground work before turning up unannounced on the ward.
- A psychologically safe learning environment is essential every time.
- Debriefing is just as important for your participants as any other situation.
- *In situ* simulation is not the first thing to do when 'testing the system'.
- Safety of patients always comes first.

Bibliography

Auerbach, M., Kessler, D. O. and Patterson, M. (2015). The use of *in situ* simulation to detect latent safety threats in paediatrics: a cross-sectional survey. *BMJ Simulation and Technology Enhanced Learning*, 1, 77–82.

Ericsson, K. A., Krampe, R. T. and Tesch-Römer, C. (1993). The role of deliberate practice in the acquisition of expert performance. *Psychological Review*, 100(3), 363.

Hollnagel, E. (2012). *The Functional Resonance Analysis Method for Modelling Non-trivial Socio-technical Systems*. Available at: http://functionalresonance.com/index.html (accessed May 2, 2017).

Kobayashi, L., Shapiro, M. J., Sucov, A., et al. (2006). Portable advanced medical simulation for new emergency department testing and orientation. *Academic Emergency Medicine*, 13(6), 691–695.

Patterson, M. D., Geis, G. L., Falcone, R. A., LeMaster, T. and Wears, R. L. (2013). *In situ* simulation: detection of safety threats and teamwork training in a high risk emergency department. *BMJ Quality and Safety*, 22, 468–471.

Wetzel, E. A., Lang, T. R., Pendergrass, T. L., Taylor, R. G. and Geis, G. L. (2013). Identification of latent safety threats using high-fidelity simulation-based training with multidisciplinary neonatology teams. *Joint Commission Journal on Quality and Patient Safety*, 39(6), AP1–AP3.

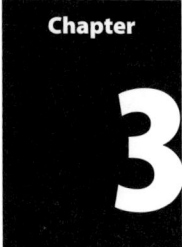

Chapter

3

Interprofessional *In Situ* Simulation

Jonathan Hurst

Interprofessional education (IPE), where 'two or more professions learn with, from and about each other to improve collaboration and the quality of care' (Barr et al., 2016), is one of the most influential health workforce interventions of the last few decades, improving healthcare systems and patient care (WHO, 2016). With the increasing complexities placed on healthcare services, effective collaboration among healthcare providers is pivotal to providing effective and comprehensive patient care (Barr et al., 2008; Reeves, 2016). Team functionality is paramount for patient safety (Künzle et al., 2010). Over the last two decades, many large-scale health reviews have called for better collaborative patient-centred practice by introducing IPE among healthcare professionals (Kohn et al., 2000; Department of Health, 2001, 2008, 2016; Steinert, 2005).

By using simulation to deliver IPE, healthcare professionals and teams can develop and strengthen essential technical and non-technical skills in real time and in a safe environment (Engum and Jeffries, 2012). Having recognised the value of simulation and technology-enhanced learning in IPE, much work has been undertaken by different healthcare professional bodies and medical royal colleges worldwide to create guidelines for its use in training. However, despite standards for practice and national guidance on using simulation-based education in healthcare (Purva et al., 2016), setting up such a programme is by no means easy. Working time directives, local service provision barriers on training time, space, financial and capacity issues all present challenges to simulation enthusiasts.

This chapter serves to discuss the issues and challenges to be considered during simulation design and execution in the healthcare setting, in line with national standards and available literature on the use of simulation for IPE.

Organisation/Management

Points to consider include:

- Organisational/educational lead buy-in
- Funding (equipment)
- Participant and Faculty time
- Location
- Training requirements

While acknowledging that the learner should be central to devising any educational material or intervention, *organisational support*, especially from senior management of all professional groups participating, is crucial to the successful, sustained implementation of interprofessional simulation-based education (Reeves et al., 2007). The scale of the simulation intervention determines which personnel should be involved. This could range from local leaders (shift coordinator and consultants) on the day of the simulation activity, to, for larger programmes, requiring sustainability and increased resources, it could include *educational leads* from each profession (e.g. college tutors, lead nurses/matrons) and departmental/directorate managers.

Clarity from the outset regarding *funding for simulation equipment, faculty time and training time for learners* is paramount and will aid the simulation design and set realistic learning outcomes. Consideration for the *location of the simulation, space and medical equipment* are explored in Chapter 2. When testing systems, actual *in situ* space, processes and equipment should be used. Consider performing simulation on days of reduced clinical work (e.g. clinical governance days) when clinical areas are less likely to be in use. When considering equipment and drugs to be used in the simulation, remember that patient safety is paramount, and when using simulated equipment in an *in situ* environment, facilitators must be meticulous to leave nothing behind at the end of the session.

Having secured time for faculty and learners, the organisational focus must now shift to the *learners' training requirements*. This needs careful consideration and planning when endeavouring to engage the interprofessional team in its entirety.

Spending time considering these organisation/management issues will promote long-term sustainability of simulation activities in the busy workplace.

Participants

Points to consider include:

- Scenario theme
- Professional group/role
- Composition of participants
- Level of experience/training requirements
- Remote senior support

The participant (Thistlewaite et al., 2010) set-up of the simulation is crucial to the scenario/programme design. In order to promote effective interprofessional interaction and increase set-up fidelity (Bland et al., 2014), the *composition and number* of participants need to closely match that of the simulated clinical team. Over-representation of any one professional group can skew the interprofessional learning (Reeves et al., 2007).

When planning the *scenario theme*, consider which participant groups would be involved in actual clinical settings. For example, a placental abruption with fetal bradycardia scenario would require midwifery, obstetric, anaesthetic and neonatal teams to be present, depending on the progression of the simulation and learning objectives.

Knowledge of *learning requirements and level of experience/skill set* of participants is key for scenario design and facilitation. Complex simulations are likely to require different levels of experience within professions, if a fully interprofessional learning experience is to be created (see 'Theories and Practice' below). Consider the availability of *remote senior support* (for all professional groups) that can be called upon during the simulation, providing advice by telephone or attending in person.

Facilitators/Faculty

Points to consider include:

- Professional representation
- Number
- Roles
- Training and faculty development

The composition of facilitators (faculty) needs careful thought. Ideally, this should mirror the *professional representation* of the participants, so as to maintain credibility during facilitation and debriefing of the simulation. Consider the *number* of facilitators

that you will need; this will be influenced by the size of the participant team. Establish facilitators' *roles* from the outset, including pastoral, emotional support for high-intensity scenarios. *Training and continuing professional development*, in both facilitation and debriefing practices, is crucial (Purva et al., 2016). This is particularly important for new faculty members. Regular peer feedback will enable faculty development. Technical faculty may also be required, if this skill set is not within the existing faculty.

Theories and Practice

IPE requires collaborative practice (Sargeant, 2009), engaging professionals to acquire the knowledge, skills and attitudes to work together for a common goal (Oandasan and Reeves, 2005; Sargeant, 2009). IPE is built on social and experiential learning. In order to construct interprofessional simulation-based education in healthcare, two specific theoretical learning perspectives are useful to consider (Sargeant, 2009): *social constructivism and complexity theory*.

Social constructivism (Lantolf and Thorne, 2006) places the emphasis on participants exploring a situation and applying an individual's prior knowledge to make sense of the clinical context – the interactivity between the participants and the influence of situational factors upon their behaviour and application of knowledge (Sargeant, 2009). Complexity theory is particularly important in the healthcare setting, where there are multiple, unpredictable system components that may have an impact on a participant's behaviour in a setting (Sargeant, 2009; Sweeney and Griffiths, 2002).

Congruent with these learning theories are the following practices, which should be incorporated into the simulation design:

- Vygotsky's zone of proximal development (Vygotsky, 1978; McLeod, 2012), where less-competent participants may develop from their more skilful peers, by using 'scaffolding' (Wood, 2001) – assistance that matches the specific needs of the participant at that time. In simulation practice, this could be highlighting a guideline or aide-memoire for the participants to work through as the clinical case becomes more complex.
- Situated and authentic learning (deliberate community of practice) (Lave and Wenger, 1991; Sargeant, 2009), where learning is seen as a social activity within a particular environment (e.g. learning within a healthcare team through

interpersonal interaction) and where practitioners work together to learn and collaboratively create new knowledge about a situation, e.g. awareness of a practice guideline, patient-specific information.

- Mentoring (Gibbons et al., 2002) between junior and senior colleagues, which occurs naturally in the workplace.

In order to create a common platform for learning and decrease cognitive load (Paas et al., 2003), a 'flipped-classroom' approach (Missildine et al., 2013), whereby information pertaining to an aspect of the simulation is given to participants prior to the event (e.g. a guideline/algorithm), can help facilitate and improve interprofessional learning. For example, if a difficult airway scenario is to be simulated, the unit guideline for this is given to participants beforehand and is available during the simulation.

With a less-experienced group of participants, a more *behavioural* learning approach may be required, which would require more input from the faculty. One or more members may need to act as confederates, otherwise known as embedded participants (INACSL Standards of Best Practice: Simulation^SM: INACSL Standards Committee, 2016), to guide the participants through a given scenario to achieve the learning objectives. In this case, it is still important that any confederate assists the participants to engage in the simulation, promoting active learning, directing them to the prior agreed learning objectives in a collaborative manner.

Design Characteristics/Learning Objectives

Points to consider include:

- Learning objectives for all IP team members
- Technical vs. non-technical factors
- Fidelity
- Space/equipment availability
- Cues
- Support mechanisms

It is important that the *learning objectives* are relevant to all participant groups involved, achievable in the set time frame and convey the process by which they are to be achieved. Focus on no more than four objectives for any given simulation, covering both technical and non-technical (human factor) skills. Within these learning objectives there may be technical issues for different participant groups that require discussion, but the main focus of interprofessional simulation should

be around how the professional groups interact with each other, the surroundings and the clinical issue. This needs to be conveyed in the learning objectives.

With the learning objectives in mind, consider the *design characteristics* of the simulation. The *fidelity* of the set-up – the degree to which the simulation replicates the real event and/or workplace – should address *physical, environmental and psychological* components (Lopreiato, 2016) of the simulation design. Physical fidelity, 'the degree to which the simulation looks, sounds and feels like the actual situation' (or the 'in-situ' nature of simulation), creates a high sense of realism, allowing participants to suspend disbelief on entering the simulation (Lopreiato, 2016). The use of monitored high-fidelity manikins, from which the participants are able to elicit clinical signs, along with using equipment identical to that used in clinical practice, increases the authenticity of the simulation – the participants' subjective interpretation/response to a constructed simulation (Bland et al., 2014). However, increasing the manikin fidelity does not automatically lead to an increase in authenticity and perceived participant learning (Bland et al., 2014). Using low-fidelity manikins, with additional moulage, in an otherwise high-fidelity environment (clinical room, with familiar equipment, following departmental system processes) can still create an authentic learning experience. A similar experience can be gained from the use of a high-fidelity manikin in a mocked-up training room, using the appliances and equipment seen in clinical practice. The design features should not detract from participants being able to achieve their learning objectives. See Chapter 5 for more information regarding fidelity.

Having an appropriate participant set-up, matching that in clinical practice, with the ability to summon senior assistance, by means of phone/bleep/crash buzzer, during the simulation further increases the environmental fidelity. Ensuring the departmental system processes are adhered to during the simulation aids the authenticity of the simulation experience and interprofessional learning. To promote psychological fidelity, each participant should perform their usual professional role and act within their clinical competencies.

The complexity of the simulation has to be appropriate to the clinical setting and participants involved (Motola et al., 2005; Reeves et al., 2007), and where the simulation is likely to extend beyond the participants' clinical capabilities, the faculty must ensure that appropriate scaffolding is in place. Senior support or supplementary information may be provided as a 'flipped-classroom' pre-simulation. *Cues* from the faculty may include altering the simulator parameters, in real time (ensuring realism of the simulated events), or questions and statements of clarification to the participants where visual cues cannot be recreated (e.g. colour or movement of a manikin).

Simulation Execution and Debriefing Practices

Points to consider:

- Pre-brief – introduction, orientation, safeguards/confidentiality
- Scenario – duration, focus, progression/problem-solving, manikin operation
- Debrief – location, safeguards, format

Simulation facilitation and debriefing should be in line with recognised standards (INACSL Standards Committee, 2016; Purva et al., 2016), including a *pre-brief, scenario facilitation* and facilitator-led *debrief* (Issenberg et al., 2005; Reeves et al., 2007).

The pre-brief information (Purva et al., 2016), given to the participants at the start of the session, should cover:

- Participant expectations
- Learning objectives
- Guidelines around conduct and confidentiality
- An introduction to the manikin and any unfamiliar equipment

In simulations where the content is deemed complex or may increase the extraneous cognitive load (Paas et al., 2003), or where systems are being tested, this pre-brief information can be provided as a separate session or in other media formats (e.g. video, e-learning, written format). Remember to allocate time for this in the simulation design.

The facilitation should be in line with the learning theory practices, allowing scenarios to progress uninterrupted to enable the participants to problem-solve independently where a constructivist style is used. The facilitator may use cues (e.g. physiological changes in the manikin's condition in line with the working diagnosis and participants' actions, blood results, phone calls) to aid the participants in achieving the learning objectives of the session, although ensuring that they do not detract from a participant-focused simulation (INACSL Standards Committee, 2016).

Debriefing is the most important component of a simulation-based learning experience (INACSL Standards Committee, 2016). This is covered, in depth, in Chapter 4.

Linked Learning Activities

Points to consider:

- Reflection (group and self)
- Evidence of participation (portfolio)
- Further reading (guidance/protocols)
- Appraisal
- Integration into clinical practice
- Further simulation participation

Following the simulation, linked learning activities allow participants to conceptualise the experiences and create new methods of encountering a problem in the future – the basis of Kolb's reflective learning cycle (Kolb, 2014). Although started during debriefing, it is important to recognise that the process of reflection extends outside the simulation experience. Participants should be directed towards where learning from this simulation sits within clinical practice/professional curricula/standards and provide sources of further reading or information. The opportunity to discuss or implement further learning may need to be provided, for example via appraisals or further simulation practice.

Evaluation/Outcomes

Points to consider:

- Participant – knowledge, skills, behaviours, critical thinking (technical and non-technical)
- Facilitator – effectiveness, confidence
- Organisation – meeting expectations, patient safety issues, systems, compliance figures

Irrespective of the type of simulation-based education performed, evaluation is crucial to aid sustainability and should take place on multiple levels in order to ensure all stakeholders' needs are met (Nestel et al., 2017).

Evaluation by participants (micro-evaluation) is commonly done in the first instance by questionnaire, in paper or electronic format, looking at the lower levels of evaluation – reaction/usefulness (level 1) and meeting learning objectives (level 2) (Kirkpatrick and Kirkpatrick, 2006). Higher levels of evaluation, looking at the effect of a simulation on knowledge, skills, behaviours and critical thinking, in the clinical area (level 3) or effects on patient care (level 4), can be powerful methods of evaluation of such an event or programme. This may involve repeated interviews with participants having undertaken similar events in clinical practice or observed behaviours in the clinical area by faculty.

Evaluation by facilitators (meso-evaluation) is useful to critically assess the effectiveness of the simulation session to adequately cover the agreed learning objectives. Evaluation of confidence and competence of facilitators, both by self-reflection, peer observation, anecdotally or by using validated observation tools, may lead to identification of training needs.

Regarding organisation evaluation (macro-evaluation), evidence on whether their expectations or requirements have been met by a simulation event or programme can be crucial to ongoing buy-in and support. Details relating to patient safety and system issues can be used to drive further content of inter-professional *in situ* simulations. If this programme was embedded in a training programme, staff compliance figures, as well as feedback, would be essential to ensure an equity of learning.

Summary

Establishing a sustained interprofessional *in situ* simulation programme requires enthusiasm, engagement and collaborative working between healthcare professionals. This chapter highlights some of the issues commonly faced by simulation enthusiasts and provides points for consideration when planning simulation strategies for the interprofessional healthcare workforce.

Bibliography

Barr, H., Hammick, M., Freeth, D. S., Reeves, S. and Koppel, I. (2008). *Effective Interprofessional Education: Argument, Assumption and Evidence (Promoting Partnership for Health)*. Oxford: Wiley-Blackwell.

Barr, H., Gray, R., Helme, M., Low, H. and Reeves, S. (2016). *Interprofessional Education Guidelines 2016*. London: CAIPE. www.caipe.org (accessed March 1, 2018).

Bland, A. J., Topping, A. and Tobbell, J. (2014). Time to unravel the conceptual confusion of authenticity and fidelity and their contribution to learning within simulation-based nurse education. A discussion paper. *Nurse Education Today*, 34(7), 1112–1118.

Department of Health. (2001). *Working Together, Learning Together*. London: Department of Health, Crown Copyright.

(2008). *A High Quality Workforce: NHS Next Stage Review*. London: Department of Health, Crown Copyright.

(2016). *Safer Maternity Care*. London: Department of Health, Crown Copyright.

Engum, S. A. and Jeffries, P. R. (2012). Interdisciplinary collisions: bringing healthcare professionals together. *Collegian*, 19(3), 145–151. doi: 10.1016/j.colegn.2012.05.005.

Gibbons, S., Adamo, G., Padden, D., et al. (2002). Clinical evaluation in advanced practice nursing education: using standardised patients in health assessment. *Journal of Nursing Education*, 41, 215–221.

INACSL Standards Committee (2016, December). INACSL standards of best practice: Simulation^{SM}.

Issenberg, S. B., McGaghie, W. C., Petrusa, E. R., Gordon, D. L. and Scalese, R. J. (2005). Features and uses of high-fidelity medical simulations that lead to effective learning: a BEME systematic review. *Medical Teacher*, 27(1), 10–28.

Kirkpatrick, D. L. and Kirkpatrick, J. D. (2006). *Evaluating Training Programs*, 3rd edition. San Francisco, CA: Berrett-Koehler Publishers.

Kohn, L. T., Corrigan, J. and Donaldson, M. S. (2000). *To Err is Human: Building a Safer Health System*. Washington, DC: National Academies Press.

Kolb, D. A. (2014). *Experiential Learning: Experience as the Source of Learning and Development*, 2nd edition. Upper Saddle River, NJ: Pearson Education.

Künzle, B., Kolbe, M. and Grote, G. (2010). Ensuring patient safety through effective leadership behaviour: a literature review. *Safety Science*, 48(1), 1–17. doi: 10.1016/j.ssci.2009.06.004.

Lantolf, J. and Thorne, S. (2006). *Sociocultural Theory and the Genesis of Second Language Development*. Oxford: Oxford University Press.

Lave, J. and Wenger, E. (1991). *Situated Learning: Legitimate Peripheral Participation*. New York, NY: Cambridge University Press.

Lopreiato, J. O. (Ed.), Downing, D., Gammon, W., Lioce, L., Sittner, B., Slot, V., Spain, A. E. (Associate Eds.) and the Terminology & Concepts Working Group. (2016). *Healthcare Simulation Dictionary*. [Online] (accessed November 13, 2016). Available from www.ssih.org/dictionary.

McLeod, S. A. (2012). Zone of Proximal Development [Online]. Available from: www.simplypsychology.org/Zone-of-Proximal-Development.html (accessed November 13, 2016).

Missildine, K., Fountain, R., Summers, L. and Gosselin, K. (2013). Flipping the classroom to improve student performance and satisfaction. *Journal of Nursing Education*, 52(10), 597–599.

Motola, I., Devine, L. A., Chung, H. S., Sullivan, J. E. and Issenberg, B. (2005). Simulation in healthcare education: best evidence practical guide. AMEE Guide No. 82. *Medical Teacher*, 35, e1511–e1530.

Nestel, D., Kelly, M., Jolly, B. and Watson, M. (2017). *Healthcare Simulation Education*, pp. 29–33. Chichester: John Wiley & Sons.

Oandasan, I. and Reeves, S. (2005). Key elements for interprofessional education. Part 1: The learner, the educator and the learning context. *Journal of Interprofessional Care*, 19(1), 21–38.

Paas, F., Renkl, A. and Sweller, J. (2003). Cognitive load theory and instructional design: recent developments. *Educational Psychologist*, 38(1), 1–4.

Purva, M., Baxendale, B., Scales, E., et al. (2016). *Simulation-based Education in Healthcare Standards Framework and Guidance*. Hull: Association for Simulated Practice in Healthcare (ASPiH).

Reeves, S. (2016). Why we need interprofessional education to improve the delivery of safe and effective care. *Interface – Comunicação, Saúde, Educação*, 20(56), 185–197. doi: 10.1590/1807-57622014.0092.

Reeves, S., Goldman, J. and Oandasan I. (2007). Key factors in planning and implementing interprofessional education in health care settings. *Journal of Allied Health*, 36(4), 231–235.

Sargeant, J. (2009). Theories to aid understanding and implementation of interprofessional education. *Journal of Continuing Education in the Health Professions*, 29(3), 178–184. doi: 10.1002/chp.20033.

Steinert, Y. (2005). Learning together to teach together: interprofessional education and faculty development. *Journal of Interprofessional Care*, 19(suppl 1), 60–75.

Sweeney, K. and Griffiths, F. (2002). *Complexity and Healthcare: An Introduction*, Chapter 1, p. 2. Oxford: Radcliffe Medical Press.

Thistlewaite, J. and Moran, M. on behalf of the World Health Organisation Study Group on Interprofessional Education and Collaborative Practice. (2010). Learning outcomes for interprofessional education (IPE): literature review and synthesis. *Journal of Interprofessional Care*, 24(5), 503–513, doi 10.3109/13561820.2010.483366.

Vygotsky, L. (1978). *Mind in Society: The Development of Higher Psychological Functions*. Cambridge, MA: Harvard University Press.

WHO. (2016). *Health workforce – nursing and midwifery*. Available from: www.who.int/hrh/nursing_midwifery/en/ (accessed February 26, 2017).

Wood, D. (2001). Scaffolding, contingent tutoring and computer-supported learning. *International Journal of Artificial Intelligence in Education*, 12, 280–292.

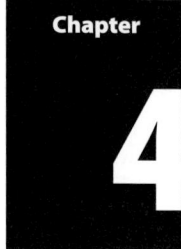

Debriefing and the Debrief

Mark Murphy and Annemarie Brown

Introduction

Debriefing can 'make or break' a simulator session and can be attributed as the 'heart and soul' of simulator training

(Rall et al., 2000)

In his attempts to accurately record events during World War II, US army Chief Historian Brigadier General Marshall performed the first historical group debrief (Shalev, 1993). Using a stepwise approach to the reconstruction of events, soldiers were interviewed as soon after action as possible. The primary aim was to obtain key information to assess performance and gather intelligence to inform future strategies. However, this method of reconstructing events following stressful combat exposure uncovered some unexpected psychological benefits.

The intention here is not to recount a historical evolution of debrief; however, this mix of fact finding, investigation, emotional responses and the development of future strategies is helpful in the formation of a definition. Put simply, in order to build upon past experience and gain knowledge, it is useful to fully perceive and make sense of them. Fanning and Gaba (2007) explain that adult learning is most successful when actively engaging and experiential, 'not only concrete events in a cognitive fashion, but also transactional events in an emotional fashion'.

The majority of healthcare education is delivered to adult learners. Such learners are usually self-motivated and attend sessions with their own learning objectives; therefore, it is crucial that they are able to participate actively in their education. There is evidence to suggest that without this, the effectiveness of the education provided is limited in this group. However, debriefing like any other skill needs to be learnt and practised and if poorly performed could actually be harmful to the learner(s), so it is important to get it right.

Fanning and Gaba (2007) go on to describe debriefing as a facilitated reflection encounter based upon an experiential learning episode. Any facilitated conversation following critical events, whether those are simulated or actual, is in essence the debrief structure. This conversation is an opportunity to identify any challenges encountered and to discuss and construct solutions. Discussions centring upon what went well are equally important to the process as those aimed at improving future performance.

The importance of debriefing as part of learning has been well documented; it is central to that process and cannot be overstated. There is considerable evidence to show that performance can be improved when debrief is utilised as part of simulation-based education (Small et al., 1999; Shapiro et al., 2004; DeVita et al., 2005; Dine et al., 2008; Morgan et al., 2009). Therefore, debrief is regarded by McGaghie et al. (2010) as the most important variable to produce effective learning from simulation-based medical education, with Rothgeb (2008) arguing that it should always be an integral part of the process. This period of facilitated reflection and discussion allows learners to become critical observers as well as active participants and is a broader description of experiential learning. Participants can 'take responsibility for their own learning; to be autonomous thinkers, to develop integrated understanding of concepts and to pose and seek to answer important questions' (Brooks and Brooks, 1993). The significance of the debrief as an essential part of the learning process can be further understood with the application of Kolb's (1984) experiential learning theory. Kolb describes a four-stage cycle of initial exposure as a 'concrete experience'. This is followed by an observational reflection of the experience by the learner(s), leading to analysis and formation of abstract concepts. Learners are then able to plan, develop and modify mental models in preparation for a repeat performance. This cycle closely mirrors the events that occur within a successful simulated experience. The simulation represents the 'concrete experience' and the actual 'learning' is provided by the subsequent debrief, where learners have the opportunity to reflect and analyse the events of the clinical encounter and make changes when returning to a new simulation and more importantly a 'real life' situation. This ongoing cycle is a 'continuous process of goal-directed action and evaluation of the consequences of that action'.

The Debrief Process

The Pre-briefing Stage (Setting the Scene and Agreeing the Agenda)

Once you have decided that a debriefing is beneficial, you then need to plan the process. First, you need to ensure that the participants understand the process, are prepared for it and that both the environment and setting are appropriate. Second, who is going to facilitate the 'debrief'? This can be more than one person, but the individuals need to plan the session together to ensure that all necessary areas are covered, without the facilitators dominating the discussions and to avoid repetition. You also need to be certain about who is being debriefed. Third, be sure of your objectives and the aspects of the experience needing to be covered. In the majority of team debriefs following a clinical simulation, the focus of the debriefing will be human factors and non-technical skills, which are discussed in detail in Chapters 6–8.

Sometimes a more thorough debrief of the technical aspects of the experience is appropriate. This will be dependent on multiple factors, including learning objectives, simulation participants and intervention location. When considering technical aspects ensure that you are prepared with up-to-date guidelines and recommendations to enable you to answer any questions or settle any disagreements accurately. Finally, you need to consider the debriefing model you are going to use.

Experiential learning requires active engagement (Chronister and Brown, 2012), meaning that in order to maximise the quality of the discussions during the debrief it is essential that those engaging in the process are equipped to do so. This necessitates securing both physical and emotional safety. Arafeh et al. (2010) support this by explaining that learners are prepared for the simulated experience by initially establishing their security.

It is important to appreciate and understand that participants may harbour fears and apprehensions surrounding the simulation and the debrief stages, particularly if they are new to the process. An awareness of the vulnerability of the participants is required (Fanning and Gaba, 2007) and it is important that the facilitator(s) create an atmosphere of trust and mutual appreciation. These fears may centre upon performance, knowledge gaps or potential error, and if not tackled may hinder the educational success of the intervention. Therefore, it is vital that ground rules about expected behaviour are agreed and that learning goals and aims are discussed. To maximise confidence in the process and minimise anxiety it is important to encourage openness and the sharing of information. This should take the form of a confidentiality agreement to which both confederate and facilitator agree, in effect 'Chatham House Rules'. In addition, it is also important to enter into a period of orientation through an interactive tour of the simulation area and equipment combined with an illustration of the methodology. This period of familiarisation to the simulation environment is an opportunity to gain acceptance to the reality that the area is a recreation and 'not real'. It is also an opportunity to request that the participants 'suspend disbelief' in order to maximise the experience. This is potentially more challenging 'in situ', although can be addressed in part by familiarity with the clinical environment. Our personal practice, where possible, would be to engage with the clinical area prior to the intervention and encourage participants to become acquainted with the team, the equipment and the methodology. This is particularly useful for those who are simulation-naïve, while also providing the simulation team with an opportunity for reconnaissance and cross-checks.

Debrief Delivery Stage

'A debriefing is a time to reflect on and discover together what happened … and what it all means' (Steinwachs, 1992). In healthcare education it has often been referred to as a 'learning' conversation and as mentioned above, according to educational theory, is stated as a time when the majority of the 'learning' occurs. To learn from a clinical exposure participants must be able to critically evaluate both the team's performance and their own. Therefore, one of the primary aims of the debrief is to aid this process through facilitation. There has been much discussion in the literature about the levels of appropriate facilitation. Some individuals and teams debrief themselves and require little facilitation, but others need guiding through the process. Fanning and Gaba (2007) suggest considering the following factors when deciding the amount of facilitation required:

1. The objective of the experiential exercise
2. The complexity of the scenarios
3. The experience level of the participants as individuals or as a team
4. The familiarity of the participants with the simulation environment
5. Time available for the session
6. The role of simulation in the overall curriculum
7. Individual personalities and relationships, if any, between participants

The authors go on to discuss the role of the facilitator and the careful balance that needs to be sought between active involvement of the participants and them taking responsibility for their own learning and ensuring that important issues are addressed. The correct balance will result in maximal learning.

The initial stage of the debriefing process should essentially provide a chance for cathartic release, when participants can express any strong emotions they are feeling following the clinical or simulated experience. It is therefore critical to provide a safe and supportive environment for the participants to ensure this occurs freely. The facilitator should then guide the participants through the various stages of the debriefing, initially stating the 'facts' and then encouraging them to explore the thought processes and emotions around their clinical decision-making. This should include any performance gaps identified, while ensuring the objectives of the session are achieved.

While the human factors involved in team resource management are usually the main focus in the debriefing sessions, technical questions should be adequately answered and can provide an opportunity to review published guidelines. Alongside processing new learning, the experience from the simulation should be linked to 'real life' situations to put the learning into context.

In a nutshell, the 'facilitated' debrief should provide a safe environment for participants to air their views openly and honestly. The facilitator guides them through a reflective process, focusing on the performance rather than the performer, reviewing their mental models and introducing new ideas, while considering changes in behaviour or approach. The facilitator should encourage candidates to relate their learning to 'real' patients and 'real' situations, with each session culminating in some 'take home messages'. The process should be neither judgemental nor non-judgemental,

but a balance between the two. Rudolph et al. (2006) describe this as 'debriefing with good judgement'.

Models of Debrief

Various models for debriefing have been described and there are many more that haven't been formally published. The majority of models are based on the theories behind psychological debriefing, which is considered to have the following phases:

1. Initial phase (Introduction). This phase is when introductions occur, the purpose of the simulation is stated, objectives are set and ground rules are agreed. During this time a climate of trust must be achieved by assuring a safe, confidential and supportive environment. It is often referred to as the 'Pre-brief'.
2. Fact phase – factual details of the experience are discussed.
3. Thought phase – exploring mental models and critical thinking behind decision-making.
4. Reaction or feeling phase – 'how did that make you feel?'
5. Symptom phase – physical and psychological effects of the experience.
6. Teaching phase – opportunity to discuss guidelines or policies and introduce new concepts/learning.
7. Re-entry or wrap-up phase – summarise, answer questions, develop plans for future actions, take home messages.

The majority of models for debriefing are based on these phases. In practice, phases 2–5 and most notably 3–5 tend to blend together to allow for a more natural flow for the discussions.

Pendleton's work is probably one of the most well-known models for feedback in medical education and is still utilised on many of the life support courses, but it has been heavily criticised for being too rigid and few would recommend its use for debriefing.

SHARP Model

The Imperial College of London describes a simple five-step debriefing tool, SHARP. These steps are subdivided into two phases; the first phase should occur before the simulation and is essentially the pre-brief, the second phase occurs after the simulation, fundamentally the debrief (Figure 4.1).

Rudolph et al. (2008) describe a step-wise approach to debriefing when discussing its role in formative

SHARP 5-STEP FEEDBACK & DEBRIEFING TOOL

BEFORE THE CASE

Set the learning objectives – What would you like to get out of this case?

AFTER THE CASE

How did it go?
What went well? Why?

Address concerns
What did not go so well? Why?

Review learning points
Were learning objectives met?
What did you learn about your technical skills?
What did you learn about your non-technical skills?

Plan ahead
What actions can you take to improve your future practice?

Figure 4.1 The SHARP five-step feedback and debriefing tool.

assessment. As you will see the steps they describe are closely related to those suggested for psychological debriefing:

- Create a context for learning.
- Have objectives in mind.
- The debriefing.
  - A. The reaction phase.
  - B. The analysis phase.
  - C. The summary phase.

GREAT Model

Owen and Follows (2006) suggest utilising the GREAT checklist to prepare and plan for the debriefing; again, the latter part of the checklist follows similar lines to the seven phases above, although it does not really touch on any of the emotional aspects of the experience, which are known to be fundamental for deeper learning.

(G) Guidelines: the facilitator must have the most recent best-evidence guidelines and local policy guidelines for managing the situation being simulated.

(R) Recommendations: if comprehensive guidelines are not available then recommendations such as those contained in published reviews should be used.

(E) Events: participants are given time to reflect on the simulation and identify the important events (e.g. the patient began fitting).

(A) Analysis: were signs identified promptly; how did treatments given compare with guidelines and recommendations; were resources used effectively, etc.?

(T) Transfer of knowledge to clinical practice: what has been learned to improve patient care? Are there any key 'take-home messages'?

As well as considering these stages and the structure you are going to utilise, the type of questioning used is also important. An open-ended questioning style should be used to encourage engagement and a learner-directed debrief, which in turn will enable participants to share their thoughts and emotions. The 'guess what I'm thinking' approach should definitely be avoided, as this will lead to frustrations on both sides and threaten any trust gained. However, in reality this is a trap that is easy to fall into and takes much practice to avoid and can affect even the most experienced debriefer.

Advocacy with Inquiry

'Advocacy with Inquiry' is a method that has become a popular style of questioning within the debrief (Rudolph et al., 2007). 'Advocacy' questions are generally statements about observations and will lead the participants to the areas or events that the facilitator wishes to discuss, while 'inquiry' questioning encourages deeper exploration of the events and emotions around them.

Examples of such questions are:

Advocacy

'I observed ...'
'I noticed ...'
'It looked a little disorganised in there. Do you know who was leading?'

Inquiry

'So, how did you feel?'
'What were you thinking at that point?'
'Were there any other options?'

Frames Model

Rudolph et al. (2006) described the 'Frames' approach to debriefing in their paper 'Debriefing with good judgement: combining rigorous feedback with genuine inquiry'. They describe cognitive 'frames', which they explain to be the participants' 'internal images of external reality'. This concept has been referred to earlier in this section as 'mental models'. These frames are obviously affected by many things, including knowledge, perceptions and feelings, and affect the actions that people take. The aim of their method is to explore the 'frames' and therefore the deeper thoughts and feelings around a performance gap. They go on to describe the instructor as a 'cognitive detective' who should work backwards from the observed performance gap to identify the frames that contributed to that gap. After identification of the frames leading to the error/event the instructor should explore new strategies with the participant to lead to a change in behaviour in the future.

Challenges to Debrief

So far, the background purpose and process of the 'debrief' have been discussed. In this section the challenges faced due to different individual personality/learning types will be reviewed and strategies for managing these different types explored. In the majority of cases the participants as adult learners will be extremely motivated, enthusiastic and willing to participate in discussion, but occasionally an individual(s) can cause challenges within the group dynamic. Bullock et al. (2015) describe three main groups in their book *Pocket Guide to Teaching for Medical Instructors*:

- Talkers
- Non-talkers
- Destroyers

Talkers

These individuals tend to be very enthusiastic to the point of being over-enthusiastic. They are very keen to impress and display their knowledge and if afforded the opportunity can potentially dominate the discussions. If they are allowed to do this, it is less likely that quieter members of the group will become involved in the discussions. Another risk is that they will go 'off-piste' and the debrief will go completely off track, resulting in objectives not being fulfilled.

If the talkers get into full flow it can be very difficult to stop them. One strategy to keep them on track is to ask them to summarise their thoughts and then deflect the focus to another participant by asking them to comment. If this is unsuccessful, micro-summaries may work. Again this moves the focus away from the individual, but also ensures the debrief remains on the right path. These strategies need to be used carefully to ensure all participants feel their contributions are of value.

Avoid ignoring the talkers or cutting them off, as this will lead to them becoming frustrated and potentially disengaging with the process.

Non-talkers

These are the quieter members of the group who may need a lot of encouragement and support; however, just because they aren't participating doesn't mean they aren't learning. Direct questioning will often make them very nervous and result in some unusual and often incorrect answers. The way this situation is dealt with is crucial to avoid them feeling ridiculed and embarrassed in front of their peers. Ideally the focus should be moved away from the individual; this can be easily achieved by simply rephrasing the question, perhaps suggesting that their answer was due to the question being unclear.

Repeating or summarising their comments or thoughts can help them feel more confident. For those who are particularly struggling, try moving them on to familiar territory, as this is where they are likely more comfortable and confident. Draw on their own experiences and ask them to relate the situation to their normal place of work and perhaps ask them to share with the group a similar 'real' event they have experienced.

Destroyers

These individuals can present themselves in different ways. They can be extremely disruptive to the group dynamics and are frequently challenging to manage. Classically they understand, or at least believe they understand, the core knowledge that is being discussed, but are reluctant to share any of that knowledge with the group. They are often extremely resistant to new concepts and remain rigid in their ideas. It is important where possible to try and help them use their knowledge constructively. In the case of particularly obstinate people, who fail to consider new ideas or the opinion of others, try to utilise the rest of the participants to draw them into the discussions, but avoid conflict developing in the group.

If a participant is complaining, it is important to identify whether their complaint is justified and, if it is, act to address it as soon as possible, and try and use these issues as constructively as possible. If complaints aren't dealt with rapidly, the situation could deteriorate and the engagement of others could be lost. It will depend on the complaint as to whether it can be dealt with within or away from the group. In the case of a very disruptive participant who is rude, aggressive and resistant to any strategies attempted to gain engagement, these participants are best dealt with outside the group situation, where their concerns and issues can be explored confidentially. If there appears to be a character clash, request another instructor to talk to the candidate. If the participant remains resistant to change and nothing can rectify the situation, the participant should be asked to leave to avoid complete disruption of the other participants' learning experience.

Video-Assisted Debrief

Video playback, as illustrated in Figure 4.2, is regularly used to assist with simulation debriefs; although Fanning and Gaba (2007) stated that the advantage over a traditional oral debrief is not consistent. Then again, they go on to state that video playback can add perspective to the simulation by allowing participants to observe how they actually performed, rather than how they thought they performed.

In our experience, video playback can be described as an art rather than a science and can take some practice to get right. The authors state that great care is required to avoid playing long sections of irrelevant segments of video, as this has a tendency to stifle the debrief. In the more inexperienced debriefer a tendency to overly rely upon event marking has been observed which can have a similar stifling effect. However, if used correctly, video playback can be a fantastic tool. It provides psychomotor and visual learning allowing the group to review the information collaboratively and discuss the decision-making and the reasons for certain outcomes; thus providing an opportunity for further reflection. It can be perfect for illustrating good practice and emphasising points, but the temptation to utilise footage to settle disagreements should be resisted.

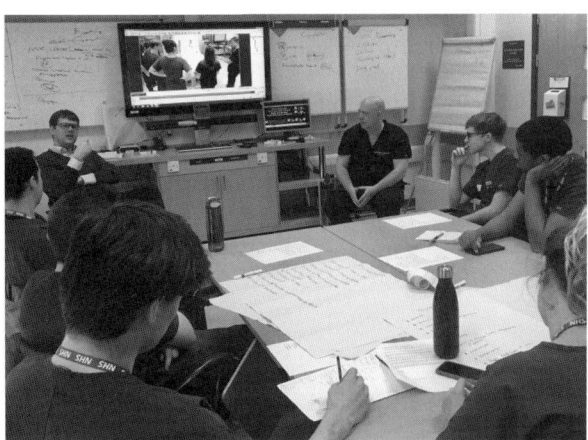

Figure 4.2 Video-assisted group debrief.

As mentioned earlier, debriefing is a skill and the skill of the debriefer is vital for delivery of a successful learning experience. Training is therefore paramount and much more important than the model chosen to use. Historically, this has been difficult to come by; some centres offer formal debriefing education, many pair a novice debriefer with an experienced one to allow for support and guidance. This situation also provides an opportunity for feedback, a 'debrief of the debrief', so to speak.

Debriefing the Debrief

This can be done informally, but there are assessment tools available for a more formal and thorough approach.

Brett-Fleegler et al. (2012) recognised the need for assessment of debriefing in healthcare simulation and developed the DASH structure to address the lack of tools appropriate for use in the healthcare setting. Their tool is based on a behaviourally anchored rating scale (BARS) and was reported to show good reliability and preliminary validity. There are six elements of the assessment and all are scored 1 to 7, with 1 being 'extremely ineffective/abysmal' and 7 'extremely effective/outstanding'.

The Imperial College of London describe their Objective Structured Assessment of the Debrief (OSAD) as a tool consisting of eight categories, which again follow the phases of debriefing. Each category is scored from 1 to 5 by the observer, with 1 being 'carried out very poorly' and 5 'carried out very well'. The authors state that it is feasible, user-friendly, evidence-based, validated and reliable.

Here are some final thoughts as you look through the 'one way mirror'.

The debrief offers a fantastic opportunity for both learning and reflection, but it also carries with it an immense responsibility.

This may well be the fiftieth occasion you have observed a particular scenario and the fiftieth occasion you have facilitated the following debrief, but remember for your candidates this could be their first time … and never forget we are all capable of becoming a victim of human factors, even you!

Bibliography

Arafeh, J. M., Hansen, S. S. and Nichols, A. (2010). Debriefing in simulated-based learning: facilitating a reflective discussion. *The Journal of Perinatal & Neonatal Nursing*, 24(4), 302–309.

Brett-Fleegler, M., Rudolph, J., Eppich, W., et al. (2012). Debriefing assessment for simulation in healthcare: development and psychometric properties. *Simulation in Healthcare*, 7(5), 288–294.

Brooks, J. G. (1999). *In Search of Understanding: The Case for Constructivist Classrooms*. Alexandria, VA: ASCD.

Brooks, J. G. and Brooks, M. G. (1993). *In Search of Understanding: The Case for Constructivist Classrooms*. Alexandria, VA: ASCD

Bullock, I., Davis, M., Lockey, A. and Mackway-Jones, K. (Eds.) (2015). *Pocket Guide to Teaching for Clinical Instructors*, 3rd edition. Chichester: John Wiley & Sons.

Chronister, C. and Brown, D. (2012). Comparison of simulation debriefing methods. *Clinical Simulation in Nursing*, 8(7), e281–e288.

DeVita, M. A., Schaefer, J., Lutz, J., Wang, H. and Dongilli, T. (2005). Improving medical emergency team (MET) performance using a novel curriculum and a computerized human patient simulator. *Quality and Safety in Health Care*, 14(5), 326–331.

Dine, C. J., Gersh, R. E., Leary, M., Riegel, B. J., Bellini, L. M. and Abella, B. S. (2008). Improving cardiopulmonary resuscitation quality and resuscitation training by combining audiovisual feedback and debriefing. *Critical Care Medicine*, 36(10), 2817–2822.

Fanning, R. M. and Gaba, D. M. (2007). The role of debriefing in simulation-based learning. *Simulation in Healthcare*, 2(2), 115–125.

Imperial College London. (2012). *The Observational Structured Assessment of Debriefing Tool (OSAD)*. London: Imperial College London, London Deanery.

Kolb, D. A. (1984). *Experiential Learning: Experience as the Source of Learning and Development*. Englewood Cliffs, NJ: Prentice Hall.

McGaghie, W. C., Issenberg, S. B., Petrusa, E. R. and Scalese, R. J. (2010). A critical review of simulation-based medical education research: 2003–2009. *Medical Education*, 44(1), 50–63.

Morgan, P. J., Tarshis, J., LeBlanc, V., et al. (2009). Efficacy of high-fidelity simulation debriefing on the performance of practicing anaesthetists in simulated scenarios. *British Journal of Anaesthesia*, 103(4), 531–537.

Owen, H. and Follows, V. (2006). GREAT simulation debriefing. *Medical Education*, 40(5), 488–489.

Rall, M., Manser, T. and Howard, S. K. (2000). Key elements of debriefing for simulator training. *European Journal of Anaesthesiology*, 17(8), 516–517.

Rothgeb, M. K. (2008). Creating a nursing simulation laboratory: a literature review. *Journal of Nursing Education*, 47(11), 489–494.

Rudolph, J. W., Simon, R., Dufresne, R. L. and Raemer, D. B. (2006). There's no such thing as 'nonjudgmental' debriefing: a theory and method for debriefing with good judgment. *Simulation in Healthcare*, 1(1), 49–55.

Rudolph, J. W., Simon, R., Raemer, D. B. and Eppich, W. J. (2008). Debriefing as formative assessment: closing performance gaps in medical education. *Academic Emergency Medicine*, 15(11), 1010–1016.

Rudolph, J. W., Simon, R., Rivard, P., Dufresne, R. L. and Raemer, D. B. (2007). Debriefing with good judgment: combining rigorous feedback with genuine inquiry. *Anesthesiology Clinics*, 25(2), 361–376.

Shalev A. (1993). Historical Group Debriefing Following Combat. US Army Medical Research & Development Command, Fort Detrick, Frederick (MD). Final Report. May 1, 1993. Available from: www.dtic.mil/cgi-bin/GetTRDoc?AD=ADA267287S (accessed November 18, 2017).

Shapiro, M. J., Morey, J. C., Small, S. D., et al. (2004). Simulation based teamwork training for emergency department staff: does it improve clinical team performance when added to an existing didactic teamwork curriculum? *Quality and Safety in Health Care*, 13(6), 417–421.

Small, S. D., Wuerz, R. C., Simon, R., Shapiro, N., Conn, A. and Setnik, G. (1999). Demonstration of high-fidelity simulation team training for emergency medicine. *Academic Emergency Medicine*, 6(4), 312–323.

Steinwachs, B. (1992). How to facilitate a debriefing. *Simulation & Gaming*, 23(2), 186–195.

Chapter

5

Fidelity in Obstetric Simulation

Shane O'Sullivan and Owen O'Sullivan

Fidelity in simulation is a term referring to the loyalty of a particular model to real life characteristics. Essentially, it refers to how 'life-like' a simulation may be. It is a concept that is often poorly defined and subject to various interpretations in the medical literature. Fidelity, or lack thereof, is an intuitively grasped property of any attempt at simulation. Maran and Glavin (2003) describe fidelity as 'the extent to which the appearance and behaviour of the simulator/simulation match the appearance and behaviour of the simulated system'.

Fidelity is often attributed to a particular simulation tool, or simulator, as a fixed variable. At times this can be set arbitrarily by manufacturers as part of marketing. Technological sophistication can be confused with fidelity. Also, it is likely that incremental enhancements of a simulator to improve its fidelity will increase the cost. Beyond a certain, ill-defined, point these enhancements will add little to the role of the simulator as an educational tool. In reality, the fidelity of the simulation (rather than the simulator) is what is important, from the perspective of the learner. A 'high-fidelity' simulator used in a certain manner can result in a low-fidelity educational experience.

With a lack of a consensus of the definition of fidelity, interpreting the body of literature looking at simulation fidelity is difficult. It is also likely that the results of certain studies cannot be easily applied in other contexts. Many papers describe high-fidelity simulation as having occurred simply due to qualities of the simulator used.

Physical vs. Psychological

Miller (1953) first made the distinction between engineering, or physical, and psychological fidelity in the context of simulation for aviation. Engineering fidelity is the extent to which the training device replicates the physical characteristics of the real-world task. Psychological fidelity is how well the simulated task captures the skills necessary for that task in the real world.

These two aspects of fidelity do not necessarily equate. For example, a simple foam model provides relatively little physical fidelity when practising suturing, but excellent functional or psychological fidelity.

Spectrum of Simulators

Simulators do not need to be physical and include mental exercises, where learners engage in imaginary activities. See Table 5.1 for a tabulated spectrum of simulation.

Table 5.1 Simulator spectrum organised by simulator type (Adapted from Gardner and Raemer, 2008).

Simulator characteristics	Fidelity	Cost	User feedback	Instructor input
Part task trainer	Low	Low to moderate	Nil	Low to moderate
Mental simulation	Low	Low	Low to moderate	Low to moderate
Computer-based system	Low to moderate	Moderate to high	Moderate to high	Nil to low
Virtual reality and haptic simulator	Moderate to high	High to very high	High	Moderate to high
Simulated patients	Low to moderate	Low	High	High
Hybrid patients	Moderate to high	Low to moderate	High	High
Integrated simulators – model-driven	High	Very high	High	Low to moderate
Integrated simulators – instructor-driven	High	Moderate to very high	Moderate to high	High

Part Task Trainers

These simulators seek to replicate only the salient portion of the environment relevant to the task at hand; for example, phlebotomy arms or static pelvic models for delivery simulation. As a consequence, they are relatively inexpensive to produce and maintain, with the most significant cost arising from the need for an instructor to teach and assess the clinical skills in question.

Computer Screen-Based Systems

Computers can be used to model different clinical scenarios, as well as faithfully replicate physiological and pharmacological data (de Wit-Zuurendonk and Oei, 2011). Students can then alter these models and the results can be observed, which enables real-time feedback to be supplied to the student while also allowing multiple attempts and therefore multiple outcomes. Moreover, as the only physical requirement for this type of simulation is an interface, multiple learners can be trained simultaneously in a semi-autonomous fashion.

Virtual Reality and Haptic Systems

Virtual reality (VR) represents the ultimate in computer-based simulation. The incorporation of a physical interface, often a part task trainer, that responds dynamically to the user and thereby attempts to replicate the physical feedback associated with a particular task allows for even further levels of interaction. This simulation method is used extensively in laparoscopic training models for surgical trainees. To date, the role for this modality has been limited in obstetric simulation.

Simulated Patients and Hybrid Simulators

Standard, or simulated, patients are already commonplace in medical education. Ranging from undergraduate history taking to communication assessment stations in objective structured clinical exams (OSCEs) at a postgraduate level, this type of simulation in isolation is almost exclusively aimed at imparting non-physical skills. Simulations involving patient actors were associated with improved perception of communication and safety compared with manikin based simulation (Crofts et al., 2008).

A standard patient can be combined with physical models such as part task trainers or even more complex integrated models (see below). These hybrid simulators allow for the integration of communication, interpersonal and psychomotor skills, as well as providing the overarching appropriate clinical context for each of these components. While lacking any specific pathology, they will potentially be able to portray symptoms accurately through verbal and non-verbal cues. This can readily change a simulation scenario from a low physical fidelity simulation into a high psychological fidelity simulation with the addition of communication skills and direct human interaction in addition to the psychomotor skills taught by a simple physical model. It is particularly significant in obstetric population, where a non-pregnant actor would likely challenge the immersion of participant involved in the simulated scenario.

The concept of hybrid simulators was first reported in 2002 for procedural skills (Kneebone et al., 2002) and has expanded to include a wide range of procedural and operative skills with simulation manufacturers designing products for this specific purpose. Higham et al. (2007) report the concept for vaginal examination and Pap smear. Cooper et al. (2012, 2016) describe a birthing suit that is worn by an SP and enables midwifery students to learn effective teamwork during delivery. Similarly, Kumar et al. (2016) describe a hybrid model of an SP and birthing model 'in situ' for supporting the development of interprofessional collaborative practice for homebirths. An alternative form of hybrid simulation developed by Pauline Lyon simply uses a life-size photograph of a woman in labour that is placed alongside the birthing model (Lyon, personal communication). Together with sound effects, the visual representation engages simulation participants differently to simplify learning on the model.

Figure 5.1 shows use of a wearable part task trainer as a hybrid solution.

Integrated Simulators

Integrated simulators combine many of the above features to be as fully immersive a simulation experience as possible. Model-driven simulators, controlled by sophisticated physiological and pharmacological algorithms that enable autonomous responses independent of instructor input, are hugely expensive. These incorporate full-body manikins capable of replicating a wide variety of clinical parameters, including speech, ECG rhythms, central venous pressure traces and chest sounds. However, they often lack non-verbal cues (e.g. changes in facial expression, muscle tone or skin colour).

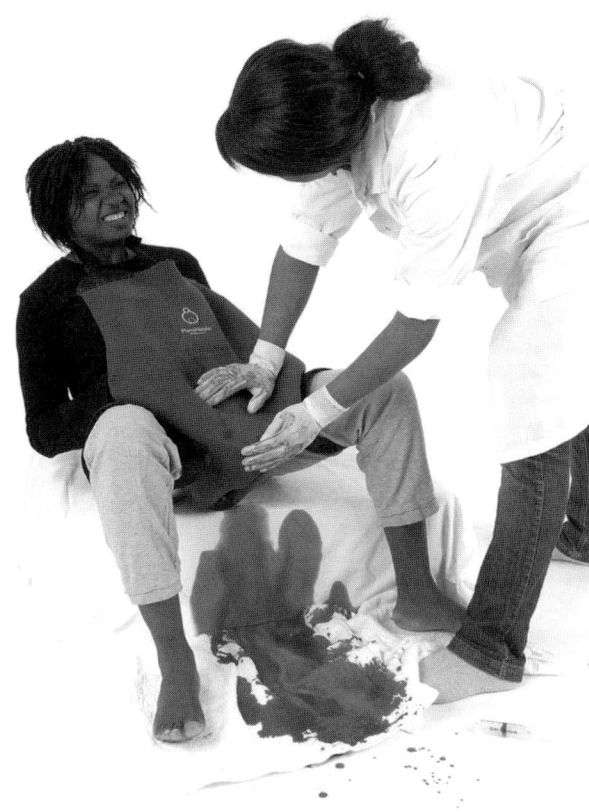

Figure 5.1 A hybrid postpartum haemorrhage simulation. A faculty member playing the part of a patient (standard patient), wearing the low-cost part task trainer MamaNatalie to facilitate a high-fidelity simulation.

(Image courtesy of Laerdal Global Healthcare)

An 'intermediate'-type simulator might have significant computer modelling built into it, but is still dependent upon instructor input to modify 'physiological' responses to learner interaction.

Used in combination with faithful location replication and simulated patients, and possibly even clinical staff, these simulators allow for both excellent physical and psychological fidelity in the hands of expert instructors, who have sufficient experience with the models to minimise delays in response and inappropriate cueing to trainees.

High vs. Low Fidelity

The fidelity of simulation (and simulators) is often arbitrarily defined along a continuum of low-, intermediate- and high-fidelity. The utility of the delineation is questionable. There is no standard which describes

how close to reality a simulation has to be to be termed high-fidelity. It is also likely that certain current simulations considered high-fidelity will be deemed lower fidelity in the future, with developments in the science of healthcare simulation. The terms are used mostly in a relative sense in that one particular simulator may be more 'realistic' and hence of higher fidelity than another. For example, a low-fidelity simulator in epidural anaesthesia may be a plastic model of the lumbar spine, while a high-fidelity model is a life-size replica of a patient's back with multiple fluid-filled compartments capable of replicating loss-of-resistance during Tuohy needle insertion.

Low-fidelity simulation is most often used for demonstration and practice of manual technical skills, e.g. suturing, urinary catheter insertion or intravenous cannulation. In this respect, it is frequently, although not exclusively, used to impart a one-dimensional skill set. The learning objective is to acquire competency in a defined set of technical skills. Moreover, instructor interaction is necessary to enable the skill acquisition – low-fidelity simulators, typically, do not respond dynamically to trainee input.

High-fidelity simulation, by comparison, is deemed a more accurate attempt at replicating 'real life', such as full clinical case scenario rather than a single skill. An example of this would be a resuscitation training scenario involving an advanced, computer-driven, patient simulator (e.g. SimMan, Laerdal Medical, Stavanger, Norway). High-fidelity simulation seeks to provide context in which a skill is not only deployed, but also examines the appropriateness of the decision to use said skill. In that regard, high-fidelity simulation also involves non-technical skills such as communication, leadership and stress management. High-fidelity simulators are characterised by their ability to respond to trainee input, either through indirect instructor input via a computer or through automatic scripted responses built into the simulation software.

At present, the evidence to favour high-fidelity over low-fidelity simulation is scant. In a small study of nursing students undergoing training in congestive cardiac failure, Kardong-Edgren et al. (2007) failed to show an improvement in post-training test scores between high- and low-fidelity arms. DeStephano et al. (2015) found that a low-fidelity hybrid spontaneous vaginal delivery model was as effective at teaching normal delivery to medical students as a high-fidelity computer-controlled manikin. Interestingly, the students felt more confident in their abilities after training on the low-fidelity hybrid model, but this may be confounded by the human interaction component this included that the remote controlled manikin lacked. Friedman et al. (2009) found no difference in the performance of anaesthesia students trained to perform epidural insertion on a high- or a low-fidelity model, and no apparent change in steepness of their learning curve over subsequent cases.

This is in contrast to a randomised controlled trial conducted by Crofts et al. (2006), which demonstrated that a high-fidelity model of shoulder dystocia, which incorporated force feedback, offered additional training benefit in terms of more successful deliveries with less force applied.

Scholz et al. (2012) found that although two groups of medical students made equivalent obstetric decisions regardless of whether they underwent training on low- or high-fidelity simulators, those that underwent high-fidelity training felt more confident in their own abilities, as well as demonstrating improved obstetric skills.

Studies need to include not only indicators that training has transferred into clinical practice, but also that alterations in clinical outcome have improved patient outcomes. However, at this point there is little evidence that high-fidelity simulation training impacts clinical outcomes. A multicentre randomised control trial by Fransen et al. (2017) failed to show a difference in a composite endpoint of obstetric complications following high-fidelity simulation team training.

Appropriateness of Fidelity

The level of fidelity required in obstetric simulation is likely not fixed. The fidelity required will depend on variables such as the type of task being taught and stage of training of the participants (Maran & Glavin, 2003). The use of simple simulators appears to be more appropriate in the training of basic skills to novices. Kardong-Edgren et al. (2007) found that students were so enthralled with the capabilities of their high-fidelity simulator that they were being repeatedly drawn back to task. Similarly, overly complex simulators that offer far more physical fidelity than that required for learning the task at hand might obscure the desired learning point.

As learners' skills increase the simulator must be able to support high-level tasks at high speed, as well as providing the necessary cues to enable appropriate decision-making. These cues must be sufficiently evident, however, to avoid 'simulator hypervigilance', whereby every small change in any given variable is falsely interpreted as being hugely significant. In teaching fine motor skills, a simulator which does not allow the accurate manoeuvres required has the potential to result in negative learning (including the automation of inappropriate behaviours).

In simulation for aviation training it is possible to reach much higher relative levels of fidelity than in healthcare simulation. The cockpit environment and computer modelling of movement, based on the laws of physics, will allow an experience closely matching flying the particular aircraft simulated. Human physiology is arguably more complex to model. It is also less predictable. A simple intervention in a flight simulator will likely produce a predictable response. Humans often respond to relatively simple interventions with much wider interindividual responses (for example, the effect of a simple fluid bolus on vital signs and urine output).

Simple Measures to Enhance Fidelity

Classically, simulation training, particularly high-fidelity training involving complex computer and audiovisual input, is carried out in clinical skills labs or dedicated simulation centres far from the clinical sites where the learned skills are supposed to be applied. One effective means of enhancing psychological fidelity is the use of *in situ* simulation (Chapter 2 explores this in detail). It should be noted that this environment may not be appropriate to novices beginning to learn a skill, where the additional cues provided by the environment may distract and detract from performance.

One of the main challenges to effective simulation is the 'buy-in' of the learner. During the orientation or pre-briefing session it is important to set ground rules and expectations in terms of the limitations of the fidelity of the tools and environment which will be used. A novice learner may perceive a simulation as realistic, while an experienced practitioner may detect inaccuracies in the same experience. For the purposes of engagement, a learner should not be concerned with exercising their limited attention capacity on how closely the simulation matches their experience. Rather, a 'suspension of disbelief' will facilitate immersion into the simulation. Without buy-in there is a risk that participants can undermine simulations by emphasising the limitations of the simulation and use them as excuses for poor performance. Psychological rather than absolute physical fidelity appears to be the ultimate determinant of learner 'buy-in', and therefore the biggest factor in knowledge transfer.

The use of hybrid simulators also allows for high levels of psychological fidelity, despite perhaps relying on relatively low levels of physical fidelity. This is perhaps the best example of the concept first described by Macedonia et al. (2003); namely, that a simulation be ARRON – 'as reasonably realistic as objectively needed'.

Engström et al. (2016) examined aspects of contextualisation on simulation. They found that interventions/interruptions of the instructor and illogical jumps in time or in space challenge the participants' immersion in simulation and can potentially negatively impact the learning experience.

Cost and Application to Low-Resource Setting

A drive to enhance fidelity of simulators, perhaps by technological advancement, will likely result in an increased cost of the tools. One result of this is that higher-fidelity simulators may be limited to centralised training centres or simulation labs. This may result in trainees having only limited access to the simulated environment, for example at training or 'sim' days (massed practice). However, there is increasing evidence that distributed practice may be more effective in meeting individual training needs (Cook et al., 2013). Distributed practice involves repetitive practice spread over a wider time span. This is arguably more likely if the training tool is more immediately available to the trainee (e.g. each department has immediate access to the simulator).

Yau et al. (2016) found that setting up a PROMPT course in their institution in the UK cost €148,806 per year. The vast majority of the expenditure arose from releasing staff to attend, either as trainers or trainees. Although only €5574 of this was related to purchasing of manikins and printing of training material, this cost would likely be prohibitive in many low-resource environments across the world.

An estimated 99% of maternal death due to obstetric haemorrhage occurs in developing regions, with almost half occurring in Sub-Saharan Africa (Say et al., 2014). Evidence from high-resource settings may not be directly applicable. Simulators deployed in this setting need to be durable, easy to maintain and sanitise, and manikins should be culturally appropriate. Specific low-cost enhancements of fidelity have been utilised to good effect. In rural Rwanda, Nathan and coworkers used local fruit juice and cornstarch to imitate blood (Nathan et al., 2016).

Walker et al. (2012) first described a pilot feasibility study of the PRONTO course in a Mexican setting. It used the 'PartoPants' simulator, a low-tech, low-cost model based on an adapted pair of scrub pants in conjunction with hybrid simulated patients to achieve a high-fidelity simulation-based obstetric training programme. Magee et al. (2013) found that low-cost simulated patients, using simple part task trainers, could be an effective way to improve family medicine resident management of postpartum haemorrhage, as well as to increase retention at 6 months. Nathan et al. (2016) also found that skills in postpartum haemorrhage management taught on a low-cost simulator in rural Rwanda were retained for up to 2 years after the intervention.

Although many of the studies have been small, and therefore markedly underpowered to demonstrate a statistically significant improvement in clinical outcomes, it may in fact take many years and wider distribution of these training programmes over both time and geography before their worth can be conclusively demonstrated. In low-resource settings, it is likely the expertise, not the physical props, that will represent the largest challenge when setting up a simulation programme.

Bibliography

Cook, D. A., Hamstra, S. J., Brydges, R., et al. (2013). Comparative effectiveness of instructional design features in simulation-based education: systematic review and meta-analysis. *Medical Teacher*, 35, e867–e898.

Cooper, S. and Biro, M. (2015). Hybrid simulated patient methodology: managing maternal deterioration. In D. Nestel and M. Bearman (Eds.), *Simulated Patient Methodology: Theory, Evidence and Practice*, pp. 120–125. Chichester: John Wiley & Sons.

Cooper, S., Bulle, B., Biro, M. A., et al. (2012). Managing women with acute physiological deterioration: student midwives performance in a simulated setting. *Women and Birth*, 25(3), e27–e36.

Crofts, J. F., Bartlett, C., Ellis, D., et al. (2006). Training for shoulder dystocia. *Obstetrics & Gynecology*, 108, 1477–1485.

Crofts, J. F., Bartlett, C., Ellis, D., et al. (2008). Patient-actor perception of care: a comparison of obstetric emergency training using manikins and patient-actors. *Quality and Safety in Health Care*, 17, 20–24.

DeStephano, C. C., Chou, B., Patel, S., et al. (2015). A randomized controlled trial of birth simulation for medical students. *American Journal of Obstetrics and Gynecology*, 213, 91.e1–91.e7.

De Wit-Zuurendonk, L. D. & Oei, S. G. (2011). Serious gaming in women's health care. *British Journal of Obstetrics & Gynaecology*, 118, 17–21.

Engström, H., Hagiwara, M. A., Backlund, P., et al. (2016). The impact of contextualization on immersion in healthcare simulation. *Advances in Simulation*, 1(1), 8.

Fransen, A., van de Ven, J., Schuit, E., van Tetering, A. A. C., Mol, B. W. and Oei, S. G. (2017). Simulation-based team training for multi-professional obstetric care teams to improve patient outcome: a multicentre, cluster randomised controlled trial. *British Journal of Obstetrics & Gynaecology*, 124, 641–650.

Friedman, Z., Siddiqui, N., Katznelson, R., et al. (2009). Clinical impact of epidural anesthesia simulation on short- and long-term learning curve: high- versus low-fidelity model training. *Regional Anesthesia and Pain Medicine*, 34, 229–232.

Gardner, R., & Raemer, D. B. (2008). Simulation in obstetrics and gynecology. *Obstetrics and Gynecology Clinics of North America*, 35, 97–127.

Higham, J., Nestel, D., Lupton, M. and Kneebone, R. (2007). Teaching and learning gynaecology examination with hybrid simulation. *The Clinical Teacher*, 4, 238–243.

Kardong-Edgren, S., Anderson, M. and Michaels, J. (2007). Does simulation fidelity improve student test scores? *Clinical Simulation in Nursing*, 3, e21–e24.

Kneebone, R., Kidd, J., Nestel, D., Asvall, S., Paraskeva, P. and Darzi, A. (2002). An innovative model for teaching and learning clinical procedures. *Medical Education*, 36(7), 628–634.

Kumar, A., Nestel, D., Stoyles, S., East, C., Wallace, E. M. and White, C. (2016). Simulation based training in a publicly funded home birth programme in Australia: a qualitative study. *Women Birth*, 29(1), 47–53.

Macedonia, C. R., Gherman, R. B. and Satin, A. J. (2003). Simulation laboratories for training in obstetrics and gynecology. *Obstetrics & Gynecology*, 102, 388–392.

Magee, S. R., Shields, R. and Nothnagle, M. (2013). Low cost, high yield: simulation of obstetric emergencies for family medicine training. *Teaching and Learning in Medicine*, 25, 207–210.

Maran, N. J. and Glavin, R. (2003). Low to high fidelity simulation – a continuum of medical education? *Medical Education*, 37, 22–28.

McGaghie, W. C., Issenberg, S. B., Petrusa, E. R. and Scalese, R. J. (2010). A critical review of simulation-based medical education research: 2003–2009. *Medical Education*, 44(1), 50–63.

Miller, R. B. (1953). *Psychological Considerations in the Design of Training Equipment*. Pittsburgh, PA: American Institutes for Research.

Nathan, L. M., Patauli, D., Nsabimana, D., et al. (2016). Retention of skills 2 years after completion of a postpartum hemorrhage simulation training program in rural Rwanda. *International Journal of Gynecology & Obstetrics*, 134, 350–353.

Say, L., Chou, D., Gemmill, A., et al. (2014). Global causes of maternal death: a WHO systematic analysis. *The Lancet Global Health*, 2, e323–e333.

Scholz, C., Mann, C., Kopp, V., et al. (2012). High-fidelity simulation increases obstetric self-assurance and skills in undergraduate medical students. *Journal of Perinatal Medicine*, 40, 607–613.

Walker, D. M., Cohen, S. R., Estrada, F., et al. (2012). PRONTO training for obstetric and neonatal emergencies in Mexico. *International Journal of Gynecology and Obstetrics*, 116, 128–133.

Yau, C. W. H., Pizzo, E., Morris, S., et al. (2016). The cost of local, multi-professional obstetric emergencies training. *Acta Obstetricia et Gynecologica Scandinavica*, 95, 1111–1119.

Chapter

6

Introduction to Human Factors and Ergonomics in Obstetric Simulation

Mark Hellaby

Human factors have seen a surge of interest in healthcare as a method to combat the unacceptably high levels of healthcare error and harm. Healthcare is very unpredictable in nature; patients have a variety of problems, or may develop new ones, there may be emergency events where healthcare staff are required to respond quickly and effectively, making potentially life-and-death decisions where an incorrect act, or an omission, can have significant consequences.

The interest in human factors stems partly from several high-profile cases, including that of Elaine Bromiley, who lost her life from a rare yet manageable airway problem. This case championed by her husband, Martin, led to the formation of the Clinical Human Factors Group (www.chfg.org), who have campaigned for change in the NHS and have a variety of resources including Elaine's story.

A recent report by the Commission on Education and Training for Patient Safety commissioned by NHS Health Education England cited that there is a need for a common language for human factors and the need for it to be embedded across education and training (HEE, 2016). This call for a common language arises from the confusion about the definition and the extent of human factors.

> **Definition of Human Factors and Ergonomics (HFE)**
> Dr Ken Catchpole describes human factors as 'enhancing clinical performance through an understanding of the effect of teamwork, tasks, equipment, workspace, culture and organisation, on human behaviour and abilities, and application of that knowledge in clinical settings'.

One of the most important things to emphasise is that humans do and always will make errors, and while effective training can reduce this, there will always be human errors – partly because of the way the human brain functions and the limitations of the human body.

We know humans are more likely to make mistakes in certain situations, for instance when we are hungry, angry, late or tired (HALT). We are also predisposed to making errors by the way we think and interact with the world around us. To an extent this cognitive vulnerability is one that can be exploited because it is predictable; however, awareness alone will not prevent these as they are subconscious and can only be captured by robust systems.

The current view of errors is that they cannot only originate in the clinical team through knowledge errors, slips and lapses and violations, but also at an organisational level through poor policies, procedures, management, etc. (Reason, 1990). Unfortunately, there is still a misconception held by a lot of people that human factors awareness just needs team training – this is only part of the issue, and really human factor awareness needs to be embedded across the system so that processes, tasks and equipment are designed to take into account how the human can and will act.

Part of the confusion stems from the myriad terms that are often incorrectly used interchangeably. To add to this confusion, there are potentially divergent views on what human factors are at an academic level, with a difference in opinion between ergonomists and behavioural psychologists. The term ergonomics, while focusing on the human–machine interaction, can also be used interchangeably with the term human factors.

Now consider that we don't just work on our own but in teams, and often multiprofessional teams or even teams across departmental or organisational boundaries. Historically we haven't trained for this teamworking component, but have had to find our way through trial and error – but without any measurement or feedback on performance, this development is very variable. Professor Eduardo Salas, who has explored team-working, says that the risk is that we concentrate on the clinical processes and not the team-working and produce a 'team of experts and not the expert team' (Salas et al., 1997). The focus of developing an effective

Table 6.1 Elements of human factors and ergonomics adapted from the SEIPS 2.0 model (Holden et al., 2013).

Element	Explanation	Obstetric example
Work system		
External environment	Influences external to the organisation, i.e. regulators, government, other organisations, companies supplying equipment	RCoG, RCoA, GMC, NHS England, OAA, Difficult Airway Society
Tools and technology	To assist in doing the task	Anaesthetic machine, CTG machine Epidural pumps
Organisation	Culture, rota, management, training, policies, team-working	Team leaders, training provided
Internal environment	Physical environment, lighting, temperature	Noise level in operating theatre during an emergency
Tasks	Specific actions	Emergency C-section, failed intubation response
Person(s)	Patient, relatives, healthcare professionals, healthcare teams and how they all work together	Mum, baby, obstetrician, anaesthetic team, theatre team
Work processes		
Physical	Patient pathways	How an expectant mum is managed in delivery unit
Cognitive	How we process information and react and human errors that occur because of the way our brain works	Decision to activate massive haemorrhage protocol
Social/behavioural	Social culture, custom and practice, professional elitism, conditioning	As the hand gel dispensers in the rooms are always empty staff now don't even check if they work

team and the processes required is often referred to as team resource management (TRM) or crew resource management (CRM). These team training programmes originate from the aeronautical industry and encompass a range of non-technical skills (NTS), which will be further discussed later in this part of the book – this is more the domain of the psychologists.

The ergonomic interpretation of human factors is completely system-focused and ergonomists use their expertise to analyse and design systems that complement the strengths and abilities of people. The aim is to make systems which are safe and work with the people. They try to design out error by analysing and redesigning the process, at all times ensuring that humans will be able to work with, rather than in spite of, the systems.

However, the two views can be seen as a spectrum of human factors and one view does support the other to improve patient safety and staff performance.

As an example of the breadth of Human Factors and Ergonomics, Table 6.1 is based on part of a human factors engineering model and looks at some elements that could affect Obstetrics.

Bibliography

HEE. (2016). *Improving Safety Through Education and Training. Report by the Commission on Education and Training for Patient Safety*. London: Health Education England.

Holden, R., Carayon, P., Gurses, A., et al. (2013). SEIPS 2.0: a human factors framework for studying and improving the work of healthcare professionals and patients. *Ergonomics*, 56(11), 1559–1686.

Reason, J. (1990). *Human Error*. Cambridge: Cambridge University Press.

Salas, E., Cannon-Bower, J. A. and Hall Johnston, J. (1997). How can you turn a team of experts into an expert team? Emerging training strategies. In C. Zsambok and G. Klien (Eds.), *Naturalistic Decision Making*, pp. 359–371. Oxford: Psychology Press.

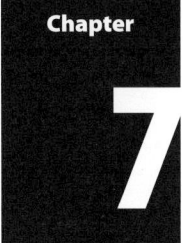

Chapter

7 Situational Awareness, Bias and Decision-Making Styles in Obstetric Simulation

Ian Parkinson and Andrew F. Smith

Situational Awareness

The obstetric delivery room, or operating theatre, are complex, dynamic environments where the transition between routine care and a potentially life-threatening emergency can be rapid. It is essential that the individual clinician tasked with working and making decisions in this situation has an effective mental representation of their changing environment. The ability to develop and maintain this understanding of one's environment (and one's place within a complex system) has been termed situational awareness and can be defined as follows:

> Situational awareness (SA) is the *perception* of elements in the environment within a volume of time and space, the *comprehension* of their meaning, and the *projection* of their status in the near future.
>
> *(Endsley, 1995)*

According to this definition, situational awareness can be divided into three levels: level 1, perception of the environment; level 2, comprehension of the current situation; and level 3, projection of the future (Figure 7.1).

Case 1

A 23-year-old primiparous female is admitted in active labour at 39 weeks with 4 cm cervical dilatation after an uncomplicated pregnancy. The patient makes normal progress in cervical dilatation, but the second stage is prolonged and is augmented by an oxytocin infusion. Delivery is ultimately by vacuum extraction (VE) of a 4600-g boy and the placenta delivered, intact, within 5 minutes. Five units of oxytocin are given IM at delivery and an IV oxytocin infusion (40 units in 500 ml at 125 ml/h) is commenced. Twenty minutes after delivery the midwife notes that the patient has passed several large clots per vaginam; on abdominal examination the uterus is soft and at the level of the umbilicus. Clinical observations show a pulse of 90 and a blood pressure of 120/80.

Individual Situational Awareness

SA Level 1: Perception

On entering the delivery room, perception of the scenario starts with scanning the room for visual cues. How does the patient look? What is connected to the patient? Who else is here? As time passes, further information can be gathered by focusing attention

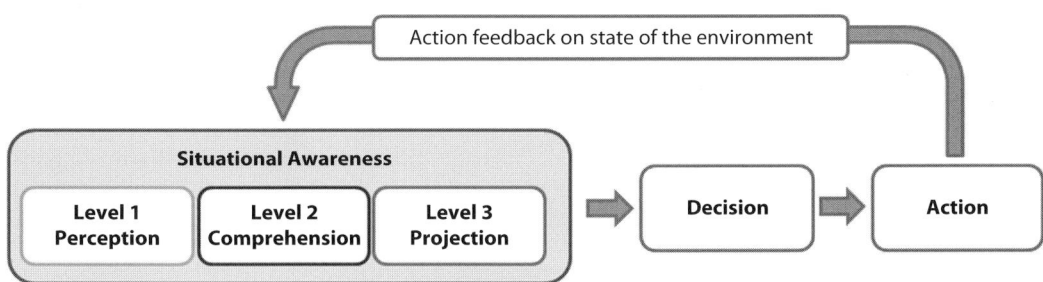

Figure 7.1 Three-level model of situational awareness in dynamic decision-making.
(Adapted with permission from Endsley, M. R. (1995). Toward a theory of situation awareness in dynamic systems. Human Factors: The Journal of the Human Factors and Ergonomics Society, 37(1), 32–64.)

elsewhere. The patient's physiological condition can be assessed by looking at the patient observations on an electronic monitor or on the patient observation chart, and also by formally physically examining the patient. The patient's clinical history is formed by talking to the patient and other clinicians responsible for the patient's care – for example, the midwife or accoucheur – and by looking at the clinical notes.

SA Level 2: Comprehension

Level 2 situational awareness encompasses the clinician's comprehension and understanding of the perceived data gathered. This level goes beyond just being 'aware' of various elements of a situation: these disparate and sometimes patchy data are integrated with medical knowledge from long-term memory; mental models of maternal physiology and how this changes during childbirth; pharmacology knowledge; obstetric guidelines and training. Perhaps most importantly, these data are compared with previous experience of similar situations to find a mental 'schema' that fits the emerging situation (Schulz et al., 2013).

In Case 1, the clinical history (prolonged second stage, augmentation with oxytocin, vacuum extraction of a large baby) fits with the model of risk factors for postpartum haemorrhage. This mental model also fits with the patient examination of a soft, atonic uterus and passing large clots per vaginum.

SA Level 3: Projection

In Level 3 the clinician projects to the future expected progress of the patient's condition. This is crucial to making early, proactive decisions about future investigations and treatments and the allocation of resources to achieving these therapeutic goals.

In this case, the clinician recognises that obstetric haemorrhage is a common (13% of maternities) and life-threatening emergency (10% of maternal deaths; Knight et al., 2014). She also recognises that a young woman will compensate well for ongoing blood loss and is not therefore falsely reassured by the reportedly normal clinical observations. This understanding allows her to plan further immediate treatment (additional uterotonic drugs) and to prepare herself and the clinical team for the probability of a developing major obstetric haemorrhage.

Team Situational Awareness

Obstetric care is usually delivered by a multidisciplinary clinical team and it is therefore important that

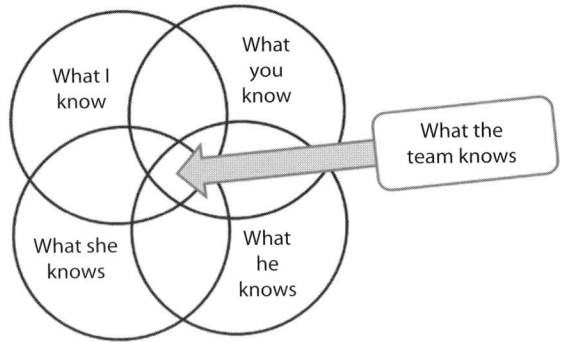

Figure 7.2 Team situational awareness.

situational awareness is maintained in the group, as well as on an individual level. The team caring for a parturient have the shared goal of maternal and neonatal well-being and it is essential that they have a shared understanding of the developing clinical situation, so that each can carry out their individual roles and responsibilities effectively (Figure 7.2).

Case 1 Continued

Despite administration of ergometrine and carboprost the patient continues to bleed heavily per vaginum. Pelvic examination by the attending obstetric speciality trainee reveals bleeding from cervical os with no tears in cervix or vagina and a 'boggy' uterus; clots are expressed per vaginum. Clinical observations, taken by the support worker, now show a BP 90/60, pulse 130.

The developing team situational awareness of a major obstetric haemorrhage is built from the observations of the midwife, the clinical support worker and the attending clinician. Not every member of the team has to understand every piece of information, but all need a shared understanding of the 'bigger picture', to avoid becoming the chain's proverbial weakest link (Endsley, 1995).

The team caring for the patient could share this understanding by declaring a 'major obstetric haemorrhage'; this communicates the shared diagnosis within the team, so that they are now all acting towards a stated common goal, and it also acts to share this information with the wider organisation. It also allows a shared projection about the patient's further course.

Distributed Situational Awareness

A further refinement of situational awareness encompasses not only people (individuals and teams) but also the equipment they use and the environment they work in. The complex, evolving interplay between people, environment and processes, where situational awareness is an emergent property of the whole system, has been termed 'distributed situational awareness' (Fioratou et al., 2010; Schulz et al., 2013). In this chapter we argue that when considering interventions to improve team performance, or incorporating new guidance or technology into our practice, it can help to explore how these impacts will play out at a system level.

Situational Awareness (SA) Errors

Case 2

The on-call anaesthetist has given a general anaesthetic to facilitate an urgent caesarean section in the operating theatre. Shortly after delivery the patient becomes tachycardic and hypotensive; the airway pressures needed to ventilate the patient increase. The obstetrician observes that the uterus is soft and it is noted that there is over 800 ml of blood in the theatre suction system. The obstetrician recommends an oxytocin infusion to treat a presumptive atonic postpartum haemorrhage and while connecting the oxytocin infusion, the anaesthetist notices redness around the intravenous cannula site on the forearm. After pulling back the surgical drapes, a widespread urticarial rash is noted over the patient's chest.

SA Level 1 Errors

The most common type of situational awareness error is at Level 1, with a failure to perceive relevant information (Endsley, 2006). This type of error can be caused by barriers to detectability; for example, a physical obstruction to sight or auditory masking from background noise. In this case the surgical drape is a visual barrier to detecting the developing urticarial rash. Another example is the misperception and misreading of the name of a medication (e.g. metronidazole for metformin), when the presentation and packaging of the drugs are similar.

A key factor in situational awareness is *allocation of attention*. In errors of this kind, the necessary information is all present, but the attention of the clinician is inappropriately focused on only part of it: for example, the accoucheur attends to the examination of the cervical dilatation and fetal head position, but neglects to notice the gradually deteriorating 'early warning' scores on the patient observation chart.

SA Level 2 Errors

Errors can also be made in the interpretation and understanding of the available cues and how they pertain to the clinical goals. A practitioner may lack the mental model to properly integrate all the available data or fail to recognise prototypical situations; they may also apply the wrong mental model to a given scenario.

In Case 2, the available information could fit with the typical picture of a haemorrhage, anaphylactic shock, an amniotic fluid or pulmonary embolus. A less-experienced clinician, through lack of experience or training, may not have all of these models, especially that of amniotic fluid embolus, for immediate recall. In the case above, the clinicians select the wrong mental model (haemorrhage) and there is a danger of then interpreting evolving signs as fitting with this existing diagnosis (a *confirmation bias*) rather than considering alternative diagnoses, such as anaphylactic shock.

SA Level 3 Errors

In errors at this level, there is a failure to predict future states completely or accurately, even though the existing situation is correctly understood. In Case 2, this could present as a comprehension that the patient has anaphylactic shock, but there is a lack of appreciation that this is an imminently life-threatening emergency that needs immediate, specific treatment (steroids, antihistamines and subcutaneous or low-dose intravenous adrenaline). Projection of different future states, depending on the action taken by the team, is crucial in clinical decision-making.

Expertise

As can be seen from the SA errors described above, developing good situational awareness is crucially dependent on expertise. While some differences in SA are due to individuals' cognitive attributes, such as spatial awareness and pattern-matching ability, the knowledge base and practical skills needed to achieve good SA are built on experience, either in clinical practice, or in training. The following factors have been identified as important in creating good SA (Endsley, 1995):

Perceptual processing and attention: experts show more efficient gaze patterns.

Working memory: can easily be 'overloaded' by the demands of situational awareness in novices or in novel situations.

Automaticity: experience brings more automatic behaviour, but also the risk of 'involuntary automaticity' where insufficient attention is paid to a routine task.

Stress: experts under stress are more likely to come to premature closure, ignoring features of the situation that conflict with their chosen mental picture.

In addition, experts are agile, switching between a *top-down, goal-driven approach* and a *bottom-up, data-driven approach* and modifying their plans 'on the fly' in response to events in their environment.

Decision-Making

Once SA is built, the clinician can begin to make decisions about diagnosis and appropriate treatments, or the course of action to be taken. This section examines first, analytical and second, more intuitive, 'real-life' cognitive models of decision-making; last, we examine the role of the patient in decision-making and methods of integrating these approaches.

Case 3

In clinical practice, a variety of cognitive and emotional factors and subjective judgements come into play in making decisions. In the following case, based on real events, these factors have deliberately been elaborated.

It has been a busy day on the labour ward and you are tired. At the lunchtime meeting there was an interesting case presentation on the expectant management of placental abruption; this afternoon, the labour ward is busy with six women in active labour. You are asked to see a 28-year-old Caucasian woman, J, because her midwife is concerned.

J is at 28 weeks gestation in her third pregnancy, having had a caesarean section with her first delivery and a successful VBAC with her second. The CTG shows a persistent bradycardia and the contractions, which were frequent, have now become constant abdominal pain. The midwife notes that the fetal head, which had been well engaged, has now moved up and is palpable abdominally.

Analytical Decision-Making

Evidence-based medicine advocates often promote a Bayesian probabilistic model to making diagnostic decisions. In principle, a constellation of clinical findings should generate a list of differential diagnoses which can then be ordered in terms of the probability of their occurrence. As treatment progresses, the results of further diagnostic tests or therapeutic interventions can be used to modify these probabilities and narrow the list of possible diagnoses, until the correct diagnosis or decision is made.

A Bayesian approach to Case 3 would be to compare the baseline risk of placental abruption (~1:200, Crowther et al., 2012) with that of a ruptured uterus (~1:500, Fitzpatrick et al., 2012) and then look at features, such as the persistent bradycardia and change of fetal station, which tend towards one diagnostic path rather than the other.

This approach suffers from assuming complete probabilistic knowledge of all potential choices and supposing that the pay-offs of each decision are known. In real-life decision-making information may be incomplete, the pay-offs can be unclear, patients and physicians may vary their ordering of preferred outcomes and trade-offs and compromises may be necessary.

Pattern-Matching, Heuristics and Biases

In this model, the remarkable human ability to identify by matching patterns is utilised. Clinical observations are grouped into 'features' to identify a particular condition and differential diagnoses are focused by compatible features or pruned by incompatible features of the presumptive diagnosis. Pattern-matching is surprisingly effective but makes extensive use of cognitive shortcuts in place of statistical logic. Tversky and Kahneman (1975) coined the term *heuristics* to describe these shortcuts which are used extensively in medicine to simplify complex situations, to make decisions quickly, or when the information used to make a decision is incomplete. Tversky and Kahneman originally described three heuristics.

Representativeness, where an existing pattern is preferred despite the chosen option being less common or likely.

Availability, referring to the tendency to make a diagnosis on the basis of a particularly memorable case, rather than the likelihood of the condition occurring. In Case 3, the case presentation of placental abruption at the lunchtime meeting means this mental schema is readily available, although not necessarily accurate, when reviewing the patient later in the afternoon.

Anchoring, which can show itself in medicine as a tendency to fixate on specific features too early in the diagnostic process and a failure to develop a broader list of options (Stiegler and Tung, 2014).

Workplace stress can lead to oxytocin 'tunnel vision' and loss of situational awareness, which combines unhelpfully with the anchoring heuristic.

Of the multitude of other heuristics and biases that have now been described (Croskerry, 2002), three of note here are as follows.

Confirmation bias (as in Case 2) of only looking at the features or test results which fit with the diagnosis that has been anchored on (haemorrhagic shock) and ignoring the features which do not fit this model (high airway pressures and urticarial rash suggest anaphylactic shock). A related phenomenon is the *task fixation* which can overtake teams or individuals in moving towards an erroneous goal. This is exemplified in the challenging case of Elaine Bromiley (Bromiley, 2008), where an anaesthetic team tended to focus on the goal of tracheal intubation to the detriment of patient oxygenation.

Two conflicting biases are those of *omission* (a tendency not to treat, often for fear of being responsible for the outcome) and *commission* (the tendency to do something, rather than do nothing). To some degree these dichotomies are related to confidence: the stereotypical underconfident trainee is less likely to perform the necessary forceps delivery; the overconfident, senior trainee is far more likely to try a difficult forceps delivery, even if they are inexperienced in this skill.

Naturalistic Decision-Making

Naturalistic decision-making has evolved from a desire to understand how experts make decisions in complex, real-life situations. Through looking at a variety of fields including firefighters, chess players, pilots and neonatal nurses this recognition-primed decision (RPD) model highlights the extensive experience in a particular field that is necessary to become a true expert (Ross et al., 2006).

In neonatal intensive care nurses, it was shown that experts recognised the subtle signs of incipient neonatal sepsis up to 24 hours before the patient's clinical signs altered and they became critically ill. These signs were not usually those described in the medical literature but an ill-defined, tacit knowledge, or 'sixth sense' that something wasn't right (Klein and Hoffman, 1993).

Experts are observed to spend more time assessing the situation and less time deliberating over the course of action to take. They have better perceptual skills and richer mental models of their domain of practice with a sense of what is typical and when there is an anomaly. They intuitively recognise a situation and, rather than comparing options, they run a mental simulation to refine their course of action.

In Case 3, the experienced consultant obstetrician immediately recognised the uterine rupture; their situational awareness focused on the length of time of the fetal distress and on the tactics best employed with this team at this time to expedite delivery. The patient was transferred to theatre for immediate caesarean section, where appropriate caution was taken over the Pfannenstiel incision, recognising that the neonate was outside the uterus, in the peritoneal cavity. The outcome was successful delivery of a live neonate.

Dual Process Decision-Making

One approach to uniting the seemingly contradictory intuitive and analytical approaches to decision-making is to see these as two possible pathways which we can toggle between as necessary (Figure 7.3). In this dual

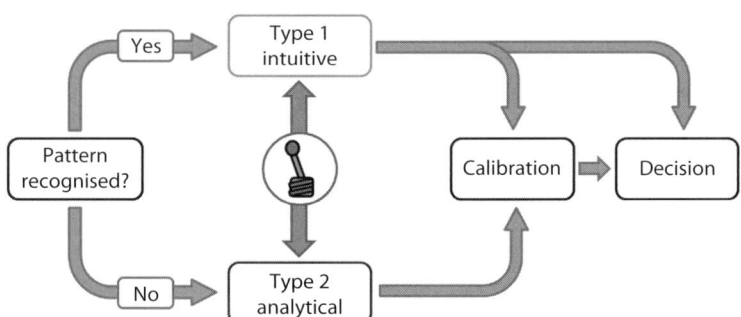

Figure 7.3 Dual process model of decision-making: intuitive (type 1) and analytical (type 2) processes can both be used to make a clinical decision. Some type 1 processes can go directly to a decision without any override or calibration. The switch in the middle represents the use of cognitive strategies to 'switch' between these two pathways.

(Adapted with permission from Croskerry, P., Singhal, G. and Mamede, S. (2013). Cognitive debiasing 1: origins of bias and theory of debiasing. BMJ Quality & Safety, 22(Suppl 2), ii58–ii64.)

process roadmap, pattern-matching is the initial junction: if a pattern of signs and features is recognised then the type 1, intuitive approach comes to the fore. If the pattern is not recognised, the slower, type 2 analytical approach process can be used to develop a list of diagnoses or possible course of action (Croskerry et al., 2013a).

By viewing type 1 and type 2 processes as acting in parallel, or considering the thought processes oscillating between these two pathways, the results of each can be compared before coming to a decision. Heuristics and biases, in this model, can be seen as failures of type 1 processing, which are either innate (thus 'hard-wired' into our neural pathways) or learned. Individual factors such as stress, fatigue and hunger can be expected to impair the type 2, executive performance which would otherwise override the type 1 pathway. More controversially, ageing can be seen to lead to a greater reliance on type 1 processes and entrenched mental schema which may have lost their validity over time (Croskerry, 2009; Croskerry et al., 2013b).

Shared Decision-Making

While cognitive theory looks at the individual clinician and their diagnostic decisions, in obstetric practice it is important to remember that patients stand at the centre of decisions made about their care. In the UK, this issue has been highlighted in the case of Montgomery vs. Lanarkshire Health Board (2015), where the appellant successfully argued that they should have been informed of the risks of shoulder dystocia when making the decision to deliver a potentially larger baby vaginally, rather than opt for a caesarean section. The GMC (2008) recommend that patients must understand 'the options open to him or her; the risks and benefits of each option; and be supported to make their choice about which treatment best meets their needs'.

Thus, the ideal situation is a comprehensible discussion of risks and benefits between the patient and the team responsible for her care, leading to a shared decision that is in the best interests of both the woman and her unborn child.

Strategies for Better Situational Awareness and Decision-Making

In this chapter we have presented a three-level model of situational awareness (perception, comprehension and projection) and several models of decision-making strategies (rational, pattern matching, naturalistic, dual purpose and shared). These psychosocial models are by their nature approximations and some will appeal more or less to the individual clinician than others. However, they are offered here mainly as aids to self-examination, self-awareness and as a structure for metacognition – thinking about the way that we think. They also provide a shared language for communicating these ideas with learners, which can be especially powerful in debriefing after a simulated scenario or reflecting on an event in clinical practice.

Below are detailed some suggestions of practical interventions, both educational and in the workplace, for promoting situational awareness and improving the quality of decision-making.

1. *Ask for help.* The first step in any crisis management algorithm invariably advocates asking for help: this will provide the practical support needed and another senior clinician with whom to review the situation. Another good reason, especially in obstetrics practice, is to get another view – a 'fresh pair of eyes' – on a situation; this could be from a colleague but could also be from a different discipline (midwifery, obstetrics or anaesthesia) with a different mindset. This should apply not only in emergencies, but also to routine practice: the authors paradoxically find that the more experienced they become, the more they ask for help. This can be especially useful when physiological stressors (hunger, fatigue, sleep deprivation, illness in the clinician) or workload stressors (interruptions and distractions, multiple tasks) cause poor situational awareness and an overreliance on heuristics and biases. It can be useful to share this introspection with a supportive team or mentor: 'today my stress bucket is full, one of my relatives is ill and I have a deadline tomorrow – can you watch my back, please?'

2. *Develop resilience.* There is an expanding body of literature on resilience for healthcare practitioners that can give practical advice on developing better coping strategies (HEENW, 2017). It has been shown that obstetricians with better coping strategies are better at dealing with ambiguous situations: in one study, their rates of vaginal deliveries in nulliparous women were higher and their patients were more likely to achieve a vaginal birth after caesarean section (Yee et al., 2015).

3. *Trust the expert instinct in yourself and others.* Two conditions in particular should cause concern. The first is where something does not 'feel

right' – expert intuition is usually right and should be followed up. The second is the opposite – where everyone agrees too readily on the reading of a situation or the decision that should be made. This may be correct, but may also be the result of 'groupthink' – a sort of collective fixation. High-reliability organisations rely on what has been called an 'intelligent wariness' among their staff; this is the state of mind we would want to promote in healthcare too. However, for those around them to understand and learn, experts should try to verbalise these 'instincts'.

4. *'Cognitive debiasing'*. Once we accept that we all use heuristics and biases in our decision-making, we can begin to use deliberate strategies to scrutinise our intuitive judgement. Unfortunately, many of our biases are hard-wired and therefore invisible to us, but we can attempt to debias our decisions using internal cognitive techniques or different ways of working (Graber et al., 2012).

   Some useful strategies are: questioning the initial diagnosis, slowing down (see below), seeking alternative diagnoses and accepting uncertainty. *'Rule out worst-case scenario'* is a strategy used in emergency department thinking which seems highly apposite to obstetric practice (Croskerry, 2002); a related military strategy is that of *'prospective hindsight'* – when I'm standing here in the future and everything has gone wrong, what was it that I missed (Endsley, 1995)?

   To be consistently useful, these strategies must either be triggered, so that one recognises and rescues oneself from a cognitive error, or, better still, they become habitual.

5. *'Slowing down' strategies*. We are often carried along by the momentum of an emerging scenario and lose our situational awareness; this is the time to slow down and re-evaluate: are there signs here that I have missed? Are there other models (additional diagnoses) that I haven't considered? How will this situation project into the future? What contingencies do I have to plan for? Do the team and patient share my understanding of the situation? How will I use the system around me to greatest advantage?

6. *Encourage reflection targeting rationale instead of behaviours*. When giving feedback, or reflecting on our own practice, we need to unpick the situational awareness and rationale underlying the actions taken. Errors in actions are easy to spot but are often specific to a situation. Errors in the underlying perceptual, cognitive and social dimensions are more difficult to explore but potentially more fruitful, because incorrect understanding here may lead to mistakes in other related situations in the future (Stiegler and Tung, 2014).

7. *Be aware of the role of patients*. We should be aware that the patients we find difficult are often the ones that provoke negative emotions in us. These patients, their partners, or their doulas or independent midwives, can elicit feelings of frustration, dislike, anger or guilt (Strachan and Baden Fuller, 2009).

   We need to be alert to the role of our own affect (emotion) on shared decision-making and the value biases and preconceptions we bring to a discussion. There is evidence to support the common-sense view that anger and regret are both unhelpful emotions to bring into medical decision-making (Steigler and Tung, 2014).

8. *Explore the possible situational awareness and decision-making effects of new interventions*. With distributed situational awareness in mind, there is a role here for simulation in piloting new guidelines, technology, physical layouts or other interventions. These simulations can be run with the team, '*in situ*' on the labour ward or in theatre, therefore testing system factors, before using these innovations in clinical practice.

Bibliography

Bromiley, M. (2008). Have you ever made a mistake. A Patient Liaison Group Debate. *Royal College of Anaesthetists Bulletin*, 48, 2442–2445.

Croskerry, P. (2002). Achieving quality in clinical decision making: cognitive strategies and detection of bias. *Academic Emergency Medicine*, 9(11), 1184–1204.

(2009). Clinical cognition and diagnostic error: applications of a dual process model of reasoning. *Advances in Health Sciences Education*, 14(1), 27–35.

Croskerry, P., Singhal, G. and Mamede, S. (2013a). Cognitive debiasing 1: origins of bias and theory of debiasing. *BMJ Quality & Safety*, 22(Suppl 2), ii58–ii64.

(2013b). Cognitive debiasing 2: impediments to and strategies for change. *BMJ Quality & Safety*, pp.bmjqs-2012.

Crowther, C. A., Dodd, J. M., Hiller, J. E., Haslam, R. R., Robinson, J. S. and Birth After Caesarean Study Group (2012). Planned vaginal birth or elective repeat caesarean: patient preference restricted cohort with nested randomised trial. *PLoS Medicine*, 9(3), e1001192.

Endsley, M. R. (1995). Toward a theory of situation awareness in dynamic systems. *Human Factors: The Journal of the Human Factors and Ergonomics Society*, 37(1), 32–64.

(2006). Expertise and situation awareness. In K. A. Ericsson, N. Charness, P. J. Feltovich and R. R. Hoffman (Eds.), *The Cambridge Handbook of Expertise and Expert Performance*, pp. 633–651. Cambridge: Cambridge University Press.

Fioratou, E., Flin, R., Glavin, R. and Patey, R. (2010). Beyond monitoring: distributed situation awareness in anaesthesia. *British Journal of Anaesthesia*, 105(1), 83–90.

Fitzpatrick, K. E., Kurinczuk, J. J., Alfirevic, Z., Spark, P., Brocklehurst, P. and Knight, M. (2012). Uterine rupture by intended mode of delivery in the UK: a national case-control study. *PLoS Medicine*, 9(3), e1001184.

GMC. (2008). *Consent: Patients and Doctors making Decisions Together*. London: GMC.

Graber, M. L., Kissam, S., Payne, V. L., et al. (2012). Cognitive interventions to reduce diagnostic error: a narrative review. *BMJ Quality & Safety*, pp.bmjqs-2011.

HEENW. (2017). *Resources|Health Education North West*. [Online]. Available from: www.nwpgmd.nhs.uk/resources (accessed April 26, 2017).

Klein, G. A. and Hoffman, R. R. (1993). Perceptual-cognitive aspects of expertise. In M. Rabinowitz (Ed.), *Cognitive Science Foundations of Instruction*, pp. 203–226. Hillsdale, NJ: Lawrence Erlbaum Associates.

Knight, M., Kenyon, S., Brocklehurst, P., Neilson, J., Shakespeare, J. and Kurinczuk, J. J. (Eds.) on behalf of MBRRACE-UK. (2014). *Saving Lives, Improving Mothers' Care – Lessons Learned to Inform Future Maternity Care from the UK and Ireland Confidential Enquiries into Maternal Deaths and Morbidity 2009–12*. Oxford: National Perinatal Epidemiology Unit, University of Oxford.

Montgomery vs. Lanarkshire Health Board (2015). UKSC 11.

Ross, L., Shafer, J. and Klein, G., (2006). Professional judgements and 'naturalistic decision making'. In K. A. Ericsson, N. Charness, P. J. Feltovich and R. R. Hoffman (Eds.), *The Cambridge Handbook of Expertise and Expert Performance*, pp. 403–420. Cambridge: Cambridge University Press.

Schulz, C. M., Endsley, M. R., Kochs, E. F., Gelb, A. W. and Wagner, K. J. (2013). Situation awareness in anesthesia concept and research. *The Journal of the American Society of Anesthesiologists*, 118(3), 729–742.

Stiegler, M. P. and Tung, A. (2014). Cognitive processes in anesthesiology decision making. *The Journal of the American Society of Anesthesiologists*, 120(1), 204–217.

Strachan, B. K. and Baden Fuller, J. (2009). Dealing with conflict and aggression in obstetrics and gynaecology. *The Obstetrician & Gynaecologist*, 11, 122–128.

Tversky, A. and Kahneman, D. (1975). Judgment under uncertainty: heuristics and biases. In *Utility, Probability, and Human Decision Making*, pp. 141–162. Dordrecht: Springer.

Yee, L. M., Liu, L. Y. and Grobman, W. A. (2015). Relationship between obstetricians' cognitive and affective traits and delivery outcomes among women with a prior cesarean. *American Journal of Obstetrics and Gynecology*, 213(3), 413–e1.

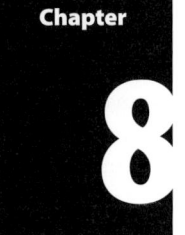

Team-Working, Communication and Use of Communication Aids and Checklists in an Emergency

Simon Mercer

Introduction

Human factors have been described as 'the science of improving human performance and well-being by examining all the effectors of human performance' (Moneypenny, 2017). There has been considerable work over the last two decades to examine how human factors theory can be adopted into clinical practice. Much of the current knowledge and opinions have been formed from key seminal papers published in the USA (Kohn et al., 2000) and the UK (Department of Health, 2000). An assurance that Human Factors are now high on the national agenda was confirmed by the recent commitment in the form of a concordat (NHS England) by key state holders such as the General Medical Council and NHS England.

Another definition of human factors by Professor Rhona Flin is 'the cognitive, social, and personal resource skills that complement technical skills, and contribute to safe and efficient task performance' (Flin et al., 2008), with key aspects including situational awareness, teamwork, leadership, followership, communication and decision-making. This is reiterated by The Clinical Human Factors Group definition of 'enhancing clinical performance through an understanding of the effects of teamwork, tasks, equipment, workspace, culture and organisation on human behaviour and abilities and application of that knowledge in clinical settings' (Catchpole). It is important that these elements, or what are also referred to as Team Resource Management (or Crew Resource Management in the Airline Industry; Civil Aviation Authority, 2003), are exercised in the management of Obstetric Emergencies.

There has been research into human factors for anaesthetists (Fletcher et al., 2003), surgeons (Yule et al., 2006) and scrub practitioners (Mitchell and Flin, 2008), and much of this work can be directly translated to the busy labour ward setting, although as yet there is no validated system for measuring non-technical skills in obstetric teams. A lack of communication and teamwork was cited as a leading cause of substandard obstetric care by the National Confidential Enquiry into Maternal Deaths (Lewis and Drife, 2004). It has also been commented that poor teamwork and suboptimal communication contribute to increased maternal and neonatal morbidity and mortality, and bad patient experience (Cornthwaite et al., 2013).

This chapter will examine the team resource management aspects of teamwork and communication and explore the importance of cognitive aids in time-critical emergencies.

Team-Working

A recent national report has demonstrated a need to increase the effectiveness and efficiency of team-working when obstetric emergencies occur (Lewis, 2007). The prospective surveillance study in one teaching hospital by Forster et al. (2006) demonstrated that 5% of obstetric patients experienced an important 'quality problem'. This was defined as an adverse event or a potential adverse event. When these were further reviewed, 87% were deemed potentially preventable and with systems issues such as teamwork being cited as causative (Forster et al., 2006). The term 'teamwork' itself has been used as a catchall to refer to a number of behavioural processes and emergent states (Valentine et al., 2015). Work has been undertaken by Salas, who defines a team as 'a distinguishable set of two or more people who interact dynamically, interdependently, and adaptively towards a common and valued goal, who have each been assigned specific roles or functions to perform, and who have a limited life-span membership' (Salas et al., 2004). Another definition by Katzenbach describes a team as 'a small number of people with complementary skills who are committed to a common purpose, performance goals, and approach for which they hold themselves mutually accountable' (Katzenbach and Smith, 1993). These definitions hold strong for the busy team working on the labour ward and in the obstetric theatres.

It is important to realise that teamwork is more than just subordinates doing what their leader tells them to do. Teamwork is about maximising the mental and physical problem-solving capabilities of the group, such that the sum of these exceeds its parts (Pierre et al., 2011). It is not surprising that poor teamwork and leadership can lead to devastating, and potentially avoidable, physical, psychological and financial consequences (Cornthwaite et al., 2013). A report by the King's Fund came to the conclusion that maternity teams required clarity about team objectives and roles and effective leadership and efficient communication (O'Neill, 2008). Black and Brocklehurst identified that the largest contributing factor to the death of babies was a delay in assembling the team and that further research related to effective team training for obstetric emergencies should be undertaken (Black and Brocklehurst, 2003). It is also thought that increased clinical exposure, learned systematic responses and a focus on teamwork could result in diminished stress and improved care (Schull et al., 2001). Observations from acute care medicine demonstrate that inadequate teamwork is one of the most common reasons for preventable error (Pierre et al., 2011).

Good teamwork is associated with improved productivity, innovation and job satisfaction (Katzenbach and Smith, 1993). It is also considered that teams who demonstrate similar mental models move quicker through the phases common to most crises. Ripley describes these as denial, deliberation and then deliberate action (Ripley, 2009). Good teamwork also relies on situational awareness, an academic definition being 'the perception of the elements in the environment within a volume of time and space, the comprehension of their meaning and the projection of their status in the near future' (Salas et al., 2004). To maintain good situational awareness, it is important the maternity staff are aware of the competencies and skills of their colleagues, the background to situations and verbalise loudly information for everyone to hear (Cornthwaite et al., 2013). A properly conducted handover is essential to ensuring good situational awareness. But equally, effective training to prepare all healthcare professionals in the maternity team to deal with high-stakes emergencies is essential for saving mothers and babies (Cornthwaite et al., 2013).

Challenging hierarchy among the team is also important in high-stakes emergency situations. Recent work has shown that 'speaking up' or the ability to effectively challenge erroneous decisions is essential to preventing harm and that despite significant multifactorial barriers, systematic training in effective 'speaking up' could improve the confidence and ability of juniors to challenge erroneous decisions (Beament and Mercer, 2016). In the field of aviation, United Airlines uses the acronym 'CUS', which stands for 'I'm concerned', 'I'm uncomfortable', and 'this is unsafe or I'm scared'. Staff, regardless of their hierarchical status, are encouraged to use this acronym to challenge senior members of staff (Leonard, 2004).

Communication

Previous work by Gawande and colleagues (2003) cited communication failures as being responsible for 43% of errors in three large teaching hospitals in the USA. Specific to obstetric practice, one review of closed obstetric malpractice claims concluded that 31% of adverse events were attributable to communication problems (White et al., 2005). In time-critical situations, it is important that there is a team leader who has the ability to impart any critical information without the potential for misinterpretation or misunderstanding, irrespective of the situation or the professional diversity of the surrounding team. Effective communication is reliant on good 'crowd control' so that excessive noise levels are kept low. During rapidly changing situations such as an obstetric emergency, continuous communication is vital and this can be facilitated by a team brief followed by regular situational updates (or SIT-REPS). Effective communication establishes and maintains a shared mental model for the team. This falls short when handovers are inadequate and the shared mental model is no longer 'shared'. Landro has referred to this as 'the Bermuda Triangle of health care' (Landro, 2006). Communication is essential, not only between the team leader and the team, but also in the reverse direction so that the multidisciplinary team can feedback important information such as physiology changes and drugs administered.

Elements of effective communication rely on clarity, 'keeping it clear', brevity, 'keeping it brief', empathy, 'how will it feel to receive this?' and ensuring there is a feedback loop. Effective communication is reliant on the following.

- Addressing statements or messages to a specific person to avoid pronouncing them into thin air. This ensures that the correct person knows that they have been asked to perform a task and there is no ambiguity among other team members.

This directed communication and closed-loop communication is particularly important when rapid response is critical. Directed communication involves specifying who is intended to receive an order or communication, usually by using a hand signal or saying the person's name (Guise and Segel, 2008).

- Closing the communication loop. An example of this would be asking a team member to repeat the instructions back to the team leader so that the instructions have been understood.
- Fostering an atmosphere of open information exchange among all team members. If this is adopted then everyone will be listened to regardless of job description or status. This culture empowers all team members to speak out to communicate to the team leader to prevent an error. Barriers to challenging and the importance of barriers to challenging have recently been reviewed (Beament and Mercer, 2016). These have included poor intraoperative communication between seniors and juniors (Belyansky et al., 2011) and poor communication skills in general (Kobayashi et al., 2006; Okuyama et al., 2014).
- Continuous re-evaluation. Periodic updating ensures that situation awareness is maintained as information is collected, summarised and shared among the team members.

Effective communication is further facilitated by a team brief and this also facilitates shared mental models and situational awareness. If time permits then this is led by the nominated team leader. This process involves the following.

- Introduction of all team members by name and role. This not only allows the use of first names during a scenario but also ensures that peripheral members of the team such as medical or nursing students can be identified and employed if necessary. The team leader is also aware of the competencies and skills of individual team members.
- Briefing of the team as to what is expected to happen. This may not be possible in an obstetric emergency, but in a trauma team situation there is often up to 10 minutes to allow a discussion of the likely events based on the team leader's mental model. This also allows a discussion of any potential problems and a highlighting of potential solutions.
- Tasks are then allocated and agreed.

During a critical emergency on the obstetric ward it will also be very important that there is effective communication with external agencies in the hospital. This will include the transfusion laboratory, critical care and the operating theatres. Additional team members may also be summoned, such as consultants and senior midwives, to ensure senior robust decisions are made in a timely manner. Often a runner will be nominated to facilitate the delivery of blood products and nominated individuals will communicate with the laboratory via the telephone. This ensures that there are direct lines of communication.

To maintain effective communication, it is vital that there is an awareness of distractions that could occur during a critical emergency. These are often caused by increased noise and the team leader has the job of maintaining 'crowd control'. It is well known that substantial extraneous noise and movement occur in the obstetric theatre environment and this is thought to create both auditory and physical distraction (Jenkins et al., 2014). A 'sterile cockpit' has been described in the airline industry during key moments in emergency care (Broom et al., 2011). An example of this is the intubation of a patient during a rapid sequence induction of anaesthesia. This requires that the noise level is kept to an absolute minimum by having only the required team members present and minimal noise. Another form of 'crowd control' practised, if noise levels inhibit communication, is for any member of the team to ASK for a pause (A, ask for a pause; S, share the mental model; K, keep communication closed loop) (Monks and Maclennan, 2016).

Communication Tools

SBAR

The communication tool SBAR is made up of the acronym **S**ituation, **B**ackground, **A**ssessment and **R**ecommendation (Haig et al., 2006). It provides a structure to a conversation where one individual is communicating information to another in a time-critical situation. This is particularly useful for conversations on the telephone.

AT-MIST

Another communication tool that is widely used by the trauma team during handover is AT-MIST. This refers to **A**ge, **T**ime of Injury, **M**echanism of injury, **I**njuries sustained, **S**igns and symptoms and **T**reatment given. It must also be noted that asking the wrong questions

Table 8.1 The STACK mnemonic used for situational updates by the UK Defence Medical Services.

S	Systolic BP
T	Temperature
A	Acidosis
C	Coagulation
K	Kit (including blood products used)

Table 8.2 The Trauma WHO.

Command Huddle	Following the primary and secondary survey a senior team use the information gleaned from the handover from the pre-hospital team, the physical examination, imaging and blood test to arrive at a decision on the next step in patient care. This is often transfer to the CT scanner, but may involve direct transfer to the operating theatre or critical care
Snap Brief	Prior to commencing surgery there is a reconfirmation of vital information to ensure the right patient is in theatre followed by a recap of the mechanism of injury, the injuries sustained, any additional radiology results and then the surgical and anaesthetic plans
Sit-Reps	Every 10–30 minutes there will be an update or 'sit-rep', usually when additional information is known. The STACK acronym described above is used here
Debrief	At a convenient moment when the case has finished there will be a debrief for all team members

can also 'get the wrong answer'. For example, during surgery, the Surgeon asking 'how are you doing' could lead to a reply from the Anaesthetist such as 'obs are stable' or 'we are keeping up'. A similar question from the Anaesthetist could lead to a response from the Surgeon such *as* 'things are a little tricky now'. Both these answers convey little information as the Anaesthetist might indeed be 'keeping up' by transfusing 400 ml/minute via a Belmont Rapid Infuser and the stable observations might be a systolic blood pressure of 70 mmHg. Equally, 'things are a little tricky' conveys no meaningful information either. In an attempt to counteract this poor communication, the Defence Medical Services have suggested a 'Trauma WHO Checklist' (Arul et al., 2015) with a situational update (Sit-Rep) using the mnemonic STACK (Table 8.1).

GAMES

To facilitate effective handover to the neonatal team, when called to a delivery in an emergency, the GAMES mnemonic can be used. **G**estation, **A**ntenatal history, **M**aternal problems/medications, **E**xamination findings (CTG, scalp pH, meconium, risk factors for sepsis) and **S**uggested actions (Maclennan et al., 2017).

Communication and Checklists

The ideal properties of cognitive aids used during anaesthetic emergencies are that they must be derived from best practice, they should be appropriate, familiar and in a format that has been used in practice and training and leads to coordinated team activity (Marshall, 2013). There is good evidence to support the impact of checklists in improving the quality of healthcare professional's handovers of care in addition to their adherence to recognised standards of care during perioperative crisis situations (Tan and Helsten, 2013; Petrovic et al., 2012). One such checklist is The World Health Organization (WHO) surgical safety checklist that was introduced in 2009 (Haynes et al., 2009; The World Health Organization; World

Alliance for Patient Safety, 2008). The primary aim of this intervention was to eliminate 'never events'.[1] This process involves a team brief and then has a series of questions to include confirmations of key aspects of the operation, any patient-specific factors and any unusual steps in the process. The WHO Checklist has recently been reported to reduce hospital mortality (Van Klei et al., 2012), and although this checklist is important, it wasn't designed to be used in a rapidly changing situation such as a massive postpartum haemorrhage, nor was it intended to be religiously adopted in a time-critical situation such as a category one caesarean section. In terms of trauma management and the WHO Checklist, a discussion paper published in 2012 sought to improve and streamline communication during the damage control resuscitation (Arul et al., 2012) and there are many similarities with acute obstetric emergencies. The Trauma WHO (Arul et al., 2015) is described in Table 8.2 with four key stages: Command Huddle, Snap Brief, Sit-Reps and Debrief.

Regarding the use of other cognitive aids, there are several used in clinical practice that are relevant to the labour ward and obstetric operating theatre. These include anaphylaxis, local anaesthetic toxicity, malignant hyperpyrexia and resuscitation council guidelines.

---

[1] Never Events are serious, largely preventable patient safety incidents that should not occur if the available preventative measures have been implemented (www.nrls.npsa.nhs.uk/neverevents/).

Marshall showed that using a linearly designed cognitive aid improves treatment of anaphylactic reactions during anaesthetic simulations (Degani and Wiener, 1993) and typical critical incidents can be practised in the relative safety and control of a simulation centre. Recently, massive haemorrhage protocols have been written to aid massive transfusions in emergency situations. These not only include the ratio of products but information on additional drugs that should be considered such as calcium. In anaesthesia, it has been suggested that during an emergency there can be an unwillingness or inability to revert to more systematic thinking (Jenkins, 2014) or the anaesthetist can become fixated (a fixation error). Under stress there is an increase in cortisol and other stress hormones which can lead to cognition and behaviour changes and may account for deficiencies in recalling information, missed treatment steps or mistakes in sequential procedures (Kuhlmann et al., 2005). In the simulation laboratory, the use of cognitive aids during scenarios around critical incidents has improved the management of anaesthetic emergencies such as malignant hyperpyrexia (Harrison et al., 2006) and local anaesthetic toxicity (Picard et al., 2009). Phipps and colleagues describe that an anaesthetist's decision to follow or indeed deviate from guidelines is influenced by the beliefs that they themselves hold about the consequence of their actions, the direct or indirect influence of others and the presence of factors that encourage or facilitate particular courses of action (Phipps et al., 2009). Gawande goes into further details on checklists and cognitive aids in his book *The Checklist Manifesto: How to Get Things Right* (Gawande, 2009).

Summary

Teamwork and communication are particularly important elements of human factors during an obstetric emergency. Cognitive aids and checklists aid coordination among the team during a critical incident.

Bibliography

Arul, G. S., Pugh, H., Mercer, S. J., et al. (2012). Optimising communication in the damage control resuscitation–damage control surgery sequence in major trauma management. *Journal of the Royal Army Med Corps*, 158, 82–84.

(2015). Human factors in decision making in major trauma in Camp Bastion, Afghanistan. *Annals of the Royal College of Surgeons of England*, 97, 262–268.

Beament, T. and Mercer, S. J. (2016). Speak up! Barriers to challenging erroneous decisions of seniors in anaesthesia. *Anaesthesia*, 71, 1332–1340.

Belyansky, I., Martin, T. R., Prabhu, A. S., et al. (2011). Poor resident-attending intraoperative communication may compromise patient safety. *Journal of Surgical Research*, 171, 386–394.

Black, R. S. and Brocklehurst, P. (2003). A systematic review of training in acute obstetric emergencies. *British Journal of Obstetrics & Gynaecology*, 110, 837–841.

Broom, M. A., Capek, A. L., Carachi, P., et al. (2011). Critical phase distractions in anaesthesia and the sterile cockpit concept. *Anaesthesia*, 66, 175–179.

Catchpole, K. Towards a working definition of human factors in healthcare. Available from: www.chfg.org/news-blog/towards-a-working-definition-of-human-factors-in-healthcare

Civil Aviation Authority. (2003). *CAP 737: Crew Resource Management (CRM) Training. Guidance for Flight Crew, CRM Instructors and CRM Instructor-Examiners*. London: CAA Safety Regulation Group.

Cornthwaite, K., Edwards, S. and Siassakos, D. (2013). Reducing risk in maternity by optimising teamwork and leadership: an evidence-based approach to save mothers and babies. *Best Practice & Research Clinical Obstetrics & Gynaecology*, 27, 571–581.

Degani, A. and Wiener, E. L. (1993). Cockpit checklists: concepts, design, and use. *Human Factors*, 35, 345–359.

Department of Health. (2000). *An Organisation with a Memory*. London: The Stationery Office.

Fletcher, G., Flin, R., McGeorge, P., Glavin, R., Maran, N. and Patey, R. (2003). Anaesthetists' non-technical skills (ANTS): evaluation of a behavioural marker system. *British Journal of Anaesthesia*, 90, 580–588.

Flin, R., O'Connor, P. and Crichton, M. (2008). *Safety at the Sharp End: A Guide to Non-Technical Skills*. Aldershot: Ashgate.

Forster, A.J., Fung, I., Caughey, S., et al. (2006). Adverse events detected by clinical surveillance on an obstetric service. *Obstetrics & Gynecology*, 108, 1073–1083.

Gawande, A. (2009). *The Checklist Manifesto: How to Get Things Right*. London: Profile.

Gawande, A., Zinner, M. J., Studert, D. M., et al. (2003). Analysis of errors reported by surgeons at three teaching hospitals. *Surgery*, 133, 614–621.

Guise, J.-M. and Segel, S. (2008). Teamwork in obstetric critical care. *Best Practice & Research Clinical Obstetrics & Gynaecology*, 22, 937–951.

Haig, K. M., Sutton, S. and Whittington, J. (2006). SBAR: a shared mental model for improving communication between clinicians. *Joint Commission Journal on Quality and Patient Safety*, 32, 167–175.

Harrison, T. K., Manser, T., Howard, S. K. and Gaba, D. M. (2006). Use of cognitive aids in a simulated anesthetic crisis. *Anesthesia & Analgesia*, 103, 551–556.

Haynes, A. B., Weiser, T. G., Berry, W. R., et al. (2009). A surgical safety checklist to reduce morbidity and mortality in a global population. *New England Journal of Medicine*, 360, 491–499.

Jenkins, A., Wilkinson, J. V., Akeroyd, M. A., et al. (2014). Distractions during critical phases of anaesthesia for caesarean section: an observational study. *Anaesthesia*, 70, 543–548.

Jenkins, B. (2014). Cognitive aids: time for a change? *Anaesthesia*, 69, 660–664.

Katzenbach, J. R. and Smith, D. K. (1993). *The Wisdom of Teams: Creating the High-performance Organization*. New York, NY: Harper Business.

Kobayashi, H., Pian-Smith, M., Sato, M., et al. (2006). A cross-cultural survey of residents' perceived barriers in questioning/challenging authority. *BMJ Quality & Safety*, 15, 277–283.

Kohn, L. T., Corrigan, J. M. and Donaldson, M. S. (2000). *To Err is Human: Building a Safer Health System*. Washington, DC: National Academies Press.

Kuhlmann, S., Piel, M. and Wolf, O. T. (2005). Impaired memory retrieval after psychosocial stress in healthy young men. *Journal of Neuroscience*, 25, 2977–2982.

Landro, L. (2006). The informed patient: hospitals combat errors at the 'hand-off': new procedures aim to reduce miscues as nurses and doctors transfer patients to next shift. *Wall Street Journal*, June 28, 2006, D1.

Leonard, M. (2004). The human factor: the critical importance of effective teamwork and communication in providing safe care. *Quality and Safety in Health Care*, 13(S1), i85–i90.

Lewis G. (2007). Saving Mothers' Lives. Available from: www.publichealth.hscni.net/sites/default/files/Saving%20Mothers%27%20Lives%202003-05%20.pdf

Lewis, G. and Drife, J. (2004). *Why Mothers Die 2000–2002. Executive Summary and Key Findings. The Sixth Report of the Confidential Enquiries into Maternal Deaths in the United Kingdom*. London: RCOG Press.

MacLennan, K., Hurst, J. and Gottstein, R. (2017). St Mary's Hospital Manchester.

Marshall, S. (2013). The use of cognitive aids during emergencies in anesthesia: a review of the literature. *Anesthesia & Analgesia*, 117, 1162–1171.

Mitchell, L. and Flin, R. (2008). Non-technical skills of the operating theatre scrub nurse: literature review. *Journal of Advanced Nursing*, 63, 15–24.

Moneypenny, M. J. (2017). When are 'human factors' not 'human factors' in can't intubate can't oxygenate scenarios? When they are 'human' factors. *British Journal of Anaesthesia*, 118, 469–469.

Monks, S. and Maclennan, K. (2016). Human factors in obstetrics. *Anaesthesia & Intensive Care Medicine*, 17(8), 400–403.

NHS England. *Human Factors in Healthcare – A Concordat from the National Quality Board*. www.england.nhs.uk/wp-content/uploads/2013/11/nqb-hum-fact-concord.pdf.

Okuyama, A., Wagner, C. and Bijnen, B. (2014). Speaking up for patient safety by hospital-based health care professionals: a literature review. *BMC Health Services Research. BioMed Central*, 14, 61.

O'Neill, O. (2008). *Safe Births: Everybody's Business: An Independent Inquiry into the Safety of Maternity Services in England*. London: King's Fund.

Petrovic, M. A., Martinez, E. A. and Aboumatar, H. (2012). Implementing a perioperative handoff tool to improve postprocedural patient transfers. *Joint Commission Journal on Quality and Patient Safety* 38, 135–142.

Phipps, D. L., Beatty, P. C. W., Parker, D., et al. (2009). Motivational influences on anaesthetists' use of practice guidelines. *British Journal of Anaesthesia*, 102, 768–774.

Picard, J., Ward, S. C., Zumpe, R., et al. (2009). Guidelines and the adoption of 'lipid rescue' therapy for local anaesthetic toxicity. *Anaesthesia*, 64, 122–125.

Pierre, M. S., Hofinger, G., Buerschaper, C. and Simon, R. (2011). *Crisis Management in Acute Care Settings*. Cham: Springer

Ripley, A. (2009). *The Unthinkable: Who Survives When Disaster Strikes – And Why*. New York, NY: Harmony.

Salas, E., Burke, C. S. and Stagl, K. C. (2004). Developing teams and team leaders: strategies and principles. In D. V. Day, S. J. Zaccaro and S. M. Halpin (Eds.), *Leader Development for Transforming Organizations: Growing Leaders for Tomorrow*. Hillsdale, NJ: Lawrence Erlbaum and Associates.

Schull, M. J., Ferris, L. E., Tu, J. V., et al. (2001). Problems for clinical judgement: 3. Thinking clearly in an emergency. *Canadian Medical Association Journal*, 164, 1170–1175.

Tan, J. A. and Helsten, D. (2013). Intraoperative handoffs. *International Anesthesiology Clinics*, 51, 31–42.

The World Health Organization. Surgical Safety Checklist. Available from: www.who.int/patientsafety/safesurgery/checklist/en/

Valentine, M. A., Nembhard, I. M. and Edmondson, A. C. (2015). Measuring teamwork in health care settings: a review of survey instruments. *Medical Care*, 53, e16–e30.

Van Klei, W. A., Hoff, R. G., Van Aarnhem, E., et al. (2012). Effects of the introduction of the WHO 'Surgical Safety Checklist' on in-hospital mortality: a cohort study. *Annals of Surgery*, 255(1), 44–49.

White, A. A., Pichert, J. W., Bledsoe, S. H., et al. (2005). Cause and effect analysis of closed claims in obstetrics and gynecology. *Obstetrics & Gynecology*, 105, 1031–1038.

World Alliance for Patient Safety. (2008). *Safe Surgery Saves Lives*. Geneva: World Health Organization. Available from: www.who.int/patientsafety/safesurgery/knowledge_base/SSSL_Brochure_finalJun08.pdf

Yule, S., Flin, R., Paterson-Brown, S., et al. (2006). Development of a rating system for surgeons' non-technical skills. *Medical Education*, 40, 1098–1104.

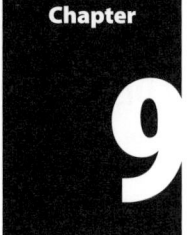

Introduction to the Scenarios

9

Kirsty MacLennan

There now follow 28 scenarios, all following the same format.

This book is designed to help you introduce or continue running obstetric simulation either in simulation centres or *in situ* at your place of work.

It is by no means prescriptive; use the chapters in whatever way works best for you and your learners. There are so many different approaches and uses of simulation; you may want to pick out an isolated skill to gain competence, rehearse rare but catastrophic emergencies, acquire skills in rare situations that are mapped to curricular requirements, or test your system or environment (existing clinical pathways, physical capacity, equipment and communication between different teams). Whatever your simulation goal, we hope that this book will be of help to you. Use it however you see fit, picking out the parts that are most relevant for you and your learners.

Scenario Chapters Explained

Every scenario chapter has the same layout, with clear subheadings, each of which is explained in turn.

Scenario in a Nutshell

This orientates the facilitator by giving a brief overview of the scenario with brief one-liners for each of the stages.

Target Learner Groups

Most commonly, the whole multidisciplinary obstetric team are the target learners, with some additional specialities depending on the scenario. Your target learners may depend on who is available. It is likely that you will need to be flexible!

Specific Learning Objectives

These should be identified at the start of the session. It is all too easy for simulation to take different, unwanted directions away from these learning goals. Ensure you set your learning objectives and achieve them. Remember, your learners are adult learners, so they need to be party to the decision regarding what the learning objectives are; constructive alignment is essential to maximise learning. Consider the use of an educational checklist at the start of your session to determine and share individual learning objectives, see www.loafnbread.com for more information.

Suggested Learners

We offer suggestions as to who could be in the simulation. We do emphasise the importance for learners to adapt their normal roles in a simulation; by adopting roles that they have no knowledge of, the fidelity of the scenario will suffer. Think ahead as to whether the simulation can be run in parallel with other care teams, including neonatal emergency response teams or full theatre teams.

If faculty are playing a role in the simulation, it is important that they are well briefed with prompts that they may need to give along the way. It is difficult to predict the direction a team simulation will take; faculty members, as plants, can help to keep the simulation heading in the direction of the planned learning objectives.

Scenario Summary for Facilitators

It is important for the facilitator to review the scenario summary in order to plan exactly what can be achieved in the time allowed with the team present.

Set boundaries for the team before they start, including: what they can do with the manikin, how to summon help, what equipment they will have access to, whether they are able to transfer to different locations, etc. This is important as simulation becomes very immersive and before you know it, the team will have gained momentum in a direction that may not be anticipated!

Set-up Overview for Facilitators

The set-up overview is a guide to how you may wish to prepare your environment for the start of the scenario. Once again, this may change depending on what space is available to you. Anticipate what equipment the learners may require and make sure it is ready – or have a plan for what to do when they request it! When running *in situ* scenarios, you may wish to use your usual equipment which aids orientation, checks availability, stock levels and ease of access. Always remember, however, that patient safety is paramount, and make certain that use of equipment has no negative impact (see Chapter 2).

Useful manikin features are also alluded to in this section. We cannot emphasise strongly enough how important it is not to get hung up on the kit. You have to start somewhere, so do not wait until you have an all-singing, all-dancing birthing simulator before you start doing simulation! There are plenty of ways of getting around the lack of simulation equipment. Fidelity comes with learner buy-in and that does not equate to expense of simulation equipment (see Chapters 1, 5 and 13).

Medical Equipment

In this chapter there is a core equipment checklist. You will not need all the equipment for every scenario, but it can be used as a prompt to remind you what to prepare. Additional equipment specific to the scenario is listed in each scenario, again as a prompt.

Information Given to the Learners

In an attempt to standardise information given and demonstrate a structured handover, most scenarios start with an SBAR handover. We have suggested who should be first responders; once again, this is a guide – if your first responding team would be different then alter this accordingly.

Scenario Schedule

The stages of the scenario are laid out clearly with columns for observations and CTG, information given and expected actions. The team may not always act as you would expect; be flexible and be prepared for this. Any clear omissions can be covered in the debrief. Our expected actions are all based (to our best knowledge) on current evidence at this time. If your local guidance differs, ensure you are clear about what expected actions you would look for in your clinical environment. The titles for each stage are for the facilitators to know what is coming in that stage – they are not to be read out to the learners!

Suggested Topics for Debrief Discussion

There are many widely practised models for the debrief (see Chapter 4) and you may or may not need to use the suggested discussion topics; however, they are there if you need them. If you find that once you have performed the scenario you do not have enough time for the debrief, then you have tried to fit too much in!

Discussion

The final part of each chapter is a discussion on current evidence on the subject covered. The useful references can be shared with the learners to further reinforce their knowledge on the topic.

We very much hope that you enjoy using the scenarios in the book.

Remember, if you are new to this, you have to start somewhere … if you are experienced in this, it is always useful to have new material!

Core Equipment Guide

Most of the scenarios require a core set of equipment as outlined below.

Any additional equipment required for each specific scenario will be outlined in the relevant chapter.

This is designed as a guide rather than an exhaustive list as equipment and drugs will vary according to the local site.

Basic monitoring (maternal and fetal)			
Pulse oximeter	ECG leads	BP cuff	CTG monitor and leads
Urinary catheter	Thermometer	Glucometer	

Basic airway/breathing equipment		
Oxygen supply	Standard Hudson face mask	Self-inflating bag valve mask
	Non-rebreathing oxygen facemask	
Oropharyngeal airways	Suction	Stethoscope

Cannulation, blood-taking, fluids and pumps			
IV cannula/ dressing/ antiseptic	Blood sample bottles to include: FBC, U+Es, LFTs, coagulation including fibrinogen screen, blood cultures, G+S/XM		Pressure bag
Gloves/apron/ tourniquet	ABG syringe/ needle	Hartmann's solution and IV giving set	Infusion pumps

For intubation or advanced airway equipment, consider the following:

Advanced airway equipment		
Anaesthetic face mask and catheter mount	HME filter	Supraglottic airways
Range of laryngoscopes	Videolaryngoscope	Endotracheal tubes – range of sizes
Bougie	Tape/tie	Capnography
Difficult airway trolley	Nasal cannula	High-flow nasal oxygen therapy (to deliver THRIVE)
Anaesthetic machine	Transfer ventilator	

Useful props			
Telephone	Patient's hand-held maternity notes	Fluid/ prescription chart	British National Formulary

A quick recap of the key physiological changes in pregnancy are summarised in the tables below (Tables 9.1–9.4).

Table 9.1 The most significant haematological changes in pregnancy.

Physiological anaemia
Neutrophilia
Mild thrombocytopenia
Increased procoagulant factors
Diminished fibrinolysis

Table 9.2 Summary of key cardiovascular changes in pregnancy.

Parameter	Change
Stroke volume	+30%
Heart rate	+15–20%
SVR	−5% (approximately)
SBP	−10 mmHg
DBP	−15–20 mmHg
MAP	−15–20 mmHg
Oxygen consumption	+20%
Cardiac output	+50–70% (increase is more dramatic in late pregnancy)

Table 9.3 Changes in lung function tests during late states (third trimester) of pregnancy.

Respiratory rate	Unchanged
FEV1	Unchanged
PEFR	Unchanged
Minute volume/ventilation	Increased by 30–50%
Tidal volume	Increased by 30–50%
FVC	Unchanged
FEVI/FVC	Unchanged
Maximum mid-expiratory flow rate (forced expiratory flow rate 25–75)	Unchanged
Functional residual volume	Decreased by 18%

Table 9.4 Example of maternity early warning scoring system.

Score	3	2	1	0	1	2	3
Temp		<35.0	35.1–36.0	36.1–37.9	38.0–38.9	≥39.0	
Systolic BP	≤70	71–80	81–100	101–139		140–159	>160
Diastolic BP				<90	90–109		≥110
HR		≤40	41–50	51–100	101–110	111–129	≥130
RR		≤8		9–20	21–24	25–29	≥30
CNS			New confusion	Alert	Voice	Pain	Unresponsive
%SpO$_2$	<86%	86–91%	92–93%	≥94%			

10

Uterine Inversion

Samantha Bonner

Scenario in a Nutshell

PPH and retained placenta in delivery room. Uterine inversion. Failed manual replacement. Transfer to theatre. Successful hydrostatic replacement of uterus. Atonic PPH follows manual removal of placenta.

Stage 1: Uterine inversion diagnosed and manual replacement attempted with simultaneous resuscitation.

Stage 2: Hydrostatic repositioning of the uterus in theatre under GA.

Stage 3. Manual removal of placenta, postpartum atonic haemorrhage.

Target Learner Groups

All members of the multidisciplinary obstetric team: midwives, obstetricians, anaesthetists, operating department practitioners/anaesthetic nurses, theatre scrub team.

Suggested learning opportunities
Recognition of symptoms and signs of uterine inversion
Effective team management of uterine inversion with concurrent attempts at uterine replacement and resuscitation
Demonstrate methods of uterine replacement – manual and hydrostatic
Knowledge of drugs and doses – tocolytic and uterotonic agents

Suggested learners (to represent their normal roles)	In the room from the start	Available when requested
Anaesthetic ST3+		√
Obstetric ST3+	√	
Midwife Coordinator		√
Operating Department Practitioner (ODP)/anaesthetic nurse		√
Scrub nurse		√
Suggested facilitators		
Faculty to play role of midwife	√	
Faculty to play role of obstetric ST1	√	

Details for Facilitators

Patient Demographics

Name: Charlotte
Age: 28
Gestation: 39+4
Booking weight: 75 kg
Parity: P3

Scenario Summary for Facilitators

A 28-year-old multiparous woman has just had a spontaneous vaginal delivery. She is now para 3 and has had two vaginal deliveries previously, for one of which she required a manual removal of the placenta. She was booked for antenatal care locally and had an uneventful pregnancy.

She is using entonox for analgesia. She had a PV bleed following delivery and the midwife had difficulty in delivering the placenta.

She called for medical help and the Obstetric ST1 attempted to remove the placenta with difficulty. No vaginal trauma was noted. The placenta was unable to be delivered. After this, the bleeding increased and a postpartum haemorrhage (PPH) was diagnosed.

On examination, the uterus is not palpable abdominally and there is a large visible mass at the introitus. This patient has an acute uterine inversion.

There is haemodynamic instability, with marked bradycardia. Attempt at manual replacement in the room fails.

The patient is transferred to theatre, requires a general anaesthetic, manual/hydrostatic and pharmacological treatment of uterine inversion and PPH with simultaneous resuscitation.

Set-up Overview for Facilitators

Clinical setting	In delivery unit, on a delivery bed
Patient position	Lithotomy

Initial monitoring in place	Pulse oximeter, NIBP
Other equipment	16G cannula dorsum of hand. Midwife is attaching 1 litre of Hartmann's to the cannula. 40 IU syntocinon: 10 IU in 500 ml normal saline running at 125 ml/h
Useful manikin functions	Birthing manikin with uterine inversion model or pelvic part task trainer with soft uterine inversion model

Medical Equipment

For core equipment checklist, see Chapter 9 including advanced airway equipment.

Additional equipment specific to scenario		
Local emergency checklists for uterine inversion/postpartum haemorrhage (if available)	Kiwi/silicone ventouse cup ± black anaesthetic face mask	Warmed saline (several litres) and giving set
Rapid IV infusor/fluid warmer	Intrauterine hydrostatic balloon device (e.g. Bakri®)	Tocolytics: eg: terbutaline, glyceryl trinitrate (GTN), magnesium sulphate (MgSO$_4$)
Cardiovascular drugs: atropine, ephedrine, phenylephrine, metaraminol	Uterotonic agents: syntometrine, syntocinon, ergometrine (Haemabate), carboprost, misoprostol	Induction agents (thiopentone and propofol), neuromuscular blockers (depolarising and non-depolarising)

Additional equipment specific to scenario		
Arterial line	Entonox mask/ mouth piece	Tranexamic acid
Prophylactic antibiotics		

Information Given to the Learners

Information given to ST3 obstetric trainee and midwife coordinator who have just been called to attend the room

This handover is given by a facilitator playing the role of the obstetric ST1.

The SBAR handover is as follows:

Situation: This is a woman who is having a PPH and I can't get the placenta out.

Background: Charlotte is a 28-year-old, previously fit and well multiparous woman who was 39+4 weeks pregnant. She had a spontaneous NVD 20 minutes ago and is now para 3. She has had 2 previous NVD, needing a manual removal of placenta last time.

She is otherwise fit and well with no known allergies.

There was a brisk loss following delivery and I got called in to assist as the midwife was having trouble delivering the placenta. She had syntometrine for 3rd stage. Now there is a big mass at the introitus and I can't palpate the uterus abdominally. I'm worried she might have a uterine inversion.

Action: I have tried to remove the placenta over the last 5 minutes but I can't. The bleeding is getting heavier. We have started a syntocinon infusion and some Hartmann's. She has lost about 600 ml so far I think.

Recommendation: Can you help me get this placenta out?

Scenario Schedule

Stage 1: Uterine inversion diagnosed and manual replacement attempted with simultaneous resuscitation	
Information given	**Expected actions**
Patient is in lithotomy with a large mass at the introitus and she is actively bleeding	State the emergency: uterine inversion with on-going PPH
	Call for help using emergency buzzer
	Locate local checklist for uterine inversion/ PPH if available
	ABCDE assessment and commence monitoring
Responding to voice but feeling very faint and nauseous. In pain. Talking.	Perform airway assessment

Observations	
A	Clear
B	RR 24/min SpO$_2$ 97%
C	HR 42 bpm BP 76/40 CRT 3s
D	A**V**PU
E	nil to note

Information given	Expected actions
	Apply Oxygen via non-rebreathing mask at 15 L/min whilst stabilising the patient (then titrate oxygen to SpO_2 94-98%)
Chest clear, bilateral air entry, no added sounds	Assess breathing
Anaesthetic ST and midwife co-ordinator arrive in response to emergency buzzer	ST3 obstetrics restates emergency and SBAR
	Continuously monitor blood pressure, heart rate, respiratory rate and SpO_2
HR and BP improve with anticholinergic	Team recognise vagally-mediated bradycardia and treat with increments of anticholinergic (atropine 300-600mcg IV increments up to 3mg)
Give repeat observations if asked	
	Rapid fluid replacement with crystalloid (warmed fluid as soon as possible)
	Secure 2nd large-bore IV access and take blood for FBC, U+E, coagulation screen including fibrinogen
	Cross match 4-6 units of blood
	Ensure bladder is empty
	Commence replacement of uterus whilst simultaneously resuscitating as above
	Call consultant obstetrician / consultant anaesthetist if not already done so
	Call theatre team to prepare in case of failure to replace uterus in the room
Using Entonox	Attempt manual replacement (Johnson manoeuvre) as soon as possible: • Ensure Syntocinon infusion is stopped • Consider further analgesia • Do not attempt to separate the placenta from the uterus • The last part of the uterus that is out (usually the fundus) should be pushed back in first and gradually the uterus should revert back into its correct position

Observations

A	Clear
B	RR 24/min SpO_2 98% on O_2
C	HR 98 bpm BP 110/68 CRT 2s
D	<u>A</u>VPU
E	nil to note

Information given	Expected actions
	Consider drugs to relax cervix, eg: • Terbutaline IV 250mcg in 5mls normal saline over 5 minutes or (can consider S/C terbutaline 250mcg but will not be absorbed quickly if patient shocked) • GTN 2 puffs (800mcg) sublingual or 100-250mcgs IV • MgSO4 4G IV over 5 minutes or as per local guidelines
Manual replacement fails	
	After attempt is not successful, decision made for immediate transfer to theatre
	Tranexamic acid 1g IV

Proceed to stage 2 once manual replacement of the uterus has been unsuccessful and the decision has been made to transfer to theatre

Stage 2: Hydrostatic repositioning of the uterus in theatre under GA

Observations	
A	Clear
B	RR 28/min SpO$_2$ 99% on O$_2$
C	HR 115 bpm BP 112/72 CRT 2s
D	**A**VPU
E	Temp 36.6°C

Information given	Expected actions
Patient is now in theatre. EBL (estimated blood loss) 1000mls	Put on monitoring
Fit and well, no previous GA, no family history of problems with GA No drug allergies, no regular medications Last ate 9 hours ago, been drinking water through labour Had ranitidine 150mg PO 2 hours ago	Focussed history from anaesthetist
Dentition all OK, good mouth opening, Mallampati 1, Calder A, good cervical spine movements	Airway assessment
	Prepare drugs and equipment for GA
	Discuss airway plan A, B and C with ODP/ anaesthetic nurse
	Discuss plan to proceed/wake in event of failed intubation (proceed as uterine inversion with ongoing haemorrhage)
	Preoxygenate with facemask and nasal cannulae at 15L/min in head-up position
Grade 1 intubation	Induction of general anaesthesia and intubation

Information given	Expected actions
	Obstetrician requests tocolytic agent (for options, see stage 1)
Manual replacement not successful	One attempt at manual replacement (Johnson manoeuvre) repeated whilst preparing equipment for hydrostatic repositioning of uterus
Hydrostatic technique is successful	Perform hydrostatic positioning of uterus: • Exclude uterine rupture • Attach an intravenous giving set to a litre of warm saline. Have several bags of warmed saline ready • The fluid needs to be higher than the patient (approximately 1-1.5m above) • Insert a silicone ventouse cup into the vagina and produce a seal by holding the vulva closed over the intra-vaginal cup • Infuse warm saline through the ventouse cup via a giving set • The process may take about 15 mins and up to 2 litres of warm saline • Alternatively, a hard, black, rubber anaesthetic facemask can also be used. This fits over the vulva. The giving set can be passed through the oxygen inlet.
PV bleeding continues – EBL now ~1500mls	Activate massive obstetric haemorrhage protocol

Proceed to stage 3 once hydrostatic replacement of the uterus is successful

Observations

A	Intubated
B	RR as per ventilator SpO$_2$ 98%
C	HR 115 bpm BP 115/82 CRT 2s
D	Anaesthetised
E	Temp 36.3°C

Stage 3: Manual removal of placenta, postpartum atonic haemorrhage

Information given	Expected actions
	Maintain uterus in place with fingers and give oxytocic: eg: 5 I.U. oxytocin
	Deliver placenta
PV blood loss worsens after placenta is delivered and uterus is atonic – EBL continues to 2000~2500mls	Manage atony:
	Bimanual compression and ensure uterine cavity empty
	Low threshold for early use of Intrauterine hydrostatic balloon device (eg: Bakri®)

Observations

A	Intubated
B	RR as per ventilator SpO$_2$ 98%
C	HR 132 BP 89/62 CRT 4s
D	Anaesthetised
E	Temp 35.9°C

Information given	Expected actions
	Start 40 IU syntocinon infusion at 10 I.U. / hr (or as per local guidelines)
	Give 500 mcg Ergometrine IM or Syntometrine 1ml IM (or as per local post-partum haemorrhage guidelines)
	Haemabate 250mcg IM and repeated every 15 mins up to a maximum of ei doses
	Consider Misoprostol 1g PR (as per lo guidelines)
	Check for vaginal trauma
	Simultaneous resuscitation should be taking place with crystalloid +/- bloo as required
	Preparation for arterial line insertion i bleeding ongoing
No coagulation products required on interpretation of TEG/ROTEM	Urgent TEG or ROTEM and arterial blc gas
ABG result: FiO2: 0.7 pH 7.32 PO$_2$ 26.0k Pa PCO$_2$ 4.1 kPa Hb 90 g/L HCO3 18 mmol/L BE -8 mmol/L lactate 3.1 mmol/L	
	Antibiotic prophylaxis given
	Ensure indwelling urinary catheter is inserted with hourly urometer
	Intrauterine hydrostatic balloon devi inserted if not done earlier
Once uterotonics given and intrauterine hydrostatic balloon device inserted, bleeding settles	

Scenario ends once uterotonics given +/- intrauterine hydrostatic balloon device inserted and bleeding settles

Observations	
A	Intubated
B	RR as per ventilator SpO$_2$ 98%
C	HR 118 bpm BP 110/62 CRT 2s
D	Anaesthetised
E	Temp 36.1°C.

Suggested Topics for Debrief Discussion

- Were attempts at replacement of the uterus made concurrently with resuscitation?
- Was the equipment required for hydrostatic replacement of the uterus readily available?

Discussion

Incidence

Acute uterine inversion is a rare complication of the third stage of labour. Its quoted incidence is variable, but the largest series to date looking at over 8 million deliveries in the USA found an incidence of 2.9 per 10,000 deliveries (data collected from 2004 to 2013) (Coad et al., 2017). Many obstetricians will never encounter this emergency in clinical practice. However, it can be associated with hypovolaemic shock and maternal mortality (Coad et al., 2017); therefore, all clinicians involved in labour care should have theoretical knowledge of its management and practise multidisciplinary team drills.

Risk Factors

Historically, uterine inversion has been related to 'mismanagement' of the third stage of labour associated with excessive cord traction, failure to guard the uterus abdominally or attempting to deliver the placenta prior to separation.

Non-iatrogenic risk factors are (Haeri et al., 2015; Witteveen et al., 2013):

- nulliparity,
- fetal macrosomia,
- rapid labour/delivery,
- short umbilical cord,
- morbidly adherent placenta,
- uterine anomalies or tumours (leiomyoma),
- connective tissue diseases: e.g. Marfan's syndrome, Ehlers–Danlos syndrome.

Risk factors are, however, absent in over 50% of cases.

Presentation

An acute inversion can occur both with vaginal delivery and at caesarean section although it is a very rare occurrence at caesarean section with an incidence of ~1 in 20,000 deliveries (Witteveen et al., 2013).

Table 10.1 Classification of uterine inversion.

1st degree (incomplete)~10%	Fundus is in the endometrial cavity
2nd degree (Complete)	The fundus protrudes through the external cervical os
3rd degree	Fundus reaches/protrudes through the introitus
4th degree	Both the uterus and vagina are inverted

There are four classifications of uterine inversion (see Table 10.1) and the clinical presentation will depend on the extent of inversion.

Clinical Symptoms and Signs

- Lump in the vagina: on vaginal examination, a round mass may be seen protruding through the cervical os (uterine fundus) or the whole uterus may be seen outside of the introitus.
- Abdominal pain and tenderness, often severe.
- Absence of uterine fundus on abdominal palpation (in milder cases an indentation may be felt per abdomen).
- Postpartum haemorrhage.
- Neurogenic shock – may have cardiovascular signs and symptoms out of proportion to the degree of blood loss. Can get marked bradycardia, secondary to increased vagal tone from stretching of the parasympathetic pelvic nerves.
- Acute urinary retention.

The placenta may or may not be separated, but it is important to replace the uterus with the placenta attached rather than attempting separation prior to replacement.

Management

The management of acute uterine inversion should be multidisciplinary and systematic. It is important to resuscitate the patient while attempting to replace the uterus as resuscitation may not be successful until the uterine position has been corrected.

It is important to remember to stop any uterotonics – the uterus has to be relaxed in order for it to be replaced.

There are three types of management for acute uterine inversion:

- manual replacement,
- hydrostatic repositioning of the uterus,
- surgical replacement.

Manual replacement is usually the quickest and most effective method. If manual replacement is unsuccessful, the patient should be transferred to theatre immediately and either manual replacement reattempted under general anaesthesia or hydrostatic repositioning of the uterus performed. If these fail then surgical replacement is required.

Manual Replacement (Johnson Manoeuvre)

If attempted immediately after diagnosis, manual replacement is usually successful. Drugs may be required to relax the cervix to ease replacement. Options include the following.

- Terbutaline IV 250 µg in 5 ml normal saline over 5 minutes or (can consider S/C terbutaline 250 µg but will not be absorbed quickly if patient shocked).
- GTN 2 puffs (800 µg) sublingual or 100–250 µg IV.
- MgSO$_4$ 4G IV over 5 minutes.

The current cardiovascular status of the patient should be considered when selecting the most appropriate tocolytic agent.

The last part of the uterus that is out (usually the fundus) should be replaced first and gradually the uterus should revert to its correct position. If successful then the clinician should keep a hand inside the uterus, ensuring that it stays in position, and administer uterotonics to aid uterine contraction.

When the uterus is replaced, only then may the placenta be manually removed. Postpartum haemorrhage due to atony is common and should be anticipated.

Uterine tamponade with an intrauterine hydrostatic balloon has been recommended (Vivanti et al., 2017). This will help with management of uterine atony and also prevent immediate recurrence of the uterine inversion.

Hydrostatic Replacement (O'Sullivan's Technique)

The theory behind hydrostatic repositioning is that large quantities of warm saline infused into the posterior fornix of the vagina while ensuring the vaginal orifice is closed will stretch the vagina, relax any cervical constriction and allow the uterus to revert to its correct position (Ogueh and Ayida, 2006).

Intrauterine Hydrostatic Balloon (Primary Treatment)

There are reported cases that have used intrauterine balloon devices (such as a Bakri® balloon) with success

as primary treatment to correct the inverted uterus (Haeri et al., 2015; Ida et al., 2015).

Surgical Replacement
Huntingdon's Procedure

Through an abdominal incision the inversion of the uterus is visualised. A clamp (Allis/Babcock) is placed on each round ligament that enters the indentation on the uterus. The myometrium may be clamped if the round ligaments cannot be accessed. Gentle upward traction on the clamps should revert the fundus of the uterus. Clamping and traction should be repeated until uterine position is corrected.

Haultain Procedure

Abdominally, a surgical incision is made on the posterior surface of the uterus. This is thought to release any constricted myometrium and aid replacement via Huntingdon's (see above). A variant of the Haultain procedure is to make a longitudinal incision posteriorly along the cervical ring, again releasing any cervical constriction preventing repositioning.

Vaginal and Laparoscopic Replacement

Occasionally, vaginal and laparoscopic replacement of the uterus has been performed with success, but there is not enough current or available literature to endorse these procedures (Vijayaraghavan and Sujatha, 2006).

Complications

A large population-based study that has been published in the United States incorporates 2427 cases of uterine inversion between 2004 and 2013 (Coad et al., 2017).

Adverse outcomes include:

- maternal death (4.1 per 10,000),
- postpartum haemorrhage, 37.7% (95% confidence interval (CI), 35.8–39.6%),
- blood transfusion, 22.4% (95% CI 20.7–24%),
- requiring surgical management, 6.0% (95% CI 5.1–7.0%),
- hysterectomy, 2.8% (95% CI 2.1–3.5%).

Summary

- Uterine inversion is a rare but potentially life-threatening obstetric emergency.
- Early recognition and prompt multidisciplinary management is essential to reduce maternal morbidity/mortality.

- Uterotonic infusions must be stopped to aid replacement of the uterus.
- Concurrent resuscitation and uterine replacement is needed as haemodynamic stability will often not be achieved until the uterine position is corrected.
- Senior obstetric, anaesthetic and midwifery staff should be involved early.
- Subsequent atonic postpartum haemorrhage should be anticipated and early use of an intrauterine balloon device is advocated.

Bibliography

Bhalla, R., Wuntakal, R., Odejinmi, F. and Khan, R. U. (2009). Acute inversion of the uterus. *The Obstetrician & Gynaecologist*, 11, 13–18.

Coad, S. L., Dahlgren, L. S. and Hutcheon, J. A. (2017). Risks and consequences of puerperal uterine inversion in the United States, 2004 through 2013. *American Journal of Obstetrics and Gynecology*, 217(3), 377.

Haeri, S., Rais, S. and Monks, B. (2015). Intrauterine tamponade balloon use in the treatment of uterine inversion. *BMJ Case Reports*, 2015. pii:brc2014206705.doi:1136/bcr-2014-206705. PubMed PMID:25564634;PubMed Central PMCID: PMC4289782.

Ida, A., Ito, K., Kubota, Y., Nosaka, M., Kato, H. and Tsuji, Y. (2015). Successful reduction of acute puerperal uterine inversion with the use of a Bakri postpartum balloon. *Case Reports in Obstetrics and Gynaecology*, 2015, 424891. doi:10.1155/2015/424891. Epub 2015.

Leal, R. F., Luz, R. M., de Almeida, J. P., Duarte, V. and Matos, I. (2014). Total and acute uterine inversion after delivery: a case report. *Journal of Medical Case Reports*, 8, 347. doi:10.1186/1752-1947-8-347

Ogueh, O. and Ayida, G. (1997). Acute uterine inversion: a new technique of hydrostatic replacement. *British Journal of Obstetrics and Gynecology*, 104, 951–952.

Paterson-Brown, S. and Howell, C. (2014). *Managing Obstetric Emergencies and Trauma (MOET)*, third edition. Cambridge: Cambridge University Press.

Vijayaraghavan, R. and Sujatha, Y. (2006). Acute postpartum uterine inversion with haemorrhagic shock: laparoscopic reduction: a new method of management? *British Journal of Obstetrics and Gynecology*, 113, 1100–1102.

Vivanti, A. J., Furet, E. and Nizard, J. (2017). Successful use of a Bakri Tamponade balloon in the treatment of puerperal uterine inversion during caesarean section. *Journal of Gynecology Obstetrics and Human Reproduction*, 46(1), 101–102.

Witteveen, T., van Stralen, G., Zwart, J. and van Roosmalen, J. (2013). Puerperal uterine inversion in the Netherlands: a nationwide cohort study. *Acta Obstetrica Gynecologica Scandinavica* 92(3), 34–37.

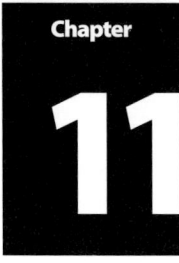

Chapter 11

Shoulder Dystocia Following Forceps Delivery for Fetal Bradycardia

Samantha Cox and Samiksha Patel

Scenario in a Nutshell

Shoulder dystocia following forceps delivery requiring internal manoeuvres.
   Stage 1: Shoulder dystocia just recognised. Help summoned and McRoberts' position.
   Stage 2: McRoberts' and suprapubic pressure unsuccessful. Internal manoeuvres required for delivery.

Target Learner Groups

Midwives, obstetricians, anaesthetists and neonatal emergency team.

Specific learning opportunities
Early recognition of shoulder dystocia and appropriate help sought
Knowledge of management of shoulder dystocia – demonstrate timely progression through the treatment algorithm
Demonstrate manoeuvres used
Demonstrate effective planning for after-coming emergencies associated with shoulder dystocia
Demonstrate effective communication between the team and to the incoming neonatal team
Demonstrate appropriate leadership and followership in different roles within the team

Suggested learners (to represent their normal roles)	In the room from the start	Available when requested
Midwife	√	
Midwifery student	√	
Midwife coordinator		√
Obstetric ST3+		√
Obstetric ST6	√	
Anaesthetic ST3+		√
Neonatal emergency team		√
Further midwives		√

Suggested learners (to represent their normal roles)	In the room from the start	Available when requested
Suggested facilitators		
Faculty to play role of patient's partner	√	

Details for Facilitators

Patient Demographics

Name: Isma

Age: 29

Gestation: 39+6

Booking weight: 78 kg

Parity: P0

Scenario Summary for Facilitators

A 29-year-old primiparous woman, Isma, attended maternity triage in spontaneous labour at 39+6 weeks pregnant. She was known to have a baby measuring above the 90th centile and she was transferred to the consultant-led unit due to a suspicious CTG.

The labour progressed at an appropriate rate and she commenced active pushing as soon as she became fully dilated.

Thirty minutes in to the active second stage, a fetal bradycardia ensued.

The obstetric registrar on call delivered the fetal head with forceps and an episiotomy in the delivery room. The head delivers slowly and the fetal chin is tight to the perineum when the forceps are removed. The head does not restitute and the body is not deliverable with axial traction. The obstetric registrar instructs for the emergency buzzer to be pushed.

Delivery suite team respond to buzzer.

McRoberts' manoeuvre and suprapubic rocking unsuccessful.

Internal manoeuvres required. Baby delivered with final internal manoeuvre attempted.

up Overview for Facilitators

al setting	In a delivery room, on a delivery bed
nt position	Lithotomy
monitoring in place	None
equipment	16G cannula dorsum left hand. Entonox mask/mouthpiece
l manikin functions	Birthing manikin or pelvic part-task trainer

cal Equipment

re equipment checklist, see Chapter 9.

tional equipment specific to scenario		
tomy scissors	Entonox mask/ mouthpiece	Local checklist for shoulder dystocia (if available)
of delivery – fetal cardia noted and quent timings of s delivery. Time very of head		

Information Given to the Learners

Information given to ST6 obstetrics, midwife and midwifery student who are in the room at the start of the scenario.

This is Isma, a 29 year old primip who is 39+6 weeks pregnant. She is known to have a baby measuring on the 90th centile. She came into triage in spontaneous labour last night. She has progressed to fully dilated overnight. ~10 minutes ago, there was a fetal bradycardia after she had been pushing for 30 minutes so the midwife caring for her activated the emergency buzzer.

To ST6 obstetrician: You attended the emergency buzzer and stayed in the room to perform a forceps delivery.

You have just delivered the head by forceps after performing an episiotomy. The head delivered slowly and the baby's chin is tight to the perineum when the forceps are removed. The head does not restitute and the body has not been deliverable by axial traction.

You have realised that it is a shoulder dystocia and have asked for the emergency buzzer to be pulled.

Information given to rest of learners

The emergency buzzer has just sounded.

From handover, you know that Isma is a 29 year old, previously fit and well primip who is 39+6 weeks pregnant, with a baby measuring on the 90th centile.

She came into triage in spontaneous labour last night. She has progressed to fully dilated overnight.

There was an emergency buzzer from this room ~10 minutes ago, when there was a fetal bradycardia. She had been pushing for 30 minutes. The ST6 obstetrician stayed in the room to perform a forceps delivery.

ario Schedule

Stage 1: Shoulder dystocia just recognised. Help summoned and McRobert's position.	
Information given	**Expected actions**
Team responding to emergency buzzer enter the room: midwife co-ordinator, ST3+ obstetrician, more midwives, anaesthetic ST3+	Obstetric ST6 to take the leadership role
Head is delivered. Woman is crying in pain and using Entonox	State the emergency to the incoming team: 'Shoulder Dystocia'
	Briefly explain what is happening to the patient and partner
	Discourage woman from pushing
	Urgently call neonatal team
	Ensure consultant obstetrician and an anaesthetist urgently contacted if have not responded to emergency buzzer
	Assess to see if episiotomy needs extending

	Information given	Expected actions
		Place 1 member of staff at each leg to place woman in McRoberts position:
		• Lie flat (remove any pillows from under back)
		• Take legs out of lithotomy
		• Ensure woman is right at the bottom of the bed
		• Hyperflex woman's hips, with thighs positioned on abdomen
		Put monitoring on (in anticipation of PPH)
		Assign a scribe who should locate the emergency checklist for shoulder dystocia, if available

Observations	
A	Clear
B	RR 28/min SpO$_2$ 98%
C	HR 128 bpm BP 126/73
D	**A**VPU
E	Nil to note

Proceed to Stage 2 once in McRoberts position

Stage 2: McRobert's and suprapubic pressure unsuccessful. Internal manoeuvres required for delivery.

Information given	Expected actions
Shoulders still not deliverable at this point	States out loud to the scribe the following manoeuvres:
	• Enters and assesses where the anterior shoulder is; communicates where to apply continuous suprapubic pressure for up to 30 seconds
	• Assistant applies suprapubic pressure from the side of the fetal back in a downward and lateral direction just above the maternal symphysis pubis
	• Rocking suprapubic pressure for up to 30 seconds (Rubin I)
	Scribe to vocalise points from checklist
	Fundal pressure should not be used
	Proceed to Internal manoeuvres (can be done in any order, but all manoeuvres must be tried):
	Try to deliver the posterior arm for up to maximum of 30 seconds
	Place fingers behind anterior shoulder and push towards fetal chest (Rubin II) for up to a maximum of 30 seconds
Shoulders still not deliverable at this point	Add fingertips to front aspect of posterior shoulder and push towards fetal back in combination with Rubin II (Woods' screw) for up to a max of 30 seconds
Head delivers with the final manoeuvre	Change direction of pushing, i.e. fingertips are applied to the front surface of the anterior shoulder and on the back wall of the posterior shoulder (reverse Woods' screw) for up to a max of 30 seconds
	Baby taken immediately for resuscitation. Should tell the neonatal team:
	• Which shoulder was anterior
	• Manoeuvres required
	• Time from head delivery to delivery of the shoulders

Information given	Expected actions
Estimated blood loss 500 mls.	Assess for bleeding and perineal trauma
	Recheck observations
Prompt from facilitator playing birth partner: 'What has just happened?', 'Is everything OK?'	Discussion with parents about delivery events

Observations	
A	Clear
B	RR 24/min SpO$_2$ 98%
C	HR 118 bpm BP 145/90
D	AVPU
E	Nil to note

Scenario ends once baby delivered and obstetrician has told parents what has happened

Suggested Topics for Debrief Discussion

- How did the group work as a team – were all members given a role?
- What would your plan be if the shoulders had not delivered at this point?

Discussion

Definition

Shoulder dystocia is defined as a vaginal cephalic delivery that requires additional obstetric manoeuvres to deliver the fetus after the head has delivered and gentle traction has failed (Crofts et al., 2012).

It most commonly results from the anterior shoulder becoming entrapped behind the symphysis pubis, although rarely the posterior shoulder can become trapped by the sacral promontory, or neither shoulder descends into the pelvis.

Incidence

Reported incidence is between 0.58% and 0.70% of vaginal deliveries.

Risk Factors

There are several risk factors associated with shoulder dystocia, but there is currently no way to predict when it will occur. There is also no robust evidence to support the use of prophylactic interventions, such as McRoberts, in deliveries judged to be at a higher risk of shoulder dystocia, meaning there are no effective intrapartum preventative measures (Athukorala et al., 2009).

The recognised risk factors for shoulder dystocia are as follows.

Maternal risk factors:
- raised BMI above 30, and
- diabetes (both pre-existing to the pregnancy and gestational).

Antenatal risk factors:
- induction of labour,
- fetal macrosomia > 4500 g,
- previous shoulder dystocia.

Intrapartum risk factors:
- prolonged first stage of labour,
- prolonged second stage of labour,
- operative vaginal delivery, and
- augmentation with oxytocin. (Crofts et al., 2012)

Most women in labour will have at least one of the above risk factors. Therefore, it is important for the delivery suite team always to be aware of the risk and be vigilant for any clinical signs of shoulder dystocia, as described below.

Signs of Shoulder Dystocia

- Slow delivery of the head.
- Chin tight to the perineum (the 'turtleneck' sign).
- Failure of restitution. (Taylor, 2010)

Management of Shoulder Dystocia

The optimum management of shoulder dystocia requires a structured approach that has been tested in emergency drills. The sequence of manoeuvres used will differ for every practitioner, but it is of benefit to have a practised sequence that can be relied upon in an emergency (see Figure 11.1).

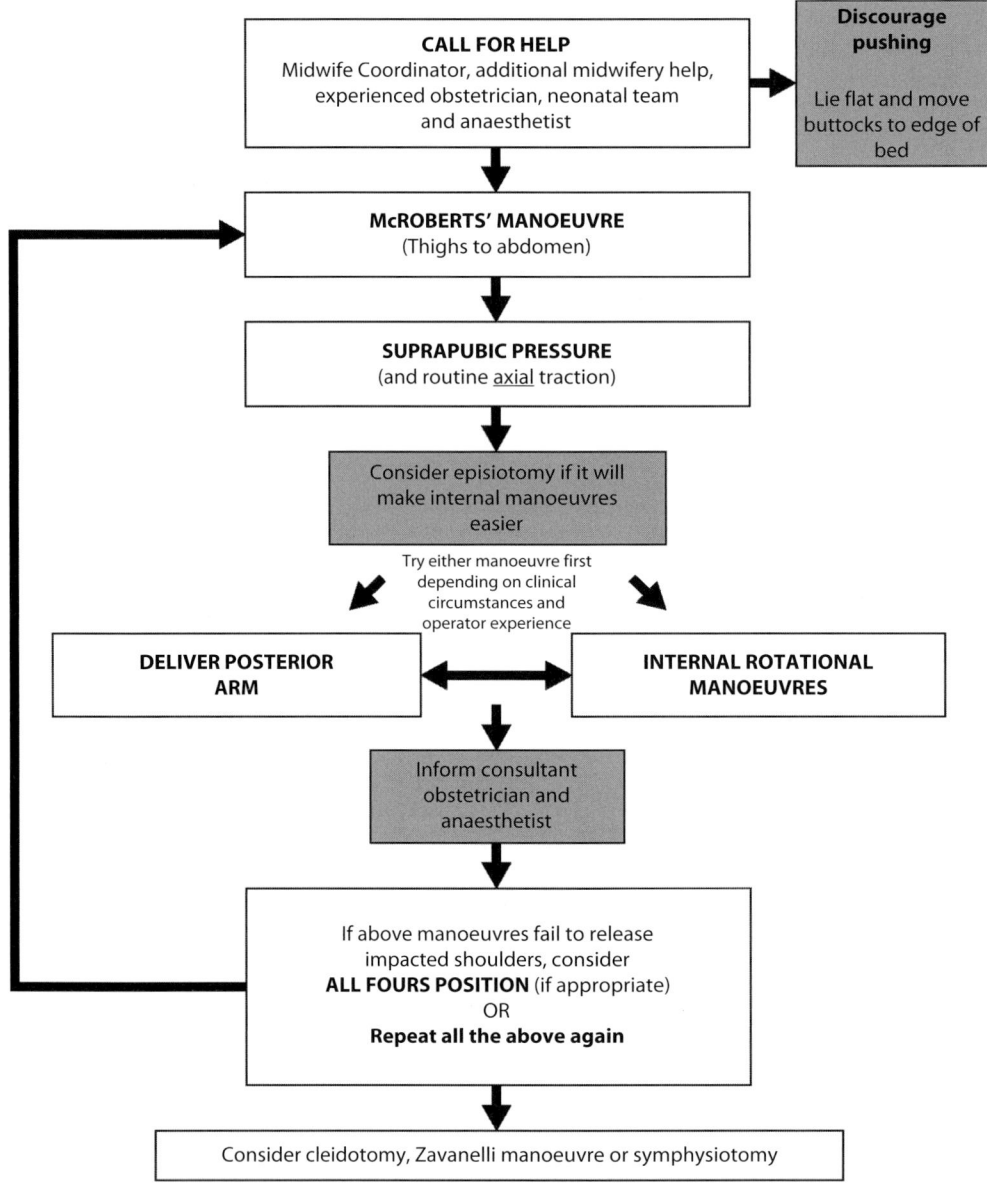

Figure 11.1 RCOG algorithm for the management of shoulder dystocia.
www.rcog.org.uk/globalassets/documents/guidelines/gtg_42.pdf

Environment

Time is a major factor when managing a shoulder dystocia with everyone working together to deliver the baby as quickly as possible. To aid team-working and accurate documentation, the team should be listening for instructions and timings from the team leader, which will be the senior obstetrician in most cases. This means limiting discussion within the room.

It is a very distressing time for the mother and birth partners. It is important to keep parents updated briefly as to what is happening throughout the delivery; a very brief introduction to who is present and the need for special manoeuvres is necessary.

Practical Manoeuvres

Expected initial steps and manoeuvres are as outlined in the 'expected actions' column of the scenario schedule.

If delivery is still not possible after these manoeuvres, place the patient (if possible) in to all fours position and try all the internal manoeuvres again.

If delivery is still not possible, then:

- consider stronger analgesia and moving to the Obstetric theatre,
- options are Zavanelli, symphysiotomy or fracture of the clavicle (final-stage manoeuvres).

Final-Stage Manoeuvres

It is incredibly difficult to decide at this point on the best course of action and the decision will be based on the balance between maternal and fetal morbidity and mortality. Therefore, at this stage, it is essential to have the most senior obstetrician present. The methods to perform these manoeuvres are beyond the scope of this chapter.

Other Techniques

Posterior axillary sling traction is a new technique that involves the passage of a small piece of suction tubing under the axilla of the posterior shoulder to form a loop. Traction applied to this loop can be used to deliver the posterior arm or to help with Woods' screw manoeuvre. It is not currently recommended due to limited evidence available to guide use and potential increased risk of fetal morbidity. A review of 19 cases showed that four babies delivered using a sling technique were complicated by transient Erb's palsy of the anterior shoulder (Cluver and Hofmeyer, 2014).

Complications

Fetal (Dajani and Magann, 2014)

- Hypoxic–ischaemic encephalopathy,
- Brachial plexus injury (2.3–16%: Crofts et al., 2012),
- Fractures of the clavicle and humerus,
- Death.

Maternal

- Perineal trauma – third- and fourth-degree perineal tears (3.8%) (Gherman et al., 1997),

- Postpartum haemorrhage (11%) (Gherman et al., 1997),
- Vaginal lacerations,
- Cervical tears,
- Bladder rupture,
- Uterine rupture,
- Symphyseal separation,
- Sacroiliac joint dislocation,
- Lateral femoral cutaneous neuropathy.

Can Anything be Done to Reduce the Risk of Shoulder Dystocia?

Induction of labour has long been investigated as a potential risk-reducing strategy for women with large for gestational age babies. A 2016 Cochrane review reported that early induction near term (between 37+0 and 38+6) appeared to reduce the risk of shoulder dystocia (Boulvain et al., 2016). The largest contributor to this meta-analysis was a single randomised control trial comparing women with babies estimated to be on the 95th centile who were randomised to either induction of labour or expectant management. This reported a reduction in the number of significant shoulder dystocia episodes in the induction group as opposed to the expectant management group, with the mean delivery weight being lower in the induction group (3831 g and 4118 g, respectively) (Boulvain et al., 2015). This finding must be balanced with the risks of inducing labour before spontaneous onset, and for this reason further research is warranted before this becomes a routine recommendation.

Women affected by gestational or pre-existing diabetes and fetal macrosomia (estimated fetal weight > 4500 g) are at a significantly increased risk of shoulder dystocia in comparison with women who do not have diabetes. Therefore, current guidance recommends consideration of elective caesarean section under these circumstances (Crofts et al., 2012).

Summary Points

- It is vital that all medical professionals working with women in labour are aware of this emergency and the steps to manage it.
- It is important to have a prepared and practised 'step-wise' approach to management – checklists can be useful.
- Contemporaneous and accurate documentation is vital; therefore, it is important to ensure the role of scribe is allocated.

Bibliography

Athukorala, C., Middleton, P. and Ca, C. (2009). Intrapartum interventions for preventing shoulder dystocia (Review). *The Cochrane Library*, 4, 24. Available at: http://onlinelibrary.wiley.com/doi/10.1002/14651858.CD005543.pub2/pdf

Boulvain, M., Senat, M. V., Perrotin, F., et al. (2015). Induction of labour versus expectant management for large-for-date fetuses: a randomised controlled trial. *The Lancet*, 385(9987), 2600–2605.

Boulvain, M., Irion, O., Dowswell, T. and Thornton, J. G. (2016). Induction of labour at or near term for suspected fetal macrosomia. *The Cochrane Database of Systematic Reviews*, 5, CD000938. Available at: www.ncbi.nlm.nih.gov/pubmed/27208913 (accessed December 28, 2016).

Cluver, C. A. and Hofmeyr, G. J. (2014). Posterior axilla sling traction for shoulder dystocia: case review and a new method of shoulder rotation with the sling. *American Journal of Obstetrics and Gynecology*, 212(6), 784.e1–784.e7. Available at: http://dx.doi.org/10.1016/j.ajog.2015.02.025.

Crofts, J., Draycott, T. J., Montague, I., Winter, C. and Fox, R. (2012). *Green-top Guideline Number 42 Shoulder Dystocia.* London: Royal College of Obstetricians and Gynaecologists.

Dajani, N. K. and Magann, E. F. (2014). Complications of shoulder dystocia. *Seminars in Perinatology*, 38(4), 201–204.

Gherman, R. B., Goodwin, T. M., Souter, I., Neumann, K., Ouzounian, J. G. and Paul, R. H. (1997). The McRoberts' maneuver for the alleviation of shoulder dystocia: how successful is it? *American Journal of Obstetrics and Gynecology*, 176(3), 656–661.

Taylor, M. (2010). Shoulder dystocia. In D. Luesley and P. Baker (Eds.), *Obstetrics and Gynecology* (pp. 419–423). London: Hodder Arnold.

Obstetric

Umbilical Cord Prolapse

Michelle MacKintosh

Scenario in a Nutshell

Umbilical cord prolapse discovered in parous woman on antenatal ward. CTG suspicious. Transferred urgently to theatre with midwife elevating presenting part per vaginum.

Stage 1: Transfer to operating table and prepare for GA category 1 caesarean section.

Stage 2: Obstetric team analyse CTG and plan for category 2 caesarean section under regional anaesthesia. Spinal inserted.

Stage 3: Deterioration of CTG requiring urgent delivery.

Target Learner Groups

All members of the multidisciplinary obstetric team: anaesthetists, midwives, obstetricians, operating department practitioners/anaesthetic nurses and theatre scrub teams.

Specific learning opportunities
Effective team management of obstetric emergency – umbilical cord prolapse
Demonstrate effective communication and decision-making, particularly around method of anaesthesia and delivery

Suggested learners (to represent their normal roles)	In the theatre from the start	Available when requested
Anaesthetic ST3+	√	
Obstetric ST3+	√	
Midwife Coordinator	√	
Midwife taking over care from ward midwife	√	
Theatre team – Operating Department Practitioner (ODP)/anaesthetic nurse	√	

Suggested learners (to represent their normal roles)	In the theatre from the start	Available when requested
Theatre team – scrub nurse	√	
Theatre team – runner	√	
Obstetric consultant		√
Anaesthetic consultant		√
Suggested facilitators		
Faculty to play role of midwife transferring patient from ward to theatre	√	
Faculty to play role of patient's partner	√	

Details for Facilitators

Patient Demographics

Name: Lucy
Age: 34
Gestation: 34+4
Booking weight: 65 kg
Parity: P2

Scenario Summary

34-year-old para 2, on antenatal ward for threatened preterm labour, 34 weeks gestation.
CTG commenced on antenatal ward as pain increased, CTG abnormal.
Vaginal examination by obstetric registrar on antenatal ward, found to have cord prolapse, cephalic, 7 cm dilated.
Transferred directly to obstetric theatre.
Transferred on bed in knee-chest position with ward midwife maintaining elevation of presenting part vaginally.

CTG recommenced in theatre, normal.

Prepare for caesarean section as cervix 7 cm dilated on ward.

Bladder filled with normal saline to maintain elevation of presenting part.

Spinal inserted in left lateral position, CTG remains acceptable – couple of decelerations, but OK on the whole.

After spinal insertion, CTG deteriorates. Fully dilated now; therefore, proceed to instrumental delivery.

Set-up Overview for Facilitators

Clinical setting	Obstetric theatre
Patient position	Wheeled in on bed in knee-chest position with midwife on bed elevating the presenting part vaginally
Initial monitoring in place	None initially
Other equipment	16G cannula dorsum left hand
Useful manikin functions	Birthing manikin

Medical Equipment

For core equipment checklist, see Chapter 9, including advanced airway equipment.

Additional equipment specific to scenario

Equipment for instilling normal saline into bladder: 500 ml bag normal saline with either giving set or 50 ml bladder syringe and kidney dish	Local emergency checklist for umbilical cord prolapse (if available)	Induction ag (thiopenton and propof neuromuscu blockers (depolarisin non-depola
Ethyl chloride spray	Theatre trolley, caesarean section tray and instrumental delivery tray	Theatre gov gloves
Spinal pack	Phenylephrine infusion	Antacids: so citrate, ranit

Information Given to the Learners

11:30 a.m. on a Tuesday morning

Handover to anaesthetic registrar and theatre team
midwife transferring patient (faculty):
(obstetric registrar to come into theatre with patient
transferring midwife – give them this information to
prior to entering theatre)
The SBAR handover is as follows:
Situation: This is Lucy, we rang just before to say that we v bringing her straight to theatre with a cord prolapse.
Background: She is a 34-year-old, para 2 who is 34+4 wee pregnant.
Assessment: She is in labour, we have just done a vaginal examination (VE) on the ward – she was 7 cm dilated with a prolapse.
Recommendation: She needs a cat 1 section.

Scenario Schedule

Stage 1: Transfer to operating table and prepare for GA category 1 Caesarean Section	
Information given	**Expected actions**
Patient is distressed with contractions	Transfer patient to operating table
	Call obstetric and anaesthetic consul
	Apply full monitoring
Allergies: penicillin	Anaesthetist takes focussed history fi patient
Medications: ferrous sulhate	
Past medical history: Fit and well, no problems with this pregnancy	
Last eaten: breakfast 3 hours ago, had water up until 20 minutes ago	
No previous GAs, no family history of problems with Gas	
No problems with pregnancy	

Observations	
A	Clear
B	RR 25/min SpO$_2$ 98%
C	HR 135 bpm BP 140/87
D	**A**VPU
E	Nil to note

Information given	Expected actions
Good mouth opening, Mallampati 2, Calder A, good cervical spine movement	Anaesthetist performs airway assessment
	Give sodium citrate and IV ranitidine 50 mg
	Pre-oxygenate with facemask and nasal cannulae in head-up position
	Check IV access and commence IV crystalloid
	Midwife recommences CTG monitoring once patient on operating table

Proceed to stage 2 once woman transferred to operating table, monitoring applied and CTG recommenced

Stage 2: Obstetric team analyse CTG and plan for category 2 Caesarean Section under regional anaesthesia. Spinal inserted

Information given	Expected actions
Obstetric consultant arrives	
	Team review CTG
	Obstetric team suggest filling bladder to elevate the presenting part to try and facilitate category 2 caesarean section
	Verbal consent from patient for caesarean section
	Anaesthetic team recognise that may have time to insert spinal in lateral position. Prepare for spinal insertion but also continue pre-oxygenation and ensure have drugs and equipment prepared for GA.
	Insert catheter into bladder. Obstetric registrar removes hand from elevating presenting part.
	Fill bladder with normal saline – either using giving set attached to catheter or 50ml bladder syringe
	Obstetric team monitor CTG and are happy for spinal in left lateral position
	Team help patient move to left lateral position
	Anaesthetic consultant arrives
Spinal insertion successful on first attempt	Anaesthetic team insert spinal in left lateral position
	Start phenylephrine infusion
	Whole team support and explain events to patient and birth partner throughout
	Obstetric team scrub
	Neonatal emergency team called to attend delivery

Proceed to stage 3 once spinal inserted

ervations

	Clear
	RR 24/min SpO$_2$ 99% on O$_2$
	HR 130 bpm BP 132/78
	AVPU
	Nil to note
	Baseline 144 bpm, baseline variability 10–15 bpm, early decelerations

Observations	
A	Clear
B	RR 20/min SpO2 99% on O$_2$
C	HR 112 bpm BP 125/67
D	**A**VPU
E	Temp 36.9°C
CTG:	Baseline 122 bpm, variability <5 bpm, deep late decelerations

Stage 3: Deterioration of CTG requiring urgent delivery	
Information given	**Expected actions**
	Obstetric team note change to CTG and review delivery plan
Dense motor block bilaterally (Bromage score = 3) Block to up to and including T6 to cold bilaterally, up to and including T8 to touch bilaterally. Sacral block present.	Anaesthetist assesses sensorimotor block
Patient now fully dilated. Vertex +1, Occipitoanterior (OA)	Repeat vaginal examination
	Proceed to instrumental delivery of live female infant
	Infant handed to neonatal team
	Paired cord gases taken
Scenario ends when infant handed to neonatal team and paired cord gases requested	

Suggested Topics for Debrief Discussion

- What was the team decision-making like?
- Was the team flexible with the obstetric and anaesthetic plan once circumstances changed, i.e. when the CTG was normal on arrival in theatre and subsequently when it deteriorated?
- Were any changes to the plan clearly communicated to the whole team and patient?

Discussion

Definition

Umbilical cord prolapse is the descent of the umbilical cord alongside (occult) or beyond (overt) the presenting part after membranes have ruptured, and is an acute obstetric emergency. It is associated with perinatal morbidity and mortality from cord compression/occlusion leading to fetal hypoxia.

Incidence

The incidence is thought to be between 0.1% and 0.6%, but is higher (1%) in breech presentation, and in 'non-frank' breech presentations, i.e. where there is a poorer fit of the presenting part in the pelvis because the legs are level with or below the buttocks rather than extended in front of the body, where it may be up to 5.6% (Broche et al., 2005).

Risk Factors

Approximately 50% of cases of umbilical cord prolapse are preceded by obstetric intervention. There are also pregnancy-related risk factors that predispose to cord prolapse, typically factors which reduce how well the presenting part fits in the maternal pelvis, e.g. low-lying placenta, footling breech, prematurity (Table 12.1).

Table 12.1 Pregnancy- and procedure-related factors that increase the risk of cord prolapse.

Pregnancy-related	Procedure-related
Malpresentation Preterm labour Multiparity Unengaged presenting part Polyhydramnios Second twin Congenital abnormality Low-lying placenta	Artificial rupture of the membranes (ARM) with high presenting part External cephalic version Internal podalic version Balloon catheter induction of labour Vaginal manipulation with ruptured membranes, e.g. instrumental, rotation, vaginal examination

Complications

The perinatal mortality rate associated with cord prolapse may be as high as 91/1000, due to birth asphyxia or prematurity or congenital malformation, which may have predisposed to cord prolapse in the first place. Delay in diagnosis to delivery appears to be a contributing factor and out of hospital cord prolapse has a 10-fold higher rate of perinatal mortality (Royal College of Obstetricians and Gynaecologists, 2014). Outcomes from cord prolapse have improved dramatically since the 1940s, and this is related to increasing use of caesarean section to deliver affected infants as well as a changing maternal demographic (fewer grand multiparous parturients) (Gibbons et al., 2014).

Reducing the Risk of Cord Prolapse

In women with transverse, oblique or unstable lie, discuss admission from 37 weeks gestation and advise women remaining in the community to present urgently if they have signs of labour or ruptured membranes. In women with preterm, pre-labour, ruptured membranes and non-cephalic presentation, inpatient care should be advised.

Artificial rupture of membranes (ARM) should be avoided if the presenting part is mobile, high or if the cord is palpable on vaginal examination (National Institute for Health and Clinical Excellence, 2008). If ARM is necessary, consider doing this in theatre so immediate recourse to caesarean section is feasible.

Diagnosis

1. Exclude at every vaginal examination in labour.
2. Vaginal examination after spontaneous rupture of membranes if high-risk.
3. Suspect if there is an abnormal fetal heart pattern, especially if this follows rupture of membranes.
4. Auscultate fetal heart after every vaginal examination in labour and after spontaneous rupture of membranes.
5. Can occur without fetal distress and be found incidentally on vaginal examination.

Management

1. Call for help.
2. Prepare for delivery in theatre if not fully dilated.
3. Avoid handling the cord to reduce vasospasm.
4. Reduce compression of cord by:
   a. manually displacing the presenting part:
      i. thought to reduce pressure on the cord and prevent vascular occlusion;
      ii. use associated with a high chance of good outcome (Murphy and MacKenzie, 1995) in a retrospective study of 132 cases where there were 11 deaths from extreme prematurity or lethal fetal abnormality and one death from asphyxia, in a patient transferred in from home;
   b. filling the bladder:
      i. using Foley catheter and giving set instill 500–750 ml normal saline into the bladder and clamp the Foley catheter;
      ii. ensure bladder is emptied prior to caesarean section;
   c. mother adopting the knee-chest or left lateral (with pillow under hip) position;
   d. consider tocolysis with 0.25 mg terbutaline SC if the fetal heart rate is abnormal and birth is not imminent.
5. Discuss with the anaesthetist the most appropriate method of anaesthesia.
6. Category 1 caesarean section if abnormal CTG, ensuring maternal safety, to deliver within 30 minutes of diagnosis.
7. Category 2 caesarean section if CTG normal, ensuring continuous monitoring.
8. If fully dilated:
   a. can attempt vaginal delivery if birth would be quick and safe, minimising impingement of cord where possible;
   b. for second twin breech extraction may be appropriate.
9. Practitioner competent in resuscitation of the newborn to be present for delivery as likely to require resuscitation.
10. Paired cord gases:
    a. strong predictive value of normal paired cord gases to exclude intrapartum hypoxic injury as a cause of brain damage.

In the Community

1. Assess risk antenatally in women requesting birth outwith a consultant-led unit.
2. Unattended women reporting cord prolapse should be advised to adopt the knee-chest face-down position and await transfer to hospital.
3. Knee-chest position is not safe for transfer by ambulance; therefore, the exaggerated Sims position should be used (left lateral with pillow under hip).
4. Transfer to consultant-led unit unless birth imminent.
5. Elevate presenting part manually or with bladder filling during transfer.
6. Promptly assess fetal viability on admission to consultant-led unit before proceeding with delivery.

At the Threshold of Viability

Between 23+0 and 24+6 weeks gestation expectant management should be discussed as an option. If the fetus is <26 weeks gestation and the CTG is pathological it is important to discuss the poor chance of healthy survival for the fetus before proceeding with caesarean section.

Clinical Governance

1. Ensure thorough and accurate documentation.
2. Debrief the patient and birth partner.
3. Complete an incident form.
4. Multidisciplinary skills drills training should include cord prolapse.

Bibliography

Broche, D. E., Riethmuller, D., Vidal, C., et al. (2005). Obstetric and perinatal outcomes of a disreputable presentation: the non frank breech. *Journal de Gynécologie Obstétrique et Biologie de la Reproduction*, 34, 781–788.

Gibbons, C., O'Herlihy, C. and Murphy, J. F. (2014). Umbilical cord prolapse – changing patterns and improved outcomes: a retrospective cohort study. *British Journal of Obstetrics and Gynaecology*, 121, 1705–1709.

Murphy, D. J. and MacKenzie, I. Z. (1995). The mortality and morbidity associated with umbilical cord prolapse. *British Journal of Obstetrics and Gynaecology*, 102, 826–830.

National Institute for Health and Clinical Excellence. (2008). *Induction of Labour. NICE Clinical Guideline 70*. Manchester: NICE.

Royal College of Obstetricians and Gynaecologists. (2014). *Umbilical Cord Prolapse. RCOG Greentop Guideline No. 50*. London: RCOG.

Obstetric

Minimising Decision to Delivery Interval (DDI) in a Category 1 Caesarean Section – Pre-Theatre Phase

Cliff Shelton and Sophie Bishop

Scenario in a Nutshell

Patient develops a non-reassuring CTG that deteriorates to a fetal bradycardia requiring a category 1 caesarean section.
- Stage 1: Recognition of non-reassuring CTG and request for review.
- Stage 2: Onset of fetal bradycardia.
- Stage 3: Review by obstetrician, decision to deliver, communicate decision and consent.
- Stage 4: Prepare patient and move to theatre.

Target Learner Groups

Members of the multidisciplinary obstetric team: midwives, anaesthetists and obstetricians.

Specific learning opportunities

- Recognition and classification of CTG – persistent fetal bradycardia
- Knowledge and implementation of intrauterine resuscitation and escalation measures
- Team decision-making for category 1 caesarean section and communication of that decision
- Safely transfer to theatre – ideally exiting the delivery room within 9 minutes of onset of bradycardia

Suggested learners (to represent their normal roles)	In the room from the start	Available when requested
Anaesthetic CT2/ST	√	
Midwifery healthcare assistant	√	
Obstetric ST3+	√	
Midwife Coordinator	√	
Midwife in room	√	

Suggested learners (to represent their normal roles)	In the room from the start	Available when requested
Operating Department Practitioner (ODP)/ anaesthetic nurse		√
Suggested facilitators		
Faculty to play role of patient (alternatively, manikin can be used)	√	
Faculty to play role of patient's partner, Richard	√	

Details for Facilitators

Patient Demographics

Name: Hayley

Age: 33

Gestation: 39+1

Booking weight: 68 kg

Parity: P0

Scenario Summary For Facilitators

Patient is a 33-year-old, 39-week pregnant primip. Transferred to delivery suite from midwifery-led birth centre due to suspected fetal bradycardia on auscultation. CTG monitoring commenced and reassuring since transfer. Commenced on oxytocin for failure to progress, just re-examined: cervix 4 cm dilated.
Fetal bradycardia on CTG – persists.
Intrauterine resuscitation commenced; escalation to senior midwife/obstetrician.
Decision for category 1 caesarean section.
Explanation and consent by obstetric and anaesthetic teams.
Safe and timely transfer to theatre.

79

Set-up Overview for Facilitators

Clinical setting	In delivery unit, on a delivery bed
Patient position	Sitting
Initial monitoring in place	CTG
Other equipment	16G cannula dorsum of hand. 10 IU syntocinon in 500 ml normal saline running at 48 ml/h (or as per local guidelines). Hartmann's running at 80 mls/h. Entonox
Useful manikin functions	This scenario is best suited to a simulated patient actor (SPA) (see discussion)

Medical Equipment

For core equipment checklist, see Chapter 9.

Additional equipment specific to scenario	
Simulated pregnant abdomen	Patient property to simulate the environment of normal labour: clothing, books, music, etc.
Drug chart showing ranitidine PO 150 mg given 2 h ago	Entonox mask/mouthpiece
Tocolytic drugs e.g. terbutaline 250 µg	

Information Given to the Learners

Time: 08:00.

This handover is given by a facilitator playing the role of the night shift midwife, who is now going home, to the midwife taking over the care of the woman.

The SBAR handover is as follows:

Situation: This is Hayley, she is in spontaneous labour and was transferred to us earlier in the night from the midwifery-led unit.

Background: Hayley is primiparous with an uncomplicated pregnancy. She was transferred to the consultant-led delivery suite from the midwifery-led birth centre 6 hours ago, as her midwife was concerned about the fetal heart rate on auscultation. However, her CTG has been reassuring since then.

She has been in active labour for 8 hours now. However, she has failed to progress and was commenced on an oxytocin infusion four hours ago. She is using entonox for pain relief.

Assessment: She is contracting 4 in 10. I have just examined her and she is 4 cm dilated.

Recommendation: Are you happy to take over Hayley's care?

Scenario Schedule

Observations	
A	Clear
B	RR 22/min SpO$_2$ 96% on air
C	HR 103 bpm BP 110/60
D	**A**VPU
E	Nil to note
CTG: Baseline FHR 130 bpm, variable decelerations with concerning characteritstics in >50% of contractions	

Stage 1: Recognition of non-reassuring CTG and request for review	
Information given	**Expected actions**
	Identify non-reassuring CTG features
	Initiate conservative measures:
	• change position – full left lateral • check BP and increase fluids if hypotensive. • seek senior / second opinion on CTG.
	Appropriate communication with patient and partner

Proceed to stage 2 when identifies needs senior review of CTG and simple measures undertaken

Stage 2: Onset of fetal bradycardia

Information given	Expected actions
Facilitator to time from onset of bradycardia to transfer of patient to theatre doors	Identify pathological CTG with fetal bradycardia.
If bradycardia not identified within 30 seconds: Prompt from patient's husband / partner, e.g.: 'is there a problem? That monitor sounds slower than before.'	Complete conservative measures: • change position • stop oxytocin infusion • increase fluids if hypotensive
	By the time the bradycardia has persisted for 3 minutes, midwife has: • informed coordinating midwife. • urgently called obstetrician • begun preparing woman for caesarean section
	Appropriate communication with patient and partner throughout

Proceed to stage 3 once senior help sought

Observations

A	Clear
B	RR 24/min SpO$_2$ 96% on air
C	HR 98 bpm BP 110/60
D	**A**VPU
E	Nil to note
CTG	Baseline FHR falls to 80 bpm

Stage 3: Review by obstetrician, decision to deliver, communicate decision and consent

Information given	Expected actions
ST6 obstetrics and midwife coordinator enter room	SBAR from midwife to co-ordinator and obstetrician
If emergency buzzer was used, ST anaesthesia and further midwives also enter room	Identify ongoing fetal bradycardia, which requires urgent delivery
	Ensure conservative measures completed: • change position – left lateral, right lateral or knee-elbow • stop oxytocin • increase fluid rate if hypotensive
	Don't offer maternal facial oxygen
No sudden worsening of abdo or back pain No PV bleeding No uterine tenderness Vaginal examination: 4 cm dilated. No cord prolapse. No change to station of presenting part	Exclude acute events with history, abdominal examination and vaginal examination: • cord prolapse • suspected placental abruption • suspected uterine rupture
	Consider tocolytic: eg: terbutaline 250 mcg SC

Observations

A	Clear
B	RR 22/min SpO$_2$ 96% on air
C	HR 100 bpm BP 110/60
D	**A**VPU
E	Nil to note
CTG	Baseline FHR persists at 80 bpm

Information given	Expected actions
	Prompt decision to deliver by catego caesarean section
	Prompt communication to anaesthe theatre team / midwife co-ordinator
If anaesthetist requests: WCC 8.3 X 10^9/L Hb 112 g/L PLTS 423 X 10^9/L	Appropriate assessment, explanatio and consent by both obstetric and anaesthetic teams: timely but safe.
	Appropriate communication with patient and partner throughout

Proceed to Stage 4 once decision made for Category 1 caesarean section explanation and consent given by both obstetrician and anaesthetist

	Observations
A	Clear
B	RR 24/min SpO$_2$ 96% on air
C	HR 104 bpm BP 110/60
D	**A**VPU
E	Nil to note
CTG	Baseline FHR persists at 80bpm

Stage 4: Prepare patient and move to theatre	
Information given	**Expected actions**
	Make ready for theatre (may include removal of jewellery, appropriate use of local pre-op checklists, etc.)
	Should leave the room within nine minutes of onset of bradycardia
	Appropriate communication with patient and partner throughout

Scenario ends when patient reached theatre doors. Facilitator stops time this point.

Suggested Topics for Debrief Discussion

- Was CTG abnormality recognised in a timely way and appropriate help sought?
- How was communication between the team and the patient/partner? Use the Patient Perception Score for patient/partner (see Discussion).
- How was the consent procedure (both obstetrician and anaesthetist)? How was the balance between amount of information given and time efficiency of the process?
- How could the process be streamlined while maintaining safety and good communicatio Get the team to list each process required fro decision made to deliver to leaving the room which of the processes was most time spent?

Discussion

Classification of Urgency of Caesarean Section

Caesarean sections are graded by urgency acc to the classification developed by Lucas et al. (

Category 1 caesarean sections are described as 'emergency' caesarean sections, and are undertaken when there is an immediate threat to the life of the woman or the fetus. The Royal Colleges of Anaesthetists and Obstetricians and Gynaecologists (RCOG) have adopted Lucas' classification, and issued guidance that the decision to delivery interval (DDI) for category 1 caesarean sections should be under 30 minutes; in practice, this often means 'as quickly as possible'. This auditable standard can be used as a target and may be used to assess performance. This culture introduces additional pressure to a situation where the stakes are already high, potentially affecting decision-making and performance.

In an Australian study of over 14,000 women, the commonest indication for immediate delivery was prolonged fetal bradycardia (53%) (Warren et al., 2018).

Factors Influencing DDI

Numerous factors have been found to influence DDI, including anaesthetic technique, available resources, time of day and the experience of the team providing medical and midwifery care.

This scenario focuses on the pre-theatre phase. If cord prolapse, placental abruption and uterine rupture are excluded, the vast majority of CTGs with prolonged fetal bradycardia are likely to recover to normal baseline within 9 minutes (Chandraharan and Arulkumaran, 2007). The 3, 6, 9, 12 guidance for the management of prolonged fetal bradycardia relates to this:

By:

3 minutes:	call for help
6 minutes:	intrauterine fetal resuscitation initiated (see below)
9 minutes:	transfer to theatre
12 minutes:	commencing delivery

Studies have found that a delay in transfer to theatre results in a significantly prolonged DDI – 82% of category 1 caesarean sections are delivered within 30 minutes if the patient leaves the room before 10 minutes are up (le Riche and Hall, 2005; Tufnell et al., 2001). They do not, however, offer explanations as to why delays in transfer may occur or what can be done to mitigate them. By simulating this process *in situ*, however, preparation for transfer can be observed and debriefed, and strategies for improvement that take into account local practices and logistics can be developed.

There is evidence to suggest that pre-operative protocols have a role in minimising the time taken to initiate transfer to theatre, with quality improvement projects by Mooney et al. (2007) and Nageotte and Vander Wal (2012) implementing various measures including the pre-emptive completion of anaesthetic questionnaires, announcement of emergencies over a public-address system, a requirement for the obstetrician to remain with the patient and assist with transfer, and algorithm-based management plans that encourage midwifery staff to initiate the transfer of the patient to theatre. *In situ* simulation could help to identify the need for such measures, and subsequently provide a method by which to trial their implementation. The effect of *in situ* simulation training on DDI has been studied by Siassakos et al. (2009a), who introduced a multiprofessional skills drill using an actor to simulate the patient. Median DDI reduced significantly following the commencement of training.

Obtaining Consent in an Emergency

Obtaining informed consent can present unique challenges in the obstetric setting. It is recognised that the effects of acute pain, drugs or pathology, combined with the emotional aspects of an unfolding emergency, can make communication difficult, and may even affect the patient's capacity to consent.

The Association of Anaesthetists of Great Britain and Ireland (AAGBI) guideline on consent for anaesthesia (2017) advises that patients are provided with explanations of analgesic techniques and operations under general and regional anaesthesia antenatally. However, this does not preclude the need to provide an explanation of the procedure at the time at which it is required.

Although consent for operative delivery under general or regional anaesthesia should ideally be in written form, in an emergency situation verbal consent is an acceptable alternative. The Royal College of Obstetrics and Gynaecology (RCOG) and NICE (National Institute for Health and Clinical Excellence) have issued guidance on obtaining valid consent, stating that in this circumstance verbal consent should be witnessed by another health professional, and that both the obstetrician and the witness should document the consent, and the reasons for proceeding without written consent, in the notes (NICE, 2014). Obtaining consent has been recognised to be a factor in prolonging the DDI in emergency caesarean section (Tufnell et al., 2001) and the debrief of this scenario should therefore focus not only on the content and format of the consent process, but its efficiency.

Intrauterine Fetal Resuscitation

Intrauterine resuscitation should be considered if the CTG is abnormal. The aim of intrauterine fetal resuscitation is to optimise both oxygen delivery to the placenta and umbilical blood flow in an attempt to reverse fetal hypoxia and acidosis and allow delivery to be expedited or labour to continue.

The obstetrician should exclude acute events, such as cord prolapse, suspected placental abruption or suspected uterine rupture (NICE, 2014).

Other measures to consider (Kither and Monaghan, 2016; NICE, 2014):

Syntocinon – switch off or reduce.

Position – relieve aortocaval compression by full left lateral position. Left lateral may not help in umbilical cord compression – right lateral or knee-elbow position should be used.

Intravenous fluids – NICE recommend IV fluids if woman is hypotensive (NICE, 2014).

Low blood pressure – treat with vasopressors if required.

Tocolysis – e.g. terbutaline 250 µg SC.

Routine maternal facial oxygen is not beneficial to the fetus and is only recommended if there are maternal indications (NICE, 2014).

Communication in an Emergency

This scenario offers the opportunity to consider the multiprofessional team's communication with the patient and her partner. In the scenario, a low-risk pregnancy transforms into an urgent clinical situation in a matter of minutes and this is likely to result in emotional trauma. In their interview-based study of 25 consecutive patients who underwent emergency caesarean section, Ryding et al. (2000) found that the experiences of women who undergo emergency caesarean section fall into four patterns:

- 'Confidence whatever happens'.
- 'Positive expectations turning into disappointment'.
- 'Fears that come true'.
- 'Confusion and amnesia'.

The latter three of these patterns (which represented 80% of Ryding's patient cohort) are clearly suboptimal and could theoretically be prevented through improved communication. The patients who reported

'confidence whatever happens' felt that they had participated in the decision to deliver by caesarean section.

The assessment of patients' satisfaction with operative birth has been addressed by a number of authors and numerous standardised tools have been developed. The Patient Perception Score (PPS), developed by Siassakos et al. (2009b), is a simple measure that has been validated in emergency deliveries by both caesarean section and instrumental techniques. It utilises a five-point Likert scale to reflect the degree of agreement with three statements, thus having a minimum score of 3 and a maximum of 15. The statements are as follows.

- I felt that I was respected by the doctor(s).
- I felt safe at all times.
- I felt well-informed due to good communication with the doctor(s).

It can be useful to base communication debrief around these areas, expanding the focus from 'doctor(s)' to include the whole multidisciplinary team.

Simulated Patient Actors (SPAs)

This scenario can be conducted using a manikin, but using simulated patient actors (SPAs) together with a simulated CTG monitor and prosthetic pregnant abdomen can provide an ideal method by which to simulate the patient communication aspects of the scenario in addition to the technical and team-working aspects.

In a pilot study of the simulation of acute care scenarios, Coffey et al. (2016) found that healthcare workers' verbal and tactile interactions differ between manikins and SPAs, with actors receiving more interactions than manikins in a manner that appeared more representative of real life. While this hybrid simulation has advantages in terms of realism, and interactivity, it does introduce challenges for the simulation facilitator; namely, that the welfare of the SPA must be safeguarded in the healthcare environment.

The following are considerations when using a simulated patient actor in a 'hybrid' simulation.

- Drug administration: scenarios involving intravenous or epidural medication can be simulated using tubing and reservoir bags attached to the patient-end of the epidural/intravenous catheter, which can then be taped to the patient's skin.
- Invasive procedures: scenarios must be designed to avoid invasive procedures. For example, if an IV cannula is required, this should be simulated and already be *in situ*, as above.

- Intimate examinations: this is of particular relevance in the obstetric setting and ideally, scenarios with SPAs should be designed where intimate examinations are not required. The learners should be briefed before entering the room that if they feel an intimate examination is required, they should state this and they will be given the result.
- Allergies: it is possible that simulated patient actors could be allergic to substances found in the healthcare environment, e.g. latex. Allergies should be discussed with the SPA prior to the date of the simulation training.
- Emotional trauma: the simulation of a potentially traumatic yet relatively common event such as emergency caesarean section means that it is possible that the SPA may have experienced something similar. We would therefore suggest a frank briefing discussion regarding the content of the scenario. Sending the SPA a copy of the simulation scenario in advance should ideally precede this.
- Halting the scenario: it can be challenging to ascertain whether an SPA is uncomfortable in a scenario, or skilfully portraying a distressed patient. We agree an unambiguous method by which the actor (or any participant) can halt the scenario at any point. This could be a gesture, word or phrase that would not be expected to occur during the scenario. Faculty should remain ready to halt the scenario promptly should the need arise.

In order to effectively debrief the patient-communication aspects of the scenario, we involve the SPAs in the debrief process, with a particular emphasis placed on how the SPA felt in the role of the patient, thus illuminating communication, consent and satisfaction with care from a patient perspective.

Bibliography

Brennand, J. E., Millins, P., Yentis, S. and Hinshaw, H. K. S., on behalf of the Joint Standing Committee of the Royal College of Anaesthetists and the Royal College of Obstetricians and Gynaecologists. (2010). *Good Practice No. 11: Classification of Urgency of Caesarean Section – A Continuum of Risk*. London: The Royal College of Anaesthetists and the Royal College of Obstetricians and Gynaecologists.

Chandraharan, E. and Arulkumaran, S. (2007). Prevention of birth asphyxia: responding appropriately to cardiotocograph(CTG) traces. *Best Practice Research Clinics in Obstetrics and Gynaecology*, 21(4), 609–624.

Coffey, F., Tsuchiya, K., Timmons, S., Baxendale, B., Adolphs, S. and Atkins, S. (2016). Simulated patients versus manikins in acute-care scenarios. *Clinical Teacher*, 13, 257–261.

Kither, H. and Monaghan, S. (2016). Intrauterine fetal resuscitation. *Anaesthesia & Intensive Care Medicine*, 17(7), 337–340.

le Riche, H. and Hall, D. (2005). Non-elective caesarean section: how long do we take to deliver? *Journal of Tropical Paediatrics*, 51, 78–81.

Lucas, D. N., Yentis, S. M., Kinsella, S. M., et al. (2000). Urgency of caesarean section: a new classification system. *Journal of the Royal Society of Medicine*, 93, 346–350.

Mooney, S. E., Ogrinc, G. and Steadman, W. (2007). Improving emergency caesarean delivery response times at a rural community hospital. *Quality and Safety in Health Care*, 16, 60–66.

Nageotte, M. P. and Vander Wal, B. (2012). Achievement of the 30-minute standard in obstetrics – can it be done? *American Journal of Obstetrics and Gynecology*, 206, 104–107.

National Institute for Health and Clinical Excellence. (2011). *Caesarean Section. NICE Clinical Guideline 132*. Manchester: NICE.

(2014). *Intrapartum Care for Healthy Women and Babies. Clinical Guideline CG190*. Manchester: NICE. Last updated: February 2017.

Ryding, E. L., Wijma, K. and Wijma, B. (2000). Emergency cesarean section: 25 women's experiences. *Journal of Reproductive and Infant Psychology*, 18, 33–39.

Siassakos, D., Hasafa, Z., Sibanda, T., et al. (2009a). Retrospective cohort study of diagnosis-delivery interval with umbilical cord prolapse: the effect of team training. *British Journal of Obstetrics and Gynaecology*, 116, 1089–1096.

Siassakos, D., Clark, J., Sibanda, T., et al. (2009b). A simple tool to measure patient perception of operative birth. *British Journal of Obstetrics and Gynaecology*, 116, 1755–1761.

Tuffnell, D. J., Wilkinson, K. and Beresford, N. (2001). Interval between decision and delivery by caesarean section – are current standards achievable? Observational case series. *British Medical Journal*, 322, 1330–1333.

Warren, M. H., Kamania, J. and Dennis, A. T. (2018). Immediate birth – an analysis of women and their babies undergoing time critical birth in a tertiary referral obstetric hospital. *International Journal of Obstetric Anaesthesia*, 33, 46–52.

Chapter

14

Amniotic Fluid Embolism

Kim Macleod and Yara Mohammed

Scenario in a Nutshell

Sudden maternal collapse with hypoxia, hypotension and haemorrhage resulting from amniotic fluid embolism during twins delivery.
    Stage 1: Maternal collapse prior to delivery of twin 2.
    Stage 2: Continued respiratory and cardiovascular deterioration.
    Stage 3: Worsening pulmonary oedema, massive haemorrhage and DIC.

Target Learner Groups

All members of the multidisciplinary obstetric team: anaesthetists, midwives, obstetricians, operating department practitioners/anaesthetic nurses, theatre team and neonatal emergency team.

Specific learning opportunities
Recognition of differential diagnosis for maternal collapse
Recognition of amniotic fluid embolism as cause of maternal collapse
Knowledge of risk factors for amniotic fluid embolism

Suggested learners (to represent their normal roles)	In the room from the start	Available when requested
Anaesthetic CT2		√
Anaesthetic ST3+		√
Obstetric ST3+	√	
Midwife Coordinator/ responding midwives		√
Midwife in room	√	
*Operating Department Practitioner (ODP)/ anaesthetic nurse/ theatre scrub team		√
*Neonatal emergency team (if simultaneous neonatal scenario planned)		√

Suggested learners (to represent their normal roles)	In the room from the start	Available when requested
Suggested facilitators		
Faculty to play role of midwife who knows patient history	√	

*From stage 3 onwards, this scenario would require a full theatre team. It can also be combined with a simultaneous neonatal resuscitation – the scenario can be fragmented depending on learning objectives and available personnel.

Details for Facilitators

Patient Demographics

Name: Amanda
Age: 39
Gestation: 37
Booking weight: 65 kg
Parity: P4 (Prev 4× NVD)

Scenario Summary for Facilitators

39-year-old, P4 parturient, 37 weeks with DCDA twins has just delivered twin 1, by forceps for a pathological CTG, on delivery suite following induction of labour for pre-eclampsia. She received two prostaglandin pessaries, followed by an ARM and IV oxytocin. She has an epidural for analgesia.
After the delivery of twin 1, the membranes of twin 2 spontaneously rupture. The woman becomes restless and agitated, complaining of difficulty breathing. Twin 2 suffers sustained fetal bradycardia.
The patient is transferred to theatre for resuscitation and caesarean section under general anaesthetic. She develops florid pulmonary oedema, hypotension, and suffers massive obstetric haemorrhage as a result of DIC and uterine atony.

Set-up Overview for Facilitators

Clinical setting	In a delivery room, on a delivery bed
Patient position	Semi-recumbent, legs in stirrups
Initial monitoring in place	Saturation, HR (from the saturation probe), NIBP
Other equipment	16G cannula in one hand, IV Hartmann's attached running at 80 ml/h and syntocinon 10 IU in 500 ml normal saline at 36 ml/h Lumbar epidural – PCEA low-dose epidural infusion infusing at 5 ml/h
Useful manikin features	Abnormal breath sounds (pulmonary oedema) Bleeding Intubation

Medical Equipment

For core equipment checklist see Chapter 9.

Additional equipment specific to scenario		
Arterial line	Rapid fluid infuser	Bakri® balloon
Epidural pump and epidural catheter	O-negative blood	Other simulated blood products

Drugs:
  Syntocinon
  Syntocinon infusion
  Haemobate
	Syntometrine
	Ergometrine
	Misoprostol
	Tranexamic acid
		Metaraminol
		Phenylephrine

Information Given to the Learners

Emergency buzzer pulled. Team arrive in delivery room. Handover given by obstetric ST3+ to emergency team (including anaesthetists, midwifery coordinator, other responding midwifery staff).

Situation:
This is an emergency, there is a fetal bradycardia in twin 2 and maternal agitation, hypotension and shortness of breath.

Background:
Amanda is 39 years old, para 4, four previous normal vaginal deliveries. She is 37 weeks with DCDA twins being induced for pre-eclampsia using syntocinon. I have delivered twin 1 by forceps for a pathological CTG. Since delivery, membranes have ruptured spontaneously for twin 2, who is now transverse lie, having a fetal bradycardia and Amanda is becoming increasingly agitated, complaining of difficulty breathing. She has good analgesia from her labour epidural.

Assessment
Her observations, SpO$_2$ 80%. Respiratory rate 30 bpm. HR 110. BP 90/50. She is very distressed.

Recommendation
Can you help with resuscitation?

Scenario Schedule

Observations	
A	Clear
B	RR 30/min SpO$_2$ 80% on air (91% on 15L/min O$_2$)
C	HR 110bpm BP 85/50 CRT 3s
D	**A**VPU
E	Temp 37°C
CTG	Fetal bradycardia 70 bpm

Stage 1: Maternal collapse prior to delivery of twin 2	
Information given	**Expected actions**
Patient restless and agitated	ABCDE approach Establish team leader Delegate tasks
	Call for consultant anaesthetist and obstetrician
	Apply oxygen via non-rebreathing mask at 15 litres/min
	Ensure manual uterine displacement
	Apply full monitoring, pulse oximeter, ECG, NIBP
Airway clear, patient talking but very distressed	Assess airway
Chest examination: fine inspiratory crackles bilaterally, trachea central, percussion note resonant	Assess breathing

Information given	Expected actions
Heart sounds: normal, tachycardic, JVP normal	Assess cardiovascular system
Assessment of epidural Sensory block to T10 cold, T12 touch bilaterally Bromage score 0 bilaterally	Assess epidural block height
No obvious signs of bleeding / rash	Expose patient
	Establish 1x further 14G IV access Take bloods for FBC, U+E, LFT, coagulation including fibrinogen and G+S. Check CBG (capillary blood glucose)
	Bolus 250 ml Hartmann's stat
Patient distressed and becoming confused / agitated	
Contracting irregularly. Twin 2 transverse lie	Assessment of stage of labour
	In view of deterioration in observations and continued fetal bradycardia team agree transfer to theatre
	Stop epidural infusion
	Stop syntocinon
Communication with theatres, they are ready to receive the patient	Communicate with theatres Urgent transfer to theatre required Maternal compromise Fetal bradycardia and transverse lie of twin 2
Portable monitoring and oxygen available for transfer	Transfer patient with portable oxygen and monitoring

Progress to stage 2 once decision made to transfer to theatre for maternal stabilisation

Observations	
A	Clear
B	RR 35/min SpO$_2$ 70% on 15L 0$_2$
C	HR 100bpm BP 80/40 CRT 4s
D	AVPU
E	Temp 36.8°C
CTG	Fetal bradycardia 60 bpm

Stage 2: Continued respiratory and cardiovascular deterioration

Information given	Expected actions
	Arrival in theatre
	Apply full monitoring
Patient markedly agitated, cyanotic, tachypnoeic, trying to sit up and coughing up pink sputum Venflon sites are oozing blood Per vaginal (PV) bleeding notices, 300 mls and ongoing	Reassess patient
	Maintain left lateral position with theatre table tilt

89

Information given	Expected actions
	Ensure 100% oxygen via anaesthetic face mask / anaesthetic machine with CPAP
Had ranitidine in labour. Unable to take sodium citrate currently	Decision to intubate and ventilate patient
Consultant anaesthetist and obstetrician attend	RSI with appropriate choice of indution agent (see chapter 24 for GA) Vasopressor on standby to support BP Fully trained assistant Consultant anaesthetist in attendance Capnography available
Grade 1 intubation Noted to have florrid pink frothy fluid in ETT	Intubate with size 7.0 ETT (at largest)
	Anaesthetist recognise pulmonary oedema Suction via ETT Alter ventilation to improve oxygenation High PEEP Alter I:E ratio to allow longer inspiratory time
	Crystalloid IV fluids to continue although cautious as note pulmonary oedema
	Decision to deliver fetus as maternal condition compromised and could be improved by delivery
	Consideration of causes for maternal collapse Hypoxia Haemorrhage
	Insert arterial line and perform ABG

Progress to stage 3 once consideration of causes discussed and decision made to intubate, ventilate and perform caesarean section

Observations	
A	Intubated
B	As per ventilator setting SpO$_2$ 92% on FiO$_2$ 1.0
C	HR 130 bpm BP 74/40 CRT 5s
D	Anaesthetised
E	Temp 36°C

Stage 3: Worsening pulmonary oedema, massive haemorrhage and DIC

Information given	Expected Actions
	Obstetricians to commence caesarean section
Following delivery bleeding noted from all sites Uterus IV cannula sites In urinary catheter	
	Repeat all observations

Information given	Expected actions
ABG result: pH 7.19 pCO_2 6 kPa pO_2 6kPa BE -15 mmol/L HCO_3^- 17 mmol/L Ca^{2+} 0.9 Lactate 8 mg/dL Hb 5 g/L	
	Manage uterine atony Syntocinon 5 iu bolus, infusion 10 IU/hr Ergometrine / syntometrine Haemabate 250 mcg IM Misprostol 1000 mcg PR
	Activate the massive obstetric haemorrhage pathway Inform consultant haematologist
	Give 2 units 0-ve RBC
	Consider vasopressors and inotropic support
TEG result See Figure 14.1	Perform TEG / ROTEM
	Resuscitate with blood / FFP / platelets / cryoprecipitate (or fibrinogen concentrate) /fluids
	Administer tranexamic acid 1 g IV over 10 mins
	Consideration for mechanical techniques: B-lynch or Bakri Balloon
	Consider hysterectomy if unable to control haemorrhage
	Cardiac output monitoring- ideally transoesophageal echocardiogram if expertise available
	Keep patient warm
	Replace calcium with 10 ml 10% calcium chloride
	Commence tranexamic acid infusion 1 g over 8 hrs
	Do not remove epidural catheter until coagulation corrected

Scenario ends with discussion with ICU

Suggested Topics for Debrief Discussion

- Did you consider the diagnosis of amniotic fluid embolism?
- How did you exclude the other potential diagnosis?
- Did you feel well able to cope with this situation?

Discussion

Introduction

Amniotic fluid embolism (AFE) is an infrequent obstetric occurrence, yet it is one of the leading causes of maternal mortality in developed countries. There are wide variations in reported incidence, risk factors and outcomes due to the rarity of the condition. Diagnosis of AFE is often made after other, more common pathologies have been excluded; this makes it very difficult to study. It is associated with significant fetal and maternal morbidity and mortality, and so prompt resuscitation and supportive management is needed to reduce risk.

Incidence and Mortality

The reported incidence of AFE ranges from 1.9 to 6.1 cases per 100,000 maternities. In the 2017 MBRRACE report, nine women died from amniotic fluid embolism, representing a mortality rate of 0.36 (95% CI 0.16–0.68).

AFE is responsible for 9% of direct maternal deaths in the UK. Reported maternal mortality rate ranges from 0.4 to 1.3 cases per 100,000 live births.

Reported neonatal mortality rates range between 10% and 30%, with an associated high risk of neurological injury secondary to neonatal acidosis. Up to 50% of surviving babies suffer neurological impairment, including hypoxic–ischaemic encephalopathy, with or without subsequent development of cerebral palsy.

Pathophysiology

AFE may arise from simultaneous tears in the fetal membranes and uterine vessels, permitting amniotic fluid to enter the uterine vein and onward into the maternal pulmonary arterial circulation. Its pathogenesis is poorly understood, but this mechanism may be precipitated by disruption of uterine vasculature, abnormal placentation, excess amniotic fluid and strong uterine contractions. It is characterised by sudden dyspnoea, cardiopulmonary collapse and coagulopathy. The clinical picture resembles anaphylaxis and findings from the US national registry highlight an association between history of allergy or atopy and development of AFE.

Risk Factors

Reported risk factors include maternal age of 35 years or older, multiple pregnancy, polyhydramnios, induction of labour, placental abnormalities (placenta praevia and placental abruption) and operative deliveries, including caesarean section.

The pathogenesis of these predisposing risk factors remains poorly understood. It has been hypothesised that the incidence of AFE increases with higher maternal age and placental abnormalities due to disruption of uterine vasculature or minor degrees of abnormal placental

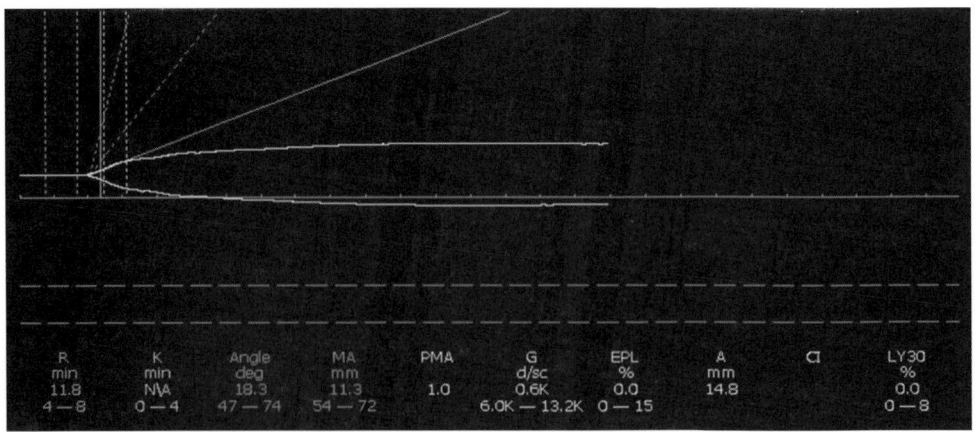

Figure 14.1 TEG result.

invasion. It has also been hypothesised that strong uterine contractions and excess amniotic fluid could increase the risk of AFE in multiple pregnancy, polyhydramnios and induction of labour. Mode of delivery is even more controversial. Most available literature does not report timing of delivery in relation to AFE, or whether operative delivery was a cause or an effect of AFE.

Diagnosis

Diagnosis is challenging, given the diagnosis is one of exclusion. Diagnosis is predominantly based on clinical signs and basic investigations as absolute confirmation is only possible at post mortem. To aid diagnosis, the UK Obstetric Surveillance System (UKOSS) has developed diagnostic criteria for AFE:

In the absence of any other clear cause:
EITHER
Acute maternal collapse with one or more of the following features:
Acute fetal compromise
Cardiac arrest
Cardiac rhythm problems
Coagulopathy
Hypotension
Maternal haemorrhage
Premonitory symptoms, e.g. restlessness, numbness, agitation, tingling
Seizure
Shortness of breath

Excluding women with maternal haemorrhage as the first presenting feature in whom there was no evidence of early coagulopathy or cardiorespiratory compromise.
OR
Women in whom the diagnosis was made at post-mortem examination with the finding of fetal squames or hair in the lungs.

Differential diagnoses include:
- Placental abruption
- Uterine rupture
- Postpartum haemorrhage
- Eclampsia
- Thrombotic embolus
- Septic shock
- Myocardial infarction

Useful investigations include clotting screen and ECG. Clotting is often abnormal prior to clinical signs

of haemorrhage, and an ECG may reveal evidence of myocardial ischaemia. CT pulmonary angiography can reveal pulmonary embolism or AFE.

Frequency of Presenting Features of AFE (UKOSS)

Signs and symptoms	Women exhibiting feature* (*n* = 60)	Women exhibiting features as the first symptom or sign of AFE (*n* = 60)
Maternal haemorrhage	39 (65%)	1 (2%)
Hypotension	38 (63%)	5 (8%)
Shortness of breath	37 (62%)	12 (20%)
Coagulopathy	37 (62%)	0 (0%)
Premonitory symptoms (e.g. restlessness, agitation, numbness, tingling)	28 (47%)	18 (30%)
Acute fetal compromise	26 (43%)	12 (20%)
Cardiac arrest	24 (40%)	5 (8%)
Cardiac rhythm problems	16 (27%)	3 (5%)
Seizures	12 (20%)	4 (7%)

*Some women presented with more than one feature.

Management

The first obstacle in managing AFE is the diagnosis, as the symptoms are non-specific. Effective management is based on prompt action when the diagnosis is suspected and early involvement of a multidisciplinary team that includes an obstetrician, an anaesthetist and a haematologist. The treatment is based on supportive management aimed at maintaining oxygenation, circulatory support and managing the coagulopathy.

The initial assessment of the patient must follow a standard ABCDE approach. An ECG may be required. Basic resuscitation involves administering high-flow oxygen and securing intravenous (IV) access with two wide-bore IV access.

Early intubation and ventilation is required to secure the airway and prevent aspiration. Manipulation of positive end expiratory pressure (PEEP), inspiratory: expiratory ratio and inspired oxygen may be required to maintain oxygenation in severe cases.

Circulatory collapse due to profound hypotension is a feature of AFE. Initial fluid replacement with crystalloid is required, although, when haemorrhage is confirmed, resuscitate with blood and required blood components. Careful fluid balance to maintain cardiac output and organ perfusion while not further exacerbating pulmonary oedema can be difficult. As the hypotension associated with AFE can be profound, early use of inotropes may be required. Monitoring of arterial ± central venous pressure and cardiac output monitoring will aid fluid and ionotropic management. Transoesophageal echocardiogram (TOE) would be valuable, if expertise allows.

Cardiac arrest should be anticipated. If the patient is still pregnant, be prepared to perform timely perimortem caesarean section to help with resuscitation (see Chapter 25).

Coagulopathy and associated haemorrhage are common in cases of AFE. In addition to laboratory coagulation screening, near patient testing of coagulation with thromboelastography (TEG) and rotational thromboelastometry (ROTEM) is useful to assess clotting function. Volume replacement with packed red blood cells is the first priority. Activation of a massive obstetric haemorrhage protocol may be required. Not only does this facilitate rapid access to blood and blood products, but it also alerts staff to the severity of the situation and prompts senior clinician involvement. Fresh frozen plasma should be administered cautiously due to the risk of volume overload. Platelets, cryoprecipitate and fibrinogen concentrate may be required based on TEG/ROTEM and clotting results. Tranexamic acid (an antifibrinolytic-given IV) aids treatment of coagulopathy. Postpartum haemorrhage due to atony should be treated aggressively with uterotonics. A hysterectomy may be required to stop the bleeding. This should not be delayed until the patient is in extremis (MBRRACE, 2017).

Bibliography

Abenhaim, H. A., Azoulay, L., Kramer, M. S. and Leduc, L. (2008). Incidence and risk factors of amniotic fluid embolism: a population-based study on 3 million births in the United States. *American Journal of Obstetrics and Gynecology*, 199(49), e1–e8.

Berg, C. J., Callaghan, W. M., Syverson, C. and Henderson, Z. (2010). Pregnancy-related mortality in the United States, 1998 to 2005. *Obstetrics & Gynecology*, 116, 1302–1309.

Clark, S. L., Hankins, G. D., Dudley, D. A., et al. (1995). Amniotic fluid embolism: analysis of the national registry. *American Journal of Obstetrics and Gynecology*, 172, 1158–1167.

Conde-Agudelo, A. and Romero, R. (2009). Amniotic fluid embolism: an evidence based review. *American Journal of Obstetrics and Gynecology*, 201(5), 445.e1–445.13.

Davies, S. (2001). Amniotic fluid embolus: a review of the literature. *Canadian Journal of Anesthesia*, 48, 88–96.

Fitzpatrick, K. E., Tuffnell, D., Kurinczuk, J. J. and Knight, M. (2016). Incidence, risk factors, management and outcomes of amniotic-fluid embolism: a population-based cohort and nested case-control study. *British Journal of Obstetrics and Gynaecology*, 123, 100–109.

Knight, M., Tuffnell, D., Brocklehurst, P., et al. on behalf of the UK Obstetric Surveillance System. (2010). Incidence and risk factors for amniotic-fluid embolism. *Obstetrics & Gynaecology*, 115, 910–917.

Knight, M., Berg, C., Brocklehurst, P., et al. (2012). Amniotic fluid embolism incidence, risk factors and outcomes: a review and recommendations. *BMC Pregnancy and Childbirth*, 12, 7.

Knight, M., Nair, M., Tuffnell, D., et al. (Eds.) on behalf of MBRRACE-UK. (2016). *Saving Lives, Improving Mothers' Care – Surveillance of Maternal Deaths in the UK 2012–14 and Lessons Learned to Inform Maternity Care from the UK and Ireland Confidential Enquiries into Maternal Deaths and Morbidity 2009–14*. Oxford: National Perinatal Epidemiology Unit, University of Oxford.

Knight, M., Nair, M., Tuffnell, D., et al. (Eds.) on behalf of MBRRACE-UK. (2017). *Saving Lives, Improving Mothers' Care – Lessons Learned to Inform Maternity Care in the UK and Ireland Confidential Enquiries into Maternal Deaths and Morbidity 2013–2015*. Oxford: National Perinatal Epidemiology Unit, University of Oxford.

Rath, W., Hofer, S. and Sincina, I. (2014). Amniotic fluid embolism: an interdisciplinary challenge epidemiology, diagnosis and treatment. *Deutsches Arzteblatt International*, 111(8), 126–132.

Tuffnell, D. J. (2005). United Kingdom Amniotic Fluid Embolism Register. *British Journal of Obstetrics & Gynaecology*, 112, 1625–1629.

Chapter

Anaphylaxis in Labour

15

Andrew Parkes and Shuayb Elkhalifa

Scenario in a Nutshell

Severe life-threatening anaphylaxis following benzypenicillin IV for intrapartum antibiotic prophylaxis for group B streptococcal colonisation.
Stage 1: Recognition of anaphylaxis and initial management.
Stage 2: Patient continues to deteriorate, with airway, respiratory and cardiovascular compromise.
Stage 3: Continuing severe life-threatening anaphylaxis.
Stage 4: Patient continues to deteriorate, requiring intubation, ventilation and referral to critical care.

Target Learner Groups

All members of the multidisciplinary obstetric team: midwives, obstetricians, anaesthetists.

Specific learning opportunities

Knowledge of common causes of anaphylaxis

Recognition of anaphylaxis

Knowledge of algorithm for treatment of severe life-threatening anaphylaxis

Orientation – knowledge of emergency equipment to treat anaphylaxis in local environment

Suggested learners (to represent their normal roles)	In the room from the start	Available when requested
Anaesthetic CT2		√
Anaesthetic ST3+		√
Obstetric ST3+		√
Midwife Coordinator		√
Suggested facilitators		
Midwife		√ (first to respond)
Faculty to play role of partner	√	

Details for Facilitators

Patient Demographics

Name: Kira

Age: 38

Gestation: 37

Booking weight: 87 kg

Parity: P3 (Prev NVD)

Scenario Summary for Facilitators

38-year-old para 3, 37 weeks pregnant, admitted to delivery suite in active labour. Spontaneous rupture of membranes (SROM) 2 hours ago, examined 1 hour ago, cervix 4 cm dilated. Receiving first dose of antibiotics for group B *Streptococcus*.
Previous baby with group B streptococcal infection as neonate. Baby spent prolonged period on NICU and parents very anxious.
Shortly after receiving first dose of IV benzylpenicillin (3 g in 100 ml normal saline running over 1 h as per guidelines) patient complains of feeling unwell – hot, light-headed and difficulty breathing.
Partner (facilitator) alerts staff to the problem. He notices that she appears rather red and flushed.
Treatment of severe life-threatening anaphylaxis ensues, requiring repeated IM/IV adrenaline boluses, bronchodilators and intubation/ventilation and delivery.

Set-up Overview for Facilitators

Clinical setting	On delivery suite in a delivery bed
Patient position	Lying semi-recumbent on bed
Initial monitoring in place	CTG monitor
Other equipment	20G venflon dorsum hand through which benzylpenicillin infusion is running (3 g in 100 ml normal saline running over 1 h or as per local guideline)
Useful manikin features	Abnormal breath sounds (wheeze) Palpable pulses Tongue swelling Intubation

Medical Equipment

For core equipment checklist see Chapter 9.

Additional equipment specific to scenario		
Nebuliser	Benzylpenicillin in 100 ml saline running through Baxter pump	
Adrenaline • 1:1000 • 1:10,000 Hydrocortisone Chlorphenamine	Metaraminol Ephedrine Noradrenaline Drugs for intubation	Salbutomol • Inhalers, nebulisers, infusion Magnesium Aminophylline

Information Given to the Learners

Patient's relative approaches passing midwife alerting her to his concerns

Time: 21:00
Please can you help? My wife doesn't look very well!
From the team midwifery handover you know:
Patient is 38 years old, otherwise fit and well. 37 weeks pregnant. G4 P3.
SROM 2 hours ago, in active labour, 4 cm dilated at last examination 1 hour ago. Previous neonatal sepsis due to Group B *Streptococcus*. Commenced on benzylpenicillin as per protocol. No known drug allergies.

Scenario Schedule

Stage 1: Recognition of anaphylaxis and initial management	
Information given	**Expected actions**
Patient says "I feeling hot and flushed, I also feel a bit dizzy and it feels hard to breath, like I have a really tight chest!" She reports that she felt fine before the antibiotics started If asked, she has had penicillin before with no problems. Nil drug allergies She is normally fit and well with no medical problems No recent medication apart from antibiotics Has not requested analgesia for labour yet	Midwife to attend the patient and take a history of the symptoms
The patient appears to be very flushed	Commence initial assessment of patient using ABCDE approach
Patient talking but you can hear that she is wheezy	Perform airway assessment
	Apply Oxygen via non-rebreathing mask at 15 L/min
	Lie patient flat in left lateral position. (If this is not possible, apply manual uterine displacement)
	Call for emergency obstetric and anaesthetic help
Emergency team will arrive in stage 2	Apply full monitoring, pulse oximetry, NIBP, ECG
	Identify anaphylaxis
	Identify benzylpenicillin infusion still running and discontinue it
Progress to stage 2 once anaphylaxis suspected, benzylpenicillin discontinued and initial management commenced	

Observations	
A	Clear
B	RR 25/min SpO$_2$ 92% on air (96% on O$_2$)
C	HR 120 bpm BP 95/55 CRT 3s
D	**A**VPU
E	Temp 36.8°C
CTG	Baseline 140 bpm. Accelerations present, no decelerations

Observations

A	Tongue and soft palate swelling
B	RR 28/min SpO$_2$ 93% on 15 L/min O$_2$
C	HR 135 bpm BP 85/40 CRT 3s
D	**A**VPU
E	Temp 36.7°C
CTG	Baseline 170 bpm, reduced variability, variable decelerations

Stage 2: Patient continues to deteriorate, with airway, respiratory and cardiovascular compromise

Information given	Expected actions
Obstetrician and anaesthetist arrive	Team delegate roles and perform initial review of patient
Partner very anxious saying "Kira is not normally this red colour and can you see the lumps on her arm near where the needle is?" (pointing out hives distal to cannula site)	Maintain supine left lateral position Continue with 15 L Oxygen Repeat all observations
Patient says "My mouth and throat are starting to feel strange. Like there is something there!" She also commences coughing Tongue and soft palate oedema noted on oral examination	Airway assessment
Patient complaining of chest feeling tight. Trachea central, diffuse audible expiratory wheeze bilaterally, percussion note resonant throughout	Breathing assessment
Normal heart sounds, tachycardic, JVP normal	Cardiovascular assessment
	Elevate legs Insert large bore cannula. Take blood for FBC, U+E, LFT, tryptase, coagulation including fibrinogen and G+S. Check CBG (capillary blood glucose)
	Commence 500 ml Hartmann's stat through clean giving set
Feels drowsy but eyes still open and responsive	Disability assessment
Gross, widespread erythema with hives around the IV cannula site	Exposure assessment
	Recognise anaphylaxis and communicate this to team
	Remove potential triggers (IV antibiotics) if not already removed
	Administer adrenaline as per ALS protocol • 50 micrograms IV or 500 micrograms IM
	Inform obstetric and anaesthetic consultants

Progress to stage 3 once 1st dose adrenaline given and IV fluids commenced

Stage 3: Continuing severe life-threatening anaphylaxis

Information given	Expected actions
Patient complaining "My chest still feels really tight and it is getting hard to breathe!" She now has marked lip, tongue and soft palate swelling	Recognise that patient continues to deteriorate
	Administer further dose of IV/IM adrenaline
	Repeat all observations
Following adrenaline there is brief improvement but then complains of feeling light headed and getting anxious with difficulty breathing	
	Administer Hydrocortisone 200 mg IV
	Administer Chlorphenamine 10 mg IV
	Consider Adrenaline infusion 0.1 mcg/kg/min and titrate to effect
	Continue IV Hartmann's
Bronchodilators help a little but RR increasing	Commence 2nd line bronchodilators Salbutomol inhaled or IV infusion (3–20 mcg/min) or IV magnesium 1.2–2g IV over 20 minutes (or inhaled ipratropium, or IV aminophylline)
	Team will need to decide whether it is safe to transfer or better to intubate, ventilate and stabilise prior to transfer Will depend on proximity of safer location
	Refer patient to critical care
	Alert theatres (if this is your closest safe location for stabilisation)

Progress to stage 4 once additional therapies given and decision to intubate

Observations

A	Marked lip, tongue and soft palate swelling
B	RR 30/min SpO$_2$ 91% on 15L O$_2$
C	HR 140 bpm BP 85/40 CRT 4s
D	A**V**PU
E	Temp 36.2°C
CTG	Baseline 170 bpm, reduced variability, variable decelerations

Observations

A	Marked lip, tongue and soft palate swelling
B	RR 33/min SpO$_2$ 88% on 15L O$_2$
C	HR 145 bpm BP 95/40 CRT 3s
D	A**V**PU
E	Temp 36.1°C
CTG	Baseline 180 bpm, reduced variability, variable decelerations

Stage 4: Patient continues to deteriorate, requiring intubation, ventilation and referral to critical care.

Information given	Expected actions
Team to decide whether to transfer pre GA – depending on local environment	
Patient markedly deteriorating Looks cyanotic Tongue swelling, voice changed Cannot talk in sentences RR increasing Marked bronchospasm Patient becoming less responsive	Reassess patient and observations

Information given	Expected actions
	Continue oxygen, IV fluids and current pharmacological management
	Recognise the need for intubation
	Explain to patient/partner the need for anaesthesia and assistance with ventilation
ODP and senior anaesthetic support available	Prepare for potential difficult airway (tongue and lip swelling + 37/40 gestation) Summon extra help and senior assistance if not already there Apply high flow nasal oxygen (THRIVE) Discuss intubation plans with team Ensure all equipment checked and ready
	Consider administration of antacid prophylaxis
	Induction of anaesthesia. RSI with induction agents of choice (Thiopentone / suxamethonium vs Propofol / Rocuronium) Vasopressors prepared and ready to administer if induction exacerbates hypotension
Difficult view – large tongue, mallampati grade 3 or 2 with videolaryngoscope Able to intubate patient (unless wish to proceed to failed intubation scenario, see chapter 24)	Oral intubation using appropriate laryngoscope Size 7.0 ETT (at largest)
	Select appropriate ventilator settings to allow time for expiration in view of profound bronchospasm
Following intubation the patient becomes more stable. Although the wheeze persists, the oxygen saturation improves	
	Insert arterial line and perform ABG
	Insert urinary catheter
	Discuss with obstetricians and critical care concerning further management Will need caesarean section for delivery of baby prior to transfer to critical care

Scenario ends when patient is safely intubated and plan agreed regarding fetal delivery and critical care admission. Further mast cell tryptase samples to be taken 1 hour and 24 hours post event. Patient should be referred to specialist Immunology / Allergy service for further investigation once recovered.

Suggested Topics for Debrief Discussion

- How confident were you managing anaphylaxis in the ward environment?
- Would you intubate and ventilate this deteriorating patient on the ward or transfer to a safer location?
- When would you check the tryptase levels?

Discussion

Introduction

Anaphylaxis is a severe, potentially life-threatening systemic hypersensitivity reaction. Although rare during pregnancy, anaphylaxis can be catastrophic for both mother and, more commonly, fetus (with neurological damage or intrauterine death). Prompt recognition and treatment is crucial.

Causes of Anaphylaxis

The incidence of anaphylaxis appears to be increasing. A Pan-European meta-analysis suggests an incidence of 1.5–7.9 per 100,000 person-years. This gives a lifetime prevalence estimated at 0.3%, although other series calculate prevalence between 0.05% and 2%. Overall, the fatality rate for anaphylaxis is low, below 0.001%, although approximately 1500 people die of suspected anaphylaxis in the USA each year. The prevalence of anaphylaxis in pregnancy has been calculated at 2.7 cases per 100,000 deliveries.

Causes of anaphylaxis in pregnant women are similar to those of the general population. Common triggers include foods (shellfish, nuts and others), venom from stinging insects (hymenoptera such as bees and wasps), medication and natural rubber latex. Food allergy is more common in children, with venom and drug allergy increasing in adults. The incidence of latex allergy is decreasing. Up to 20% of all anaphylaxis cases may not have an obviously identifiable cause.

The most common peripartum cause of anaphylaxis are drugs allergies. Allergies to antibiotics are responsible for approximately half of the reported cases of anaphylaxis during this time, with the majority of those being to penicillins or cephalosporins prescribed prophylactically at caesarean section or to prevent neonatal group B streptococcal infection. Other common causes are muscle relaxants used during surgery performed under general anaesthesia, latex, chlorhexidine and oxytocin. Allergy to local anaesthetics is extremely uncommon, with only a handful of cases proven worldwide.

Recognition of Anaphylaxis

The clinical diagnosis of anaphylaxis relies on the recognition of a sudden onset and rapid progression of signs and symptoms after exposure to a known (or likely) allergen. See Box 15.1.

Symptoms and signs of anaphylaxis specific to pregnancy may include intense vulval or vaginal itching, lower back pain, uterine cramps and premature labour.

Anaphylactic reactions can present with a wide spectrum of symptoms and signs, and not all reactions have all of these. In a recent study describing a cohort of

---

Box 15.1 Criteria for Anaphylaxis

Anaphylaxis is highly likely when any **one** of the following three criteria is fulfilled:

1. Acute onset (minutes to several hours) with involvement of the skin, mucosal tissue, or both (e.g. generalised hives, pruritus or flushing, swollen lips/tongue/uvula **AND** at least one of the following:
   a. Respiratory compromise (dyspnoea, wheeze/bronchospasm, stridor, hypoxia)
   b. Reduced BP or associated symptoms of end-organ dysfunction (hypotension, tachycardia, reduced GCS, GI disturbance).

2. Two or more of the following that occur rapidly after exposure to **a likely** allergen for that patient (minutes to several hours):
   a. Involvement of the skin or mucosal tissue (hives, pruritus, flushing, angioedema)
   b. Respiratory compromise (dyspnoea, wheeze/bronchospasm, stridor, hypoxia)
   c. Reduced BP or associated symptoms (hypotension, tachycardia, bradycardia (rarely), reduced GCS)
   d. Persistent gastrointestinal symptoms (e.g. crampy abdominal pain, vomiting, diarrhoea).

3. Reduced BP after exposure to **known** allergen for that patient (minutes to several hours): (systolic BP < 90 mmHg)

Applying the above criteria demonstrates a sensitivity of (96.7%) and specificity of (82.4%) for the diagnosis of anaphylaxis.

paediatric and adult patients with anaphylaxis, systems affected included:

- skin (84%),
- cardiovascular (72%),
- respiratory (68%),
- gastrointestinal (45%),
- central nervous (15%).

Anaphylaxis can present with any combination of these. Symptoms and signs usually occur within 2 hours of exposure to the allergen, within 30 minutes of exposure to food allergens and even faster with parenteral medication or insect stings. In a large case series of fatal anaphylaxis, the median time from symptoms to arrest has been reported as 30, 15 and 5 minutes for food, insect venom, and parenteral medication, respectively. Study of simulation in anaesthetists has shown that recognition of anaphylaxis in a scenario can take up to 10 minutes.

Differential Diagnosis of Anaphylaxis in Pregnancy

Many conditions can mimic anaphylaxis (Box 15.2). Specific to the obstetric population, other conditions that can mimic an allergic reaction include amniotic fluid embolism, problems related to regional anaesthesia (sympathetic blockade, high block, total spinal or local anaesthetic toxicity), major haemorrhage, rapid administration of synthetic oxytocin analogues and pregnancy-related laryngeal dysfunction.

Management of Anaphylaxis

The management of anaphylaxis in pregnancy should follow established algorithms published by the Resuscitation Council (UK) (Figure 15.1) and, in theatre, the Association of Anaesthetists of Great Britain and Ireland. There are caveats specific to pregnancy, especially at or approaching full-term, to remember. Avoid aortocaval compression by ensuring left lateral tilt or manual uterine displacement. Ideally, early continuous fetal monitoring should be established. An emergency caesarean section may be indicated in severe anaphylaxis if unresponsive to treatment, or there are signs of fetal distress. Hypotension and hypoxia are poorly tolerated by the fetus.

Investigation of Suspected Anaphylaxis

Following suspected anaphylaxis, it is useful to send blood samples for mast cell tryptase levels. The first

Box 15.2 Differential Diagnoses of Anaphylaxis

Skin or mucosal
  Chronic remittent or physical urticaria and angioedema
  Pollen food syndrome

Respiratory diseases
  Acute laryngotracheitis
  Tracheal or bronchial obstruction (e.g. foreign substances, vocal cord dysfunction)
  Status asthmaticus (without involvement of other organs)

Cardiovascular diseases
  Vasovagal syncope
  Pulmonary embolism
  Myocardial infarction
  Cardiac arrhythmias
  Hypertensive crisis
  Cardiogenic shock

Pharmacological or toxic reactions
  Ethanol
  Histamine, e.g. scombroid fish poisoning, opiates, other histamine-releasing drugs
  Hoigné's syndrome (pseudoanaphylaxis)

Neuropsychiatric diseases
  Hyperventilation syndrome
  Anxiety and panic disorder, somatoform disorder (e.g. psychogenic dyspnoea, vocal cord dysfunction)
  Dissociative disorder and conversion (e.g. globus hystericus)
  Epilepsy
  Cerebrovascular event
  Psychogenic aetiology
  Trauma

Endocrinological diseases
  Hypoglycaemia
  Thyrotoxic crisis
  Carcinoid syndrome
  Tumours (e.g. phaeochromocytoma, VIPoma)

sample should be sent as soon as possible after suspected anaphylaxis, followed by another sample 1–2 hours later. These should be compared with a baseline level taken 24 hours after the reaction. A dynamic rise in tryptase may be significant, even if the highest value remains within a reported normal range. A raised mast cell tryptase level has a high positive predictive value for anaphylaxis but a poor negative

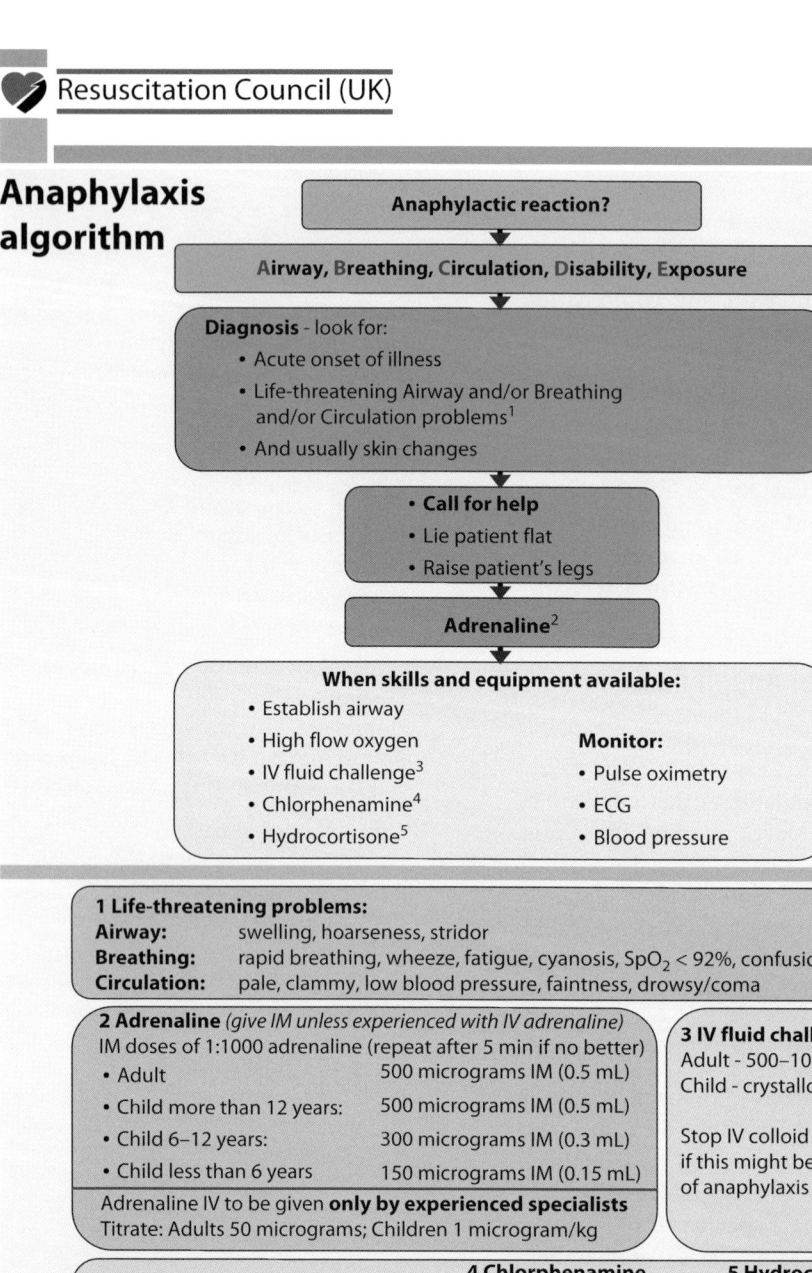

Resuscitation Council (UK)

Anaphylaxis algorithm

Anaphylactic reaction?

↓

Airway, Breathing, Circulation, Disability, Exposure

↓

Diagnosis - look for:
- Acute onset of illness
- Life-threatening Airway and/or Breathing and/or Circulation problems[1]
- And usually skin changes

↓

- **Call for help**
- Lie patient flat
- Raise patient's legs

↓

Adrenaline[2]

↓

When skills and equipment available:
- Establish airway
- High flow oxygen
- IV fluid challenge[3]
- Chlorphenamine[4]
- Hydrocortisone[5]

Monitor:
- Pulse oximetry
- ECG
- Blood pressure

1 Life-threatening problems:
Airway:	swelling, hoarseness, stridor
Breathing:	rapid breathing, wheeze, fatigue, cyanosis, SpO_2 < 92%, confusion
Circulation:	pale, clammy, low blood pressure, faintness, drowsy/coma

2 Adrenaline *(give IM unless experienced with IV adrenaline)*
IM doses of 1:1000 adrenaline (repeat after 5 min if no better)
- Adult	500 micrograms IM (0.5 mL)
- Child more than 12 years:	500 micrograms IM (0.5 mL)
- Child 6–12 years:	300 micrograms IM (0.3 mL)
- Child less than 6 years	150 micrograms IM (0.15 mL)

Adrenaline IV to be given **only by experienced specialists**
Titrate: Adults 50 micrograms; Children 1 microgram/kg

3 IV fluid challenge
Adult - 500–1000 mL
Child - crystalloid 20 mL/kg

Stop IV colloid
if this might be the cause
of anaphylaxis

	4 Chlorphenamine (IM or slow IV)	5 Hydrocortisone (IM or slow IV)
Adult or child more than 12 years	10 mg	200 mg
Child 6–12 years	5 mg	100 mg
Child 6 months to 6 years	2.5 mg	50 mg
Child less than 6 months	250 micrograms/kg	25 mg

March 2008

5th Floor, Tavistock House North, Tavistock Square, London WC1H 9HR
Telephone (020) 7388-4678 • Fax (020) 7383-0773 • Email enquiries@resus.org.uk
www.resus.org.uk • Registered Charity No. 286360

Figure 15.1 Anaphylaxis poster.

predictive value. Normal mast cell tryptase levels do not exclude anaphylaxis. Blood may also be obtained for specific IgE levels to likely causes, although these tests are poorly sensitive. The patient should be referred to a specialist Immunology/Allergy service for further investigation. Reactions related to anaesthesia should be referred to a combined Anaesthesia/Immunology clinic.

The mainstay of investigation is performing skin tests using likely culprit substances and comparing the results with both positive and negative controls (histamine and 0.9% saline, respectively). Interpretation of skin tests along with careful review of the patient's history and records hopefully allow a culprit drug or substance to be found. Unfortunately, skin tests to many antibiotics and other drugs are not entirely reliable and the gold standard of investigation is to perform a graded challenge test with the drug in an appropriate clinical setting.

Investigation of suspected reactions in pregnancy is difficult as, even though the risks to the unborn child and mother are small, skin tests and certainly challenge tests are not recommended. Ideally these tests should be deferred until after delivery. Specific IgE blood tests can be taken, although they may be unhelpful.

Penicillin Allergy

Allergy to a penicillin or cephalosporin is the most common drug-related cause of anaphylaxis in pregnancy. Many women will offer a history of penicillin allergy, although studies have shown that perhaps only 10% of people with a declared penicillin allergy are truly allergic. Anybody with a history of anaphylaxis or a severe reaction (respiratory distress, urticaria, angioedema) should avoid all penicillins and cephalosporins. Women with a more benign history may receive a cephalosporin, if required, as cross-reactivity is unlikely in these cases. Current NICE guidance recommends that people who declare a penicillin allergy and are likely to need regular antibiotics going forward should be investigated at a local allergy clinic to clarify their allergy status.

Bibliography

Adriaensens, I., Vercauteren, M., Soetens, F., Janssen, L., Leysen, J. and Ebo, D. (2013). Allergic reactions during labour analgesia and caesarean section anaesthesia. *International Journal of Obstetric Anaesthesia*, 22, 231–242.

EAACI Food Allergy and Anaphylaxis Guidelines Group. (2014). Anaphylaxis: guidelines from the European Academy of Allergy and Clinical Immunology. *Allergy*, 69(8), 1026–1045. doi: 10.1111/all.12437. Epub 2014 Jun 9.

Hughes, R. G., Brocklehurst, P., Steer, P. J., Heath, P. and Stenson, B. M. on behalf of the Royal College of Obstetricians and Gynaecologists. (2017). Prevention of early-onset neonatal group B streptococcal disease. Green-top Guideline No. 36. *British Journal of Obstetrics and Gynaecology*, 124, e280–e305.

Johansson, S. G. O., Bieber, T., Dahl, R., et al. (2004). Revised nomenclature for allergy for global use: Report of the Nomenclature Review Committee of the World Allergy Organization, October 2003. *Journal of Allergy and Clinical Immunology*, 113, 832–836.

Naisbitt, D. J., Gordon, S. F., Pirmohamed, M. and Park, B. K. (2000). Immunological principles of adverse drug reactions: the initiation and propagation of immune responses elicited by drug treatment. *Drug Safety*, 23(6), 483–507.

NICE. (2011). *Clinical Guideline [CG134]*. Manchester: NICE.

Panesar, S. S., Javad, S., De Silva, D., et al. (2013). The epidemiology of anaphylaxis in Europe: a systematic review. *Allergy*, 68, 1353–1361.

Pichler, W. J. (2003). Delayed drug hypersensitivity reactions. *Annals of Internal Medicine*, 139(8), 683–693.

Pumphrey, R. S. H. (2000). Lessons for management of anaphylaxis from a study of fatal reactions. *Clinical and Experimental Allergy*, 30, 1144–1150.

Rich, R., Fleisher, T., Shearer, W., Schroeder, H., Frew, A. and Weyand, C. (2013). *Clinical Immunology Principles and Practice*; 4th edition (part five, pp. 491–578). Philadelphia, PA: Elsevier Saunders.

Sampson, H. A., Munoz-Furlong, A., Campbell, R. L., et al. (2006). Second symposium on the definition and management of anaphylaxis: summary report – Second National Institute of Allergy and Infectious Disease/Food Allergy and Anaphylaxis Network Symposium. *Journal of Allergy and Clinical Immunology*, 117, 391–397.

Simons, F. E. R., Ardusso, L. R. F., Bilo, M. B., et al. (2011). World Allergy Organization guidelines for the assessment and management of anaphylaxis. *Journal of Allergy and Clinical Immunology*, 127, 587–593.

Simons, F. E. R. and Schatz, M. (2012). Anaphylaxis in pregnancy. *Journal of Allergy and Clinical Immunology*, 130, 597–606

Worm, M., Edenharter, G., Rueff, F., et al. (2012). Symptom profile and risk factors of anaphylaxis in Central Europe. *Allergy*, 67, 691–698.

Chapter

16

Acute Pulmonary Embolism in Pregnancy

Louise Simcox and David Simcox

Scenario in a Nutshell

Patient presents with acute pulmonary embolism, with signs progressing to acute massive pulmonary embolism.

Stage 1: Patient presents with shortness of breath to triage – initial assessment and transfer to obstetric HDU.

Stage 2: Discussion of investigations and treatment required – patient not keen for X-rays/CTPA or V/Q because of possible harm to baby.

Stage 3: Patient becomes cardiovascularly unstable with signs of acute massive pulmonary embolism.

Target Learner Groups

Obstetricians, anaesthetists and midwives.

Specific learning opportunities
Knowledge of differential diagnosis of acute shortness of breath in a pregnant woman and planning of appropriate investigations
Knowledge of management of likely pulmonary embolism in pregnancy
Appropriate use of senior involvement of obstetric, anaesthetic and other specialities, particularly when patient deteriorates

Suggested learners (to represent their normal roles)	In the room from the start	Available when requested
Anaesthetic ST3+		√
Obstetric ST1	√	
Obstetric ST3+		√
Midwife Coordinator		√
Midwife in room	√	
Suggested facilitators		
Faculty to play role of patient's partner	√	

Details for Facilitators
Patient Demographics

Name: Toni

Age: 37

Gestation: 31+1

Booking weight: 92 kg

Parity: P0

Scenario Summary for Facilitators

37-year-old, 31-week pregnant primiparous woman. Attended obstetric triage with shortness of breath. Been under follow-up in Fetal Medicine Unit (FMU) for polyhydramnios.

BMI 39.

Two-day history of shortness of breath, sudden onset, progressively worsening. No chest pain.

Found to be tachypnoeic, tachycardic and hypoxic. Transferred to obstetric HDU from triage.

Assessed by Obstetric and Anaesthetic Registrar.

Portable CXR unremarkable.

ECG sinus tachycardia and right bundle branch block.

Plan further investigations. Patient not keen for CTPA or V/Q – needs further explanation of the risks involved.

Treatment with unfractionated/low molecular weight heparin.

Patient then deteriorates cardiovascularly with BP falling. Massive acute PE. Need consultant involvement from obstetrics, anaesthetics, medicine/respiratory, radiology and cardiothoracic surgery to aid decision-making for treatment options of acute massive PE in pregnancy.

Set-up Overview for Facilitators

Clinical setting	On a trolley in triage
Patient position	Sitting upright
Initial monitoring in place	Pulse oximeter NIBP cuff CTG

Medical Equipment

For core equipment checklist, see Chapter 9.

Additional equipment specific to scenario		
Low molecular weight heparin Unfractionated heparin	Arterial line	Thrombolysis according to local guidelines
Local guidelines for IV heparin therapy/ thrombolysis		

Information Given to the Learners

Handover to obstetric ST1 from triage midwife.

Situation: This is Toni, who has just arrived in triage feeling short of breath.

Background: 37-year-old otherwise fit and well. BMI 39. 31 weeks pregnant, first pregnancy.

Attending FMU for follow-up scans for polyhydramnios – conservative management.

She has been feeling short of breath for the last 2 days but had attributed this to late pregnancy and polyhydramnios. Partner reports she struggled to catch her breath walking to the unit.

Assessment: I am just doing her first set of observations. She feels quite short of breath so I came to get you.

Recommendation: Would you mind reviewing her please?

Scenario Schedule

Observations	
A	Clear
B	RR 26/min SpO$_2$ 93% on air
C	HR 120bpm BP 106/64 CRT 1s
D	**A**VPU
E	Temp 36.9°C
CTG	normal

Stage 1: Patient presents with shortness of breath to triage – initial assessment and transfer to obstetric HDU

Information given	Expected actions
	Commence ABCDE approach to patient and perform observations
Speaking – short of breath but can complete sentences	Assess airway. Administer 15 L/min O$_2$ via non-rebreathing mask whilst stabilising the patient (then titrate oxygen to SpO$_2$ 94–98%)
	Call for senior obstetric/anaesthetic assistance
	Considers differential diagnosis of acute shortness of breath in pregnancy such as pulmonary embolism (PE), asthma, pneumonia, other systemic sepsis, peripartum cardiomyopathy, pre-existing cardiac pathology
If asked: Usually fit and well. No problems with pregnancy up until now. Sudden onset of shortness of breath 2 days ago. Thought may be due to bump getting bigger and had been told had 'lots of fluid around baby'.	Take history from patient
Partner (facilitator) interjects: he is worried. Says that she has definitely been more short of breath in the last 2 days. Had to rest on way in from car park.	

105

Information given	Expected actions
No cough, no sputum, no haemoptysis. No sore throat or upper respiratory tract infection symptoms. No family members or close contacts unwell. No cardiac history. No chest pain. No other positive symptoms on systems review.	
Chest clear, good air entry bilaterally Heart sounds 1+2+0 Mild bilateral ankle oedema. No calf tenderness/redness/swelling.	Examine respiratory and cardiovascular systems
	Secure IV access and take blood for FBC, U+E, LFT, CRP, coagulation screen including fibrinogen, group and save (G+S), troponin
	Don't request d-dimers or thrombophilia screen
ABG result(results given on air): pH: 7.47 pO$_2$: 9.2 kPa pCO$_2$: 3.0 kPa HCO$_3$: 21 mmol/L Lactate: 2 mmol/L BE: -1.6 mmol/L	Perform arterial blood gas (ABG)
	Transfer patient to delivery unit/obstetric HDU bed.

Progress to stage 2 when taken history and made decision to transfer to delivery unit/obstetric HDU

Stage 2: Discussion of investigations and treatment required – patient not keen for X-rays/CTPA or V/Q because of possible harm to baby

Observations	
A	Clear
B	RR 25/min SpO$_2$ 99% on O$_2$
C	HR 123 bpm BP 110/62 CRT 1s
D	**A**VPU
E	Temp 37.2°C
CTG: normal	

Information given	Expected actions
Patient is now in obstetric HDU room	Continue with 15L/min O$_2$ (then titrate oxygen to SpO$_2$ 94–98%)
	Repeat observations
Obstetric ST3+ and anaesthetic ST3+ arrive	SBAR handover from obstetric ST1 to anaesthetic ST3+ and obstetric ST3+
	Recognise pulmonary embolism high on list of differential diagnoses
	Inform obstetric and anaesthetic consultants
	Initiate investigations (blood tests already sent):
12 Lead ECG – right bundle branch block (RBBB), tachycardic (see Figure 16.1)	12-lead ECG

Information given	Expected actions
CXR – normal	CXR
	Commence therapy with treatment dose low-molecular-weight heparin. Unfractionated heparin would be an appropriate alternative treatment option
	Discuss V/Q scan or CTPA with patient (as per local guidelines – RCOG guidance would be for V/Q scan in this example)
Patient very concerned about further tests – wants more information, what are risks to baby? Are there alternatives? Can she opt not to have it?	Outline risks of V/Q and CTPA to mother and fetus
Once discussed risks/benefits of investigations, patient starts to feel unwell, dizzy.	

Progress to stage 3 once have outlined risks/benefits of investigations for PE and patient becomes dizzy.

Stage 3: Patient becomes cardiovascularly unstable with signs of acute massive pulmonary embolism

Observations	
A	Clear
B	RR 30/min SpO$_2$ 94% on O$_2$
C	HR 132 BP 75/45 CRT 3s
D	AVPU
E	T. 36.8°C

CTG: Baseline FHR 165 bpm, baseline variability 5 bpm, no decelerations

Information given	Expected actions
Patient still conscious and talking but feels more short of breath Feels dizzy and sick	Repeat observations and start rapid IV fluids
	Request urgent consultant obstetric and anaesthetic involvement
	Request urgent senior review from acute medicine
Still talking but feels very faint Trachea central, good air entry bilaterally, no added sounds HS 1+2+0 Abdomen soft, non-tender No PV bleeding	Reassess patient with ABCDE approach and reconsider differential diagnosis: • acute PE • decompensated cardiac failure • sepsis • haemorrhage
	Site second large-bore IV cannula
	Consider IV antibiotics for community-acquired pneumonia and complete sepsis 6 while looking for definitive diagnosis
	Acute PE still most likely, also need to rule out cardiac cause

Information given	Expected actions
	Ensure urgent initiation of treatment if not already done so – unfractionated heparin (UFH) most appropriate option now (fixed dose, eg: 5,000 units IV followed by 1000 units/hr or weight-based dose according to local guidelines). Use booking weight.
Call from Radiology to say they are ready for V/Q scan or CTPA	Discuss whether patient stable enough for transfer to Radiology
Echo result: Small LV cavity size with normal LV systolic function. Septal flattening consistent with RV pressure overload. Severely dilated RV with severely reduced systolic function No valvular abnormalities	Bedside echo good option - request cardiologist to attend to perform echo. Don't delay start of treatment for PE while waiting for investigations.
	Diagnosis of massive PE
	Need consultant multidisciplinary discussion regarding thrombolysis/ surgical thrombectomy/catheter thromboembolectomy with acute medicine/ respiratory, cardiothoracic surgery, radiology, obstetrics and anaesthesia.
	Arterial line insertion by anaesthetist
	If decide on thrombolysis, administer as per local guidance then commence IV heparin infusion (omit loading dose).

End scenario once options for treatment of massive pulmonary embolism are considered and senior multidisciplinary opinions urgently requested

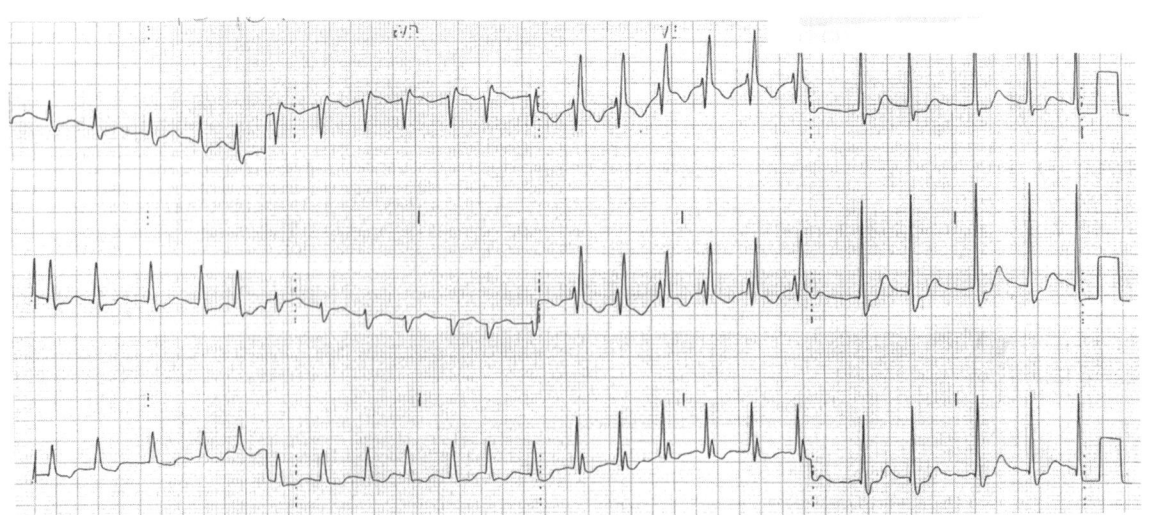

Figure 16.1 ECG

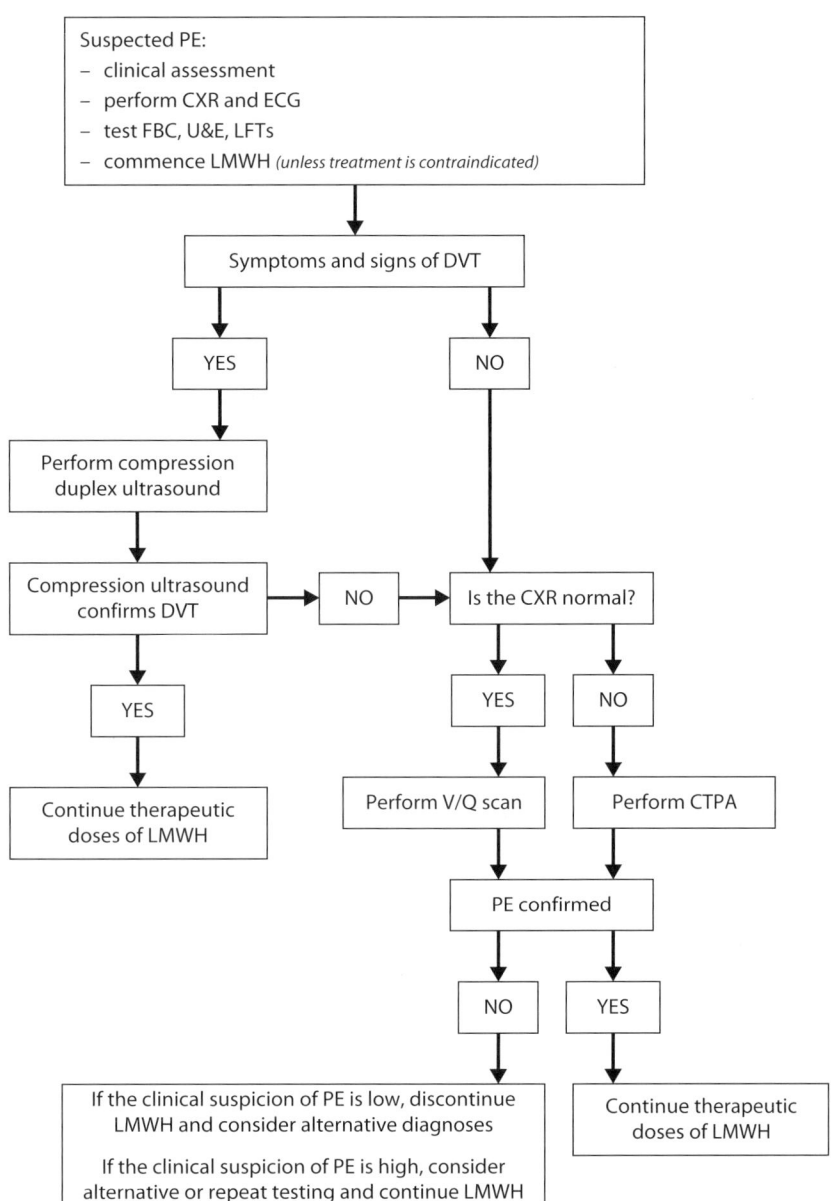

Figure 16.2 Algorithm for the investigation and initial management of suspected PE in pregnancy and the puerperium (reproduced with kind permission from the RCOG) Green-top Guideline No 37a: Reducing the risk of thromboembolism during pregnancy and the puerperium. Nelson-Piercy, C., MacCallum, P. and MacKillop, L. London: Royal College of Obstetricians and Gynaecologists, 2015.
For original see: www.rcog.org.uk/globalassets/documents/guidelines/gtg-37b.pdf, p. 29

Suggested Topics for Debrief Discussion

- Was treatment for suspected PE started early?
- How easy was it/would it be to locate LMWH, unfractionated heparin and thrombolysis on your delivery unit?

Discussion

Incidence

Venous thromboembolism (VTE) remains a leading cause of direct maternal death in developed countries. It complicates 1 in 1000 pregnancies, and is approximately 10 times more common in the pregnant than non-pregnant state.

Risk Factors

As in this scenario, many women with pregnancy-associated pulmonary thromboembolism (PTE) will have identifiable antenatal risk factors such as obesity, maternal age (>35 years) and multiparity (see Table 16.1).

Clinical Presentation

Diagnosis of acute VTE in pregnancy can be difficult with the physiological symptoms of pregnancy often mimicking those of VTE. Data from the RIETE registry (an international, observational registry of patients with objective evidence of acute venous thromboembolism) found that most women with a PE in pregnancy present with dyspnoea (87%) or chest pain (61%) (Blanci-Molina et al., 2010).

Venous thromboembolism can occur at any stage of pregnancy, although the risk is highest in the puerperium.

The majority of deep vein thromboses (DVTs) in pregnancy are left-sided (90% in pregnancy vs. 55% in those non-pregnant). This observation is partly explained by compression of the left common iliac vein which is crossed by the right common iliac. Ileo-femoral DVTs are more common in pregnancy (72% in pregnancy vs. 9% in the non-pregnant). Overall,

Table 16.1 Table of risk factors for PE in pregnancy (Nelson-Piercy et al., 2015).

Risk factors for PE in pregnancy
Previous VTE
Hospital admission
Thrombophilia
Medical comorbidities (e.g. cancer, heart failure, active SLE, inflammatory bowel disease, inflammatory polyarthropathy, nephrotic syndrome, Type I diabetes with nephropathy, sickle cell disease, current IVDU)
Any surgical procedure
Ovarian hyperstimulation syndrome (first trimester only)
Obesity
Age > 35 years
Parity ≥ 3
Smoker
Gross varicose veins
Current pre-eclampsia
Immobility (e.g. paraplegia, symphysis-pubis dysfunction)
First-degree relative with history of unprovoked or oestrogen-provoked VTE
Multiple pregnancy
Assisted reproductive therapy (e.g. IVF)
Hyperemesis gravidarum

the increased ileo-femoral distribution in pregnancy probably predisposes to pulmonary embolism (PE).

Investigations

Clinical Probability Scores and D-Dimers

Investigation of VTE in pregnancy differs from the non-pregnant state. Whereas outside pregnancy the use of D-dimer assays in conjunction with pre-test probability scores (such as the Wells score) are almost universally used to identify a low-risk cohort where no further investigation is required, no such parallels exist in pregnancy. The physiologically elevated D-dimer level in pregnancy makes this investigation of no utility, and there have been no pretest probability risk scores validated for widespread use in pregnancy or the postpartum period.

ECG

An ECG should be performed on all women with suspicion of acute PE as it may show signs of PE or indicate an alternative diagnosis.

Data from the RIETE registry found that the ECG was abnormal in 39% of pregnant women with acute PE; the most common abnormalities were T-wave inversion (21%), S1,Q3,T3 pattern (15%) and right bundle branch block (18% during pregnancy and 4.2% in the puerperium). Twenty-nine percent of pregnant women with acute PE had sinus tachycardia (36% of women in the postpartum period).

Chest X-Ray

CXR was normal in 69% of pregnant women with acute PE. CXR abnormalities seen with acute PE in pregnancy were (Blanco-Molina et al., 2010):

Pulmonary effusion	23%
Lung infarction	14%
Atelectasis	9%
Infiltrate	9%
Cardiomegaly	4.5%

Compression Duplex Ultrasound

If there is a clinical suspicion of DVT in pregnancy, compression duplex ultrasound is the primary diagnostic test.

It should also be done if the woman has symptoms or signs of a PE with symptoms or signs of a DVT as if the duplex ultrasound is positive, treatment can be commenced and the radiation of V/Q scanning or CTPA can be avoided.

CT Pulmonary Angiography (CTPA) and V/Q Scanning

In women with suspected PE without symptoms or signs of DVT it is appropriate to proceed to objective testing using CTPA or Ventilation/Perfusion (V/Q) scanning without preliminary scanning of the legs.

The choice between CTPA and V/Q scan will depend on local guidelines, availability and clinician/patient preference. CTPA performs better in situations where the chest radiograph is abnormal. However, it may not identify peripheral PTE (up to 30% of peripheral emboli are not identified on CTPA).

Regarding V/Q scanning during pregnancy, the ventilation component can often be omitted, thus reducing the radiation dose to the fetus. When comparing Q scans with CTPA for the detection of PE in pregnancy, both have comparable negative predictive values (100% Q scan vs. 99% CTPA). On balance, most UK hospitals will proceed to Q scan to assess for PTE antenatally if available. This is guided by the low incidence of pulmonary comorbid disease in pregnancy, similar negative predictive values and lower breast cancer risk (the radiation dose estimate to the breast for CTPA is 20–100 times greater than for V/Q scanning, resulting in an increase from background breast cancer risk of 1 in 200 to 1.1 in 200 with CTPA).

Management

It is important that treatment is implemented at clinical suspicion of PE. Low molecular weight heparin (LMWH) is now the treatment of choice given its excellent safety profile and low associated bleeding risk. Dose calculation is based on the maternal booking weight.

The treatment of non-massive PTE in pregnancy involves therapeutic anticoagulation with LMWH (usually for a minimum total duration of 3 months and for at least 6 weeks postnatally). This should be commenced immediately following clinical suspicion of PTE until this is excluded by definitive imaging unless treatment is contraindicated for another reason. One of the advantages of LMWH over unfractionated heparin, particularly in pregnancy, is the potential reduced risk of bleeding. Monitoring of Anti-Xa activity is not usually required, apart from in women at extremes of body weight (< 50 kg or > 90 kg) or with other complicating factors such as renal impairment (creatinine clearance < 30ml/min).

Acute, Massive PE
Unfractionated Heparin
Acute massive PTE, presenting with shock/haemodynamic compromise, should be treated with unfractionated heparin due to its rapid onset of action.

Thrombolysis
Thrombolysis can be considered in women with life-threatening PE or in the context of subsequent cardiac arrest. Intravenous unfractionated heparin should be commenced promptly following thrombolysis, and this can be converted to LMWH once stability is achieved, with dosage and monitoring based on local guidelines.

There have been no maternal deaths or intracranial bleeds reported in pregnant women receiving thrombolytic therapy to date and complication rates appear similar to those in the non-pregnant population. In a report of 172 pregnant women treated with thrombolytic therapy, there were five maternal bleeding complications (2.9%) and three fetal deaths (1.7%) (Ahearn et al., 2002).

Embolectomy
The Royal College of Obstetrics and Gynaecology guidelines (UK) (Nelson-Piercy et al., 2015) recommend that embolectomy is reserved for moribund patients or where thrombolysis is unsuitable.

Planning Delivery
When VTE occurs close to term, the risk of recurrent thrombosis may be increased if anticoagulation is interrupted for planned induction or caesarean section. The risk of recurrent VTE is highest in the first 2 weeks following the thrombotic event, and where VTE occurs within the 4 weeks prior to delivery the use of an IVC filter should be strongly considered (in discussion with local haematology and interventional radiology colleagues).

It seems reasonable to allow spontaneous labour in women who are therapeutically anticoagulated with LMWH, with instructions not to inject any further LMWH at this point and seek specialist review. Consideration should be made to de-intensifying anticoagulation during labour (to prophylactic doses of LMWH) and then recommencing therapeutic anticoagulation following delivery. Consideration can also be given to the use of IV unfractionated heparin which can be more easily manipulated and due to its shorter half-life minimises the duration without therapeutic anticoagulation. However, there are issues in monitoring unfractionated heparin in pregnancy with the APTT due to the physiological changes of pregnancy.

Further Counselling

With regard to the longer term, consideration should be made to reducing the risk of future thromboembolic events in women who develop pregnancy-associated VTE. Women who have suffered a VTE in a previous pregnancy should be offered prophylactic LMWH during future pregnancies and for 6 weeks postnatally, and should be counselled to avoid oestrogen-containing contraceptives.

Bibliography

Ahearn, G. S., Hadjiliadis, D., Govert, J. A. and Tapson, V. F. (2002). Massive pulmonary embolism during pregnancy successfully treated with recombinant tissue plasminogen activator: a case report and review of treatment options. *Archives of Internal Medicine*, 162, 1221–1227.

Blanco-Molina, A., Rota, L., Di Micco, P., et al. (2010). Venous thromboembolism during pregnancy, postpartum or during contraceptive use. Findings from the RIETE Registry. *Thrombosis and Haemostasis*, 103, 306–311.

Greer, I. A. and Nelson-Piercy, C. (2005). Low-molecular-weight heparins for thromboprophylaxis and treatment of venous thromboembolism in pregnancy: a systematic review of safety and efficacy. *Blood*, 106, 401–407.

Greer, I. and Thomson, A. J. (2015). *Green-top Guideline No. 37b – Thromboembolic Disease in Pregnancy and the Puerperium: Acute Management*. London: Royal College of Obstetricians and Gynaecologists.

Grüning, T., Mingo, R. E., Gosling, M. G., et al. (2016). Diagnosing venous thromboembolism in pregnancy. *The British Journal of Radiology*, 89(1062), 20160021. doi:10.1259/bjr.20160021.

Nelson-Piercy, C., MacCallum, P. and MacKillop, L. (2015). *Green-top Guideline No. 37a – Reducing the Risk of Thromboembolism During Pregnancy and the Puerperium*. London: Royal College of Obstetricians and Gynaecologists.

Ramsay, R., Byrd, L., Tower, C., et al. (2015). The problem of pulmonary embolism diagnosis in pregnancy. *British Journal of Haematology*, 170, 727–728.

Simcox, L. E., Ormesher, L., Tower, C., et al. (2015). Pulmonary thrombo-embolism in pregnancy: diagnosis and management. *Breathe*, 11, 282–289.

Chapter

17

Eclampsia

Stephanie Worton, Emma Shawkat and Jenny Myers

Scenario in a Nutshell

Patient has a seizure in triage. Emergency treatment of seizure, treated as eclampsia while considering other causes. When recovers, is in active labour.
    Stage 1: Patient just admitted to triage and has a tonic–clonic seizure.
    Stage 2: Immediate post-seizure care and treatment of severe hypertension.
    Stage 3: Patient in active labour – plan made for labour and delivery.

Target Learner Groups

All members of the multidisciplinary obstetric team: anaesthetists, midwives and obstetricians.

Specific learning opportunities
Demonstrate effective team management of eclampsia
Demonstrate knowledge of the differential diagnosis of a seizure in pregnancy
Demonstrate timely management of acute, severe hypertension

Suggested learners (to represent their normal roles)	In the room from the start	Available when requested
Anaesthetic ST3+		√
Obstetric ST1-2/FY2	√	
Obstetric ST3+		√
Midwife coordinator		√
Midwife in room	√	
Suggested facilitators		
Faculty to play role of midwife finishing shift (can be played by facilitator running scenario)	√	
Faculty to play role of patient's partner (comes in at start of stage 2)	√	

Details for Facilitators

Patient Demographics

Name: Sarah
Age: 19
Gestation: 38+4
Booking weight: 62 kg
Parity: P0

Scenario Summary for Facilitators

Nulliparous 19-year-old, 38 weeks gestation. Attended with abdominal pain and headache and felt suddenly unwell upon arrival.
Seizure in triage room lasting 2 minutes.
Severe systolic hypertension requiring intravenous therapy.
Once stabilised found to be in labour (8 cm). Plan made for labour and delivery.

Set-up Overview for Facilitators

Clinical setting	Triage room
Patient position	Semi-recumbent on triage trolley
Initial monitoring in place	None
Other equipment	None
Useful manikin functions	Seizures

Medical Equipment

For core equipment checklist see Chapter 9.

Additional equipment specific to scenario		
Eclampsia box as per local guidelines including MgSO$_4$	Antihypertensive drugs according to local guidelines: labetalol, hydralazine	Pen torch
Tendon hammer	Arterial line	Local checklist for eclampsia

Information Given to the Learners

Information given to ST2 obstetric trainee and midwife.

Time: 23.00

This handover is given by a facilitator playing the role of the midwife in the room already with the patient.

The SBAR handover is as follows:

Situation: This is Sarah – I've had to bring her straight round from the waiting area as she was feeling very unwell and getting a bit agitated.

Background: 19-year-old, previously fit and well primip who is 38+4 weeks pregnant with no allergies. She rang about an hour ago to say that she had a bad headache and abdominal pain. Her partner has her handheld notes – he is just parking the car.

Action: I've literally just got her on to the trolley so I haven't had a chance to do anything yet.

Recommendation: Are you able to take over her care?

Scenario Schedule

Observations

A	Noisy, obstructed
B	RR 25/min SpO$_2$ poor trace
C	HR 132bpm BP 190/110
D	AVP**U**
E	Nil to note
CTG:	If put on, unable to get trace during seizure

Stage 1: Patient just admitted to triage and has a tonic-clonic seizure

Information given	Expected actions
As midwife and ST2 obstetrics enter room, patient starts having a tonic-clonic seizure	Call for help using emergency buzzer
	Commence ABCDE approach to patient
	Keep patient safe (bed sides up, limit self harm)
Noisy, snoring sounds which resolve on head-tilt/chin lift or jaw thrust. If tries to use oropharyngeal airway, jaw is tightly clenched while fitting.	Perform airway assessment and airway-opening manoeuvres
	Apply oxygen via non-rebreathing mask at 15 L/min
	Turn patient to left lateral position when safe to do so
	Apply full monitoring (BP, ECG leads, pulse oximeter)
Other staff arrive responding to emergency buzzer No other details available at this stage as no notes	State the emergency when team arrive: tonic-clonic seizure in a patient presenting with headache and abdo pain
	Secure wide-bore IV access (x2) Take blood for FBC, U+E, LFT, coagulation (including fibrinogen) and G+S
CBG 6.1 mmol/L	Check capillary blood glucose (CBG)
	Designate a 'scribe'
	Call obstetric and anaesthetic consultants
	Team consider differential diagnosis of seizure in pregnancy (see Discussion) Decision to treat as eclampsia while also considering other potential causes of seizure

Information given	Expected actions
	Locate eclampsia box or trolley and eclampsia emergency checklist (if available)
	Prepare and commence loading dose of magnesium sulphate; 4g IV over 5 minutes or according to local protocol
Seizure self-terminates after 2 minutes, following which the patient is post-ictal/drowsy - GCS=13 E=3 – eye opening to speech V=4 – saying a few words but a little confused M=6 – obeying commands	Repeat observations post-seizure
	Commence treatment for severe hypertension as per local pre-eclampsia guidelines. Aim to achieve SBP <150mmHg whilst maintaining DBP >80mmHg. For example: • Labetolol 50mg slow IV bolus over 5 minutes. If required, repeat at 10 minute intervals up to 200mg ± maintenance infusion (20mg/hr, if required double every 30 minutes up to maximum 160mg/hr) *or* • Hydralazine 2.5mg slow IV bolus over 5 minutes. If required repeat at 20 minute intervals up to maximum of 20mg, ± maintenance infusion if required (1-5mg/hr)
Proteinuria +++ on dipstick	Insert urinary catheter. Check urine sample for proteinuria (+/- urine sample to lab for protein:creatinine ratio according to local guidelines) and monitor hourly urine output.

Observations

A	Clear
B	RR 28/min SpO$_2$ 96% on O$_2$
C	HR 110bpm BP 195/112
D	A<u>V</u>PU
E	Temp 36.7°C

CTG: Fetal bradycardia if put on immediately after seizure, normalises after a couple of minutes.

Proceed to stage 2 once magnesium sulphate bolus commenced and antihypertensive given

Stage 2: Immediate post-seizure care and treatment of severe hypertension

Information given	Expected actions
Patients' partner (facilitator) arrives with hand-held notes. Patient remains post-ictal.	Maintain left lateral position until GCS 15
	Commence maintenance dose of magnesium sulphate once loading dose is complete (1g/hr) – made up as per local guidelines

115

Information given	Expected actions
Maternity notes indicate a low risk pregnancy No history of epilepsy No history of high BP or proteinuria in the pregnancy Her partner informs you that she has complained of swelling of hands and legs over the last few days and tonight developed a severe headache She has had period pains and 'niggles' on-and-off today	Take history
	Assess for complications of pre-eclampsia and other pathologies with clinical examination, including:
Less drowsy - GCS 15:talking and opening eyes now Cranial nerves intact No neurological deficit – normal power and sensation upper and lower limbs 4 beats of clonus present Brisk reflexes	Neurological examination
Trachea central, good chest expansion bilaterally good air entry bilaterally chest clear	Respiratory examination
Abdomen soft, non-tender	Abdominal examination
	Communicate events to patient and partner
	Transfer patient from triage to obstetric HDU once safe to do so
Facilitator may prompt that 15 minutes have passed since first dose antihypertensive	Reassess BP 15 mins after first dose of antihypertensive –remains high
	Administer further antihypertensive treatment as per local protocol
	Anaesthetist plans to insert arterial line

Proceed to stage 3 once history and examination complete and further antihypertensive given

Observations 15 mins after first dose antihypertensive	
A	Clear
B	RR 20/min SpO$_2$ 100% on O$_2$
C	HR 118bpm BP 188/105
D	**A**VPU
E	Temp 36.7°C
CTG	Normal

Stage 3: Patient in active labour - plan made for labour and delivery	
Information given	**Expected actions**
Patient is now fully alert and reporting contractions.	Commence continuous fetal monitoring
Cervix is fully effaced, 8cm dilated	Perform vaginal examination
If needed, partner could prompt: 'What happens next then? Is it safe to go through labour now?"	Plan for on-going care: Obstetric HDU care with continuous intra-arterial BP monitoring Maintain BP <150mmHg/80-100mmHg
	Continue magnesium sulphate infusion until 24 hours after delivery (or until 24 hours after seizure, whichever is latest)
	Fluid restriction 80ml/hr with strict input-output fluid monitoring
	Frequency of blood tests and assessment of deep tendon reflexes as per local protocol (e.g: bloods 6-hourly, deep tendon reflexes 4-hourly)
	Consider options for analgesia: ansaesthetist to check blood results prior to consideration of regional analgesia/anaesthesia
	VTE risk assessment
	Antacid prophylaxis
	Plan for delivery in conjunction with woman and senior obstetric team –no contraindication to vaginal delivery
	Plan for management of the 3rd stage –avoid ergometrine, give syntocinon.
	Use concentrated syntocinon regime if 40 IU syntocinon infusion is required postpartum
Scenario ends when plan for ongoing care is discussed with Sarah and her partner	

Observations	
A	Clear
B	RR 16 SpO$_2$ 99% on O$_2$
C	HR 103bpm BP 161/88 CRT 2s
D	**A**VPU
E	Temp 36.5°C
CTG	Normal

Suggested Topics for Debrief Discussion

- Did the team consider causes other than eclampsia for the seizure?
- How easy was it to access: emergency checklist (if available locally), eclampsia box/trolley, syringe driver, antihypertensive drugs? Could this be improved?

Discussion

Acute Seizure Management in Pregnancy

A seizure occurring in pregnancy is an obstetric emergency requiring prompt management to avert or reduce maternal and fetal morbidity. Although the cause may not be immediately known, clinical management should always proceed via a systematic approach (ABCDE prioritisation) and include actions to minimise self-inflicted harm. Due to altered physiology in pregnancy – which increases the likelihood of aspiration, increases the metabolic oxygen demand and necessitates displacement of the gravid uterus from the vena cava – the risks associated with seizures are increased in pregnancy.

Acute management of a maternal seizure must include investigation to determine the likely cause. Some potential causes of seizures in pregnancy are provided in Table 17.1 but also, any pathology causing

Table 17.1 Differential diagnosis of maternal seizure (alphabetical).

Amniotic fluid embolus	Hyponatraemia
Cerebral venous sinus thrombosis	Infection
Dural puncture (iatrogenic – postpartum)	Intracerebral mass lesion
Eclampsia	Non-epileptic attack disorder
Epilepsy (primary, secondary or gestational)	Stroke: ischaemic or haemorrhagic
Hypocalcaemia	Thrombotic thrombocytopenic purpura
Hypoglycaemia	Withdrawal from substance of abuse

Table 17.2 Investigation of a seizure in pregnancy.

Investigation	Indication
Maternal observations, including BP	All
Urine for proteinuria	All
Capillary blood glucose (CBG)	All
Blood tests; for FBC, U+E, LFT, Coagulation screen (including fibrinogen) and G+S	All
Serum blood glucose	Diabetes, liver failure, hypopituitarism, abnormal CBG
Sepsis screening	Pyrexia, history, clinical symptoms/signs
CT/MRI head or venogram (discuss with radiologist)	Focal neurological deficit, atypical seizures or recovery, altered consciousness, red-flag headache
EEG (non-acute)	In conjunction with CT head for the investigation of first seizure in pregnancy where epilepsy is considered as diagnosis

severe hypoxia or hypotension can present with a seizure due to inadequate oxygen delivery to the brain.

Due to its background population incidence (1 in 200), epilepsy is the commonest cause of seizures in pregnancy. Eclampsia must always be considered in women with new-onset seizures in the second half of pregnancy, except where there is a clear history and clinical findings indicating an alternative cause; urgent treatment with magnesium sulphate should be administered in the first instance while investigations continue to determine the cause.

Acute investigations required for all women with seizure (unless known epileptic cause) are listed in Table 17.2. Interpretation of these preliminary investigations in their clinical context will direct

further investigations to confirm or refute suspected causes.

Pre-eclampsia

Worldwide, hypertensive disorders of pregnancy are the second largest contributor to direct maternal mortality (after haemorrhage), accounting for around 14% of all maternal deaths (Say et al., 2014).

Definition

Pre-eclampsia has historically been defined as new onset hypertension (systolic blood pressure (SBP) >140 mmHg or diastolic blood pressure (DBP) >90 mmHg) after 20 weeks gestation with proteinuria (>0.3 g/24 h). With a better understanding of the disease process, the International Society for the study of Hypertension in Pregnancy (ISSHP) have revised the definition (Tranquilli et al., 2014).

Pre-eclampsia is now diagnosed when there is de novo hypertension > 20 weeks gestation with one or more of the following:

1. Proteinuria (protein:creatinine ratio (PCR) ≥ 30 mg/mmol or ≥ 300 mg/day or 2+ protein on dipstick)
2. Maternal organ dysfunction (renal insufficiency, liver involvement, neurological complications or haematological complications)
3. Fetal growth restriction (FGR)

Classification of hypertension (NICE, 2010):

Mild: BP < 150/100 mmHg

Moderate: BP 150–159/100–109 mmHg

Severe: BP 160/110 mmHg or higher

Eclampsia

Definition

Eclampsia is the new onset of grand mal seizure activity during pregnancy or postpartum in a woman with pre-eclampsia (although for many women the seizure may precede documentation of symptoms and signs of pre-eclampsia – 2/3 of women in the UK who develop eclampsia do not have hypertension and proteinuria documented in the preceding week (Nelson-Piercy, 2015).

Incidence

The incidence of eclampsia varies from 0.1% in Europe to 2.7% in Africa (Abalos et al., 2013). Eclampsia is three times more likely in teenagers.

Clinical Presentation

Eclampsia may arise in the antenatal (~45%), intrapartum (~20%) or postnatal (~35%) period. Eclamptic seizures are typically short-lasting, tonic–clonic seizures followed by a brief period of post-ictal drowsiness.

The most common symptom that immediately precedes eclamptic seizures is a headache, with or without visual disturbance.

Neurological examination following eclamptic seizures is usually normal, apart from clonus or brisk reflexes. In women with a seizure fitting this description with history and/or clinical findings in support of a diagnosis of pre-eclampsia, no further investigation may be required to confirm the diagnosis. It should not be forgotten that pre-eclampsia can cause or coexist with intracerebral pathologies; therefore, any focal neurological signs, altered consciousness/confusion, an atypical presentation or severe headache should be an indication for neuroimaging. The choice of imaging should be made in conjunction with a radiologist according to local service availability and suspected pathology.

The fetal heart rate is likely to show abnormalities at the time of a seizure due to maternal hypoxia or reduced venous return. A bradycardia in this scenario should not warrant urgent intervention to deliver as maternal well-being remains the primary concern and maternal stabilisation is the most likely recourse to fetal resuscitation. There is no evidence of long-term morbidity resulting from *in utero* hypoxia related to an isolated seizure.

Management

Management of eclampsia should focus on:

- emergency management of the fitting patient including IV magnesium sulphate for seizure treatment and secondary prevention,
- acute treatment of severe hypertension if present (see discussion – Chapter 18),
- multidisciplinary planning of delivery once stable,
- ongoing management of severe pre-eclampsia (see discussion – Chapter 18).

Magnesium Sulphate

Magnesium sulphate is the drug of choice for treating eclampsia and prevention of further seizures. Administration of magnesium sulphate to women with severe pre-eclampsia significantly reduces the incidence of eclampsia compared to other anticonvulsants (Duley et al., 2010). Magnesium sulphate is administered as a

Table 17.3 NICE-recommended protocol for administration of magnesium sulphate (NICE, 2010).

Loading dose	4 g magnesium sulphate over 5 minutes
Maintenance	1 g/h until 24 h post-delivery or 24 h post the most recent fit (whichever is later)
First fit on magnesium or recurrent fit	Further 2–4 g bolus and increase infusion to 2 g/h

loading bolus followed by a maintenance infusion as described in Table 17.3.

Women commonly feel flushed and unwell during magnesium sulphate bolus infusion; they should be reassured that this is common and temporary.

Mechanism of Action

The mechanism of magnesium sulphate as an anticonvulsant is incompletely understood. Possible modes of action include the following (Euser et al., 2009).

- Competitive antagonist to the glutamate N-methyl-D-aspartate receptor (thereby increasing the seizure threshold).
- Cerebral vasodilator (but effects on cerebral vasculature more modest than vasculature elsewhere).
- Decreasing the release of acetylcholine at motor end plates within the neuromuscular junction.
- Decreasing permeability of the blood–brain barrier (possibly by calcium antagonism), thereby decreasing cerebral oedema formation.
- Inhibition of platelet aggregation.

Monitoring of Magnesium Therapy

Therapeutic serum magnesium levels required to prevent eclampsia were thought to be > 2 mmol/L (suggested therapeutic range 2–3.5 mmol/L), but the relationship between serum level and clinical effect may not be that simple, as some studies have demonstrated effective prevention of seizures with regimes that result in serum magnesium of < 2.0 mmol/L (Okusanya et al., 2016) and conversely, there are also reports of clinical failure among patients with serum magnesium levels in what was thought to be the therapeutic range.

As magnesium levels increase into the toxic range, progressive neuromuscular depression may result in (Idama et al., 1998):

- loss of deep tendon reflexes (~5 mmol/L);
- slurred speech, drowsiness, nausea, double vision, facial paraesthesia (~3.8–5 mmol/L);

- ECG changes (increased PR interval, wide QRS, T-wave changes);
- severe muscle weakness (6–8 mmol/L);
- respiratory depression (>6 mm/L);
- sinoatrial and atrioventricular node blockade leading to complete heart block (>7.5 mmol/L);
- cardiac arrest (>12 mmol/L).

Magnesium is renally excreted and in the presence of normal urine output serum levels do not need to be monitored. Clinical signs of magnesium toxicity should be observed by continuous oxygen saturation monitoring and regular monitoring of respiratory rate and assessment of deep tendon reflexes.

Monitoring of serum magnesium levels is indicated in women with renal impairment or in the presence of oliguria. Magnesium toxicity is treated by stopping the infusion and administering 10 ml 10% calcium gluconate IV in severe cases.

Delivery

The multifactorial decision to deliver a preterm baby in pre-eclampsia is discussed further in Chapter 18. In the context of eclampsia, or severe pre-eclampsia with other end-organ dysfunction, the maternal risks associated with ongoing pregnancy necessitate urgent delivery. Delivery should not be attempted until the maternal condition is stabilised, including control of BP.

There is no clear evidence favouring caesarean section or vaginal delivery in severe pre-eclampsia (NICE, 2010). An assessment of individual factors by a senior obstetrician, in conjunction with the woman's wishes, is required to determine the most appropriate mode of delivery. Any pre-existing absolute or relative contraindications to vaginal delivery or induction of labour should be weighed in accordance with the fetal condition, the favourability of the cervix and the urgency of delivery.

Following delivery, ergometrine should be avoided due to the risk of an acute elevation of BP. If syntocinon infusion is required postpartum, this should also be administered as a concentrated regime to limit the volume infused.

For further discussion of pre-eclampsia, including anaesthetic considerations, see the discussion in Chapter 18.

Bibliography

Abalos, E., Cuesta, C., Grosso, A. L., Chou, D. and Say, L. (2013). Global and regional estimates of preeclampsia and eclampsia: a systematic review. *European Journal of Obstetrics, Gynecology and Reproductive Biology*, 170(1), 1–7.

Aya, A. G. M., Ondze, B., Ripart, J. and Cuvillon, P. (2016). Seizures in the peripartum period: epidemiology, diagnosis and management. *Anaesthesia Critical Care & Pain Medicine*, 35, S13–S21.

Duley, L., Gulmezoglu, A. M., Henderson-Smart, D. J. and Chou, D. (2010). Magnesium sulphate and other anticonvulsants for women with pre-eclampsia. In L. Duley (Ed.), *Cochrane Database of Systematic Reviews*. Chichester: John Wiley & Sons.

Euser, A. and Cipolla, M. (2009). Magnesium sulphate therapy for the prevention of eclampsia: a brief review. *Stroke*, 40(4), 1169–1175.

Idamo, O. and Lindow, S. (1998). Magnesium sulphate: a review of clinical pharmacology applied to obstetrics. *British Journal of Obstetrics and Gynaecology*, 105, 260–268.

National Institute for Health and Care Excellence. (2010). *Hypertension in Pregnancy: Diagnosis and Management.* London: NICE.

Nelson-Piercy, C. (2015). Hypertension and pre-eclampsia. In C. Nelson-Piercy (Ed.), *Handbook of Obstetric Medicine*, 5th edn. Boca Raton: CRC Press.

Okusanya, B. O., Oladapo, O. T., Long, Q., et al. (2016). Clinical pharmacokinetic properties of magnesium sulphate in women with pre-eclampsia and eclampsia. *British Journal of Obstetrics and Gynaecology*, 123, 356–366.

Say, L., Chou, D., Gemmill, A., et al. (2014). Global causes of maternal death: a WHO systematic analysis. *Lancet Global Health*, 2(6), e323–e333.

Tranquilli, A., Dekker, G., Magee, L., et al. (2014). The classification, diagnosis and management of the hypertensive disorders of pregnancy: a revised statement from the ISSHP. *Pregnancy Hypertension*, 4, 97–104.

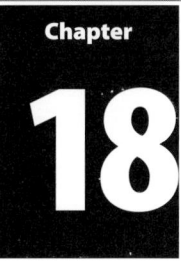

Chapter

18

HELLP Syndrome with Fetal Compromise Requiring an Emergency GA Caesarean Section

Emma Shawkat, Stephanie Worton and Jenny Myers

Scenario in a Nutshell

Woman presents with severe hypertension, headache and epigastric pain. Probable HELLP syndrome from blood results and clinical picture. Needs urgent category 1 GA caesarean section.

Stage 1: Initial assessment of hypertensive, pregnant woman with headache and epigastric pain.

Stage 2: Stabilisation prior to delivery and consideration of differential diagnosis.

Stage 3: Preparation and induction of general anaesthesia for category 1 caesarean section with attempts to attenuate the response to laryngoscopy.

Target Learner Groups

All members of the multidisciplinary obstetric team: midwives, obstetricians, anaesthetists, operating department practitioners/anaesthetic nurses, theatre scrub team.

Suggested learning opportunities
Demonstrate thorough assessment and investigation of pregnant woman presenting with acute hypertension, headache and epigastric pain
Consideration of differential diagnosis of thrombocytopenia in this presentation and likely diagnosis of HELLP syndrome
Effective team management of pre-eclampsia and HELLP
Demonstrate adapting anaesthetic induction technique to attenuate response to laryngoscopy and intubation in hypertensive patient

Suggested learners (to represent their normal roles)	In the room from the start	Available when requested
Midwife	√	
Anaesthetic ST3+		√
Anaesthetic consultant		√ at home
Obstetric ST3+	√	
Midwife Coordinator		√
Operating Department Practitioner (ODP)/anaesthetic nurse		√

Suggested learners (to represent their normal roles)	In the room from the start	Available when requested
Scrub nurse		√
Suggested facilitators		
Faculty to play role of midwife handing over	√	

Details for Facilitators

Patient Demographics

Name: Hannah

Age: 32

Gestation: 35+1

Booking weight: 78 kg

Parity: P1

Scenario Summary

A 32-year-old multip is 35 weeks pregnant. She presents to antenatal triage with a headache, epigastric pain and reduced fetal movements.

On triage she is found to be hypertensive with ++ protein on urine dipstick.

Fetal heart (FH) auscultated.

Labile BP with a pathological CTG; however, BP responds to second-line antihypertensives.

Blood results abnormal: thrombocytopenia, anaemia and abnormal LFTs.

Delivery required due to suspected fetal compromise.

Requires a GA due to thrombocytopenia.

Set-up Overview for Facilitators

Clinical setting	In a triage room, on a trolley
Patient position	Sitting
Initial monitoring in place	Pulse oximeter, NIBP
Other equipment	CTG
Useful manikin functions	Intubation

Medical Equipment

For core equipment checklist, see Chapter 9 including advanced airway equipment.

Additional equipment specific to scenario

IV antihypertensive agents according to local guidance	Local emergency checklist for severe pre-eclampsia (if available)	Arterial line
Drugs to attenuate response to laryngoscopy/intubation, e.g. Opioids: alfentanil, remifentanil, fentanyl Magnesium sulphate Lidocaine GTN Labetalol Esmolol	Induction agents (thiopentone and propofol) Neuromuscular blockers (depolarising and non-depolarising)	Magnesium sulphate and diluent
Antacids: sodium citrate, ranitidine		

Information Given to the Learners

Information given to ST3+ obstetric trainee who has been asked to review the patient and the midwife who is taking over care of the patient.

Time: 21:00

This handover is given by a facilitator playing the role of the current midwife.

The SBAR handover is as follows:

Situation: This is Hannah, she arrived in triage a few minutes ago with high blood pressure, headache, abdominal pain and reduced fetal movements.

Background: Hannah is a 32-year-old para 1, gravida 4. She is 35 weeks pregnant. She has had 2 previous first-trimester miscarriages and 1 normal vaginal delivery at 36 weeks following induction of labour (IOL) for pre-eclampsia. Her booking BP was 112/78 mmHg. She feels her fetal movements have been reduced over the last 24 hours.

Assessment: We have done a set of observations: her last BP was 172/101. We have dipped her urine: she has 2+ of protein. I am just getting the CTG on now.

Recommendation: Would you be able to review her and make a plan please?

Scenario Schedule

Observations	
A	Clear
B	RR 21/min SpO$_2$ 97% on air
C	HR 110bpm BP 188/110
D	**A**VPU
E	Temp 36.7°C
CTG	Suspicious: baseline 140bpm, variability >5bpm with unprovoked decelerations

Stage 1: Initial assessment of hypertensive, pregnant woman with headache and epigastric pain	
Information given	**Expected actions**
Patient complaining of severe headache	Initial systematic ABCDE approach to patient and apply full monitoring
	Acute, severe hypertension noted
	CTG commenced Concern regarding CTG but realise Hannah needs full assessment and stabilisation as priority
	Call for senior obstetric and anaesthetic help and inform midwife co-ordinator

Information given	Expected actions
Feeling generally unwell for ~3 days, with a headache today and a couple of days' history of swollen ankles. No visual symptoms. Feels fetal movements have been reduced over the past 24 hours. On further questioning also has epigastric pain. No vomiting. No shortness of breath. On examination: Resp: trachea central, chest clear, good air entry bilaterally, no added sounds. CVS: HS 1+2+0, bilateral oedema to knees Abdo: soft, epigastric tenderness, bowel sounds present CNS: normal power and tone of upper and lower limbs, 4 beats of clonus, reflexes normal.	Take a history and perform examination while treating the hypertension
	Secure IV access x2 Take blood for FBC, U+E, LFT, Coagulation including fibrinogen and G+S.
CBG 6.0 mmol/L	Check CBG
	Urgent BP control as per local severe pre-eclampsia guidelines. Local example: • Labetalol 50mg IV bolus slowly, repeat after 10 mins (up to dose 200mg) +/- Infusion of neat labetalol (5mg/ml): 20mg/hr double every 30 mins to maximum up to 160mg/hr • Hydralazine 2.5mg IV slowly. Repeat at 20 min intervals if necessary up to max of 20mg. Infusion if required 1mg/ml at rate of 1-5ml/hr
	Commence loading dose of 4g IV magnesium sulphate, made up and infused according to local guidance
	Keep patient safe and transfer to obstetric HDU
	Fluid restrict to 80mls/hr and commence meticulous fluid balance documentation

123

Information given	Expected actions
If asks to dip urine, remind that sample in triage showed proteinuria++	Catheterise and send urine for uPCR (urinary protein:creatinine ratio)
	IM steroids for fetal lung maturation (however delivery not to be delayed for 2nd dose)
	Inform neonatal intensive care unit (NICU)
	Apply mechanical thromboprophylaxis (TED stockings or intermittent pneumatic compression devices)

Proceed to Stage 2 once initial assessment complete and treatment has been initiated for acute, severe hypertension

Stage 2: Stabilisation prior to delivery and consideration of differential diagnosis

Information given	Expected actions
Patient is now in obstetric HDU and it is ~15 minutes after 1st dose of antihypertensive was given.	
Anaesthetic ST3+ arrives	SBAR from ST3+ obstetrics
Prompt that loading dose of MgSO4 almost complete	Maintenance dose of MgSO4 1g/hour commenced (prepared according to local guidance)
	Repeat all observations
	As BP remains high 15 minutes after 1st dose of antihypertensive, give second dose of antihypertensive or change to second agent as per local guidelines
	Obstetricians concerned regarding CTG and wish to perform caesarean section but appreciate need to stabilise patient first
	Anaesthetist states that need to stabilise mother prior to delivery but preparations for theatre can be made concurrently Call theatre team Call anaesthetic consultant in from home Transfer to theatre for further stabilisation prior to caesarean section Consider an arterial line

Observations	
A	Clear
B	RR 18/min SpO$_2$ 97% on air
C	HR 108bpm BP 170/103
D	**A**VPU
E	Temp 36.8°C
CTG	Pathological: baseline 150bpm, variability <5bpm and decelerations

Information given	Expected actions
Initial blood results are available: WCC 11.8 X 10^9/L Hb 89 g/L Plts 71 X 10^9/l Fibrinogen 4 g/L PT 11.2s APTT 26s Bili 41 µmol/L AST 212 I.U./L ALT 256 I.U./L Albumin 28 g/L	
Raised reticulocyte count on peripheral bood film LDH 620 IU/L haptoglobin 0.18 g/L(low)	Recognise likely diagnosis of microangiopathic haemolytic anaemia (MAHA) Request tests to confirm haemolysis: peripheral blood film, LDH +/- haptoglobin (liaise with local lab)
If asked: Headache today but no CNS symptoms such as confusion, irritability, agitation No history of bloody diarrhoea (HUS)	Look for other signs/symptoms to help narrow differential diagnosis of MAHA (see discussion in Chapter 19 and Table 19.1)
CBG 6.2mmol/l	Check CBG if not done earlier
	Recognise likely diagnosis of HELLP
	Anticipate haemorrhage during caesaraen section: Cross match 4-6 units blood Ensure 2 X large bore IV access Have fluid warming and rapid fluid infusor available Discuss with haematologist on call
	BP now stabilising: team aiming for a systolic BP<160mmHg prior to surgery
	Team decision that mother is now stable enough to proceed with urgent caesarean section
	Anaesthetist considers risks of regional anaesthesia versus GA – in view of low PLTS, prepares for GA

Progress to stage 3 once second antihypertensive dose has been given, BP has stabilised and team are preparing for GA

Observations	
A	Clear
B	RR 22/min SpO$_2$ 97% on air
C	HR 100bpm BP 154/95
D	**A**VPU
E	Temp 36.9°C
CTG	Pathological: baseline 150bpm, variability <5bpm and decelerations

Stage 3: Preparation and induction of general anaesthesia for category 1 caesarean section with attempts to attenuate the response to laryngoscopy

Information given	Expected actions
Fit and well no regular medications, no drug allergies No previous GAs or family history of problems with Gas Last eaten 7 hours ago	Anaesthetist takes a focussed history
Mallampati 2, Calder A, good range of cervical spine movements. Some facial oedema, no hoarseness or altered voice	Perform airway assessment
	Ensure correct positioning – 15° left lateral tilt, head-up for preoxygenation and position optimised for intubation
	Brief explanation of procedure including cricoid pressure and consent for GA including mention of risk of awareness
	Check patency of IV cannula and ensure fluid attached and running (but doesn't administer large volumes)
	Antacid prophylaxis: Sodium citrate and IV ranitidine (if not received PO ranitidine earlier)
	Suction available, switched on
	Prepare drugs for induction of anaesthesia – have 2 syringes of induction agent available
	Consider the need to attenuate the response to laryngoscopy and use appropriate drugs and doses (see discussion)
	Once history taken, commence preoxygenation with facemask and nasal cannulae for 2-3 mins or ETO2 >0.9.
	Meanwhile, theatre team, obstetrican and midwife are preparing for caesarean section
	Neonatal team called to attend

Observations	
A	Intubated
B	RR as per ventilator SpO$_2$ 99%, FiO2 1.0
C	HR and BP dependent on drugs and doses given at induction. BP dangerously high if no attempt to attenuate response to laryngoscopy.
D	Anaesthetised
E	Temp 36.7°C

Information given	Expected actions
	WHO checklist undertaken as per local guidance. As part of this, the anaesthetist should clearly verbalise: • Plan A, B and C of their airway strategy (including checking a range of smaller endotracheal tubes (ETT) are available and asking for a size 7.0 ETT as first-line) • Who their emergency anaesthetic assistance is and how they can be contacted in case of difficult airway • Plan made to either continue surgery using a supraglottic airway or wake the patient up in the event of a failed intubation (see fig 24.2, chapter 24)
Grade 2b intubation	Induction and intubation – anaesthetist should adapt anaesthetic technique to attenuate pressor response to laryngoscopy and intubation (see discussion)
Scenario ends once patient successfully intubated and Caesarean Section is about to proceed	

Suggested Topics for Debrief Discussion

• Was acute severe hypertension treated appropriately by the team?
• Anaesthetist: taking into account the cardiovascular response to intubation in the scenario, were you happy with the measures that you used to attenuate the response to laryngoscopy or is there anything you would alter if doing it again?

Discussion

Pre-eclampsia

For definition of pre-eclampsia and classifications of hypertension, see Discussion, Chapter 17.

Features of Severe Pre-eclampsia (SPE)

• Severe hypertension and proteinuria **or**
• Mild or moderate hypertension and proteinuria with one or more of the following:
  · symptoms of severe headache
  · problems with vision, such as blurring or flashing before the eyes
  · severe pain just below the ribs or vomiting
  · papilloedema
  · signs of clonus ($\geq$ 3 beats)
  · liver tenderness
  · HELLP syndrome
  · platelet count falling to below 100×10^9 per litre
  · abnormal liver enzymes (ALT or AST rising to above 70 IU/l).

Incidence

Pre-eclampsia complicates 2–8% of pregnancies (Duley, 2009) with severe pre-eclampsia occurring in 0.5% of pregnancies.

Aetiology

Pre-eclampsia (PE) is a pregnancy-specific disorder, with unknown aetiology. It is a heterogeneous disease that is believed to be either placental or maternal in origin (Ness and Roberts, 1996). Placental PE is due to abnormal invasion of the trophoblast cells and maladaptation of the maternal spiral arteries that results in uteroplacental hypoxia and a systemic inflammatory response producing the clinical signs of PE (Redman, 1991). Maternal

127

PE is due to an exacerbated maternal response to the systemic inflammatory process of normal pregnancy, with a normal placenta (Redman and Sargent, 2004).

Risk Factors for Pre-eclampsia

Several maternal factors are known to increase the risk of developing PE including (Duckitt and Harrington, 2005):

- previous history of pre-eclampsia
- pre-existing diabetes
- chronic hypertension
- chronic kidney disease
- autoimmune disease such as antiphospholipid syndrome or systemic lupus erythematosus
- nulliparity
- multiple pregnancy
- family history of PE
- body mass index (BMI) > 35
- maternal age $\geq$ 40

Clinical Presentation

Symptoms and complications of pre-eclampsia reflect the underlying pathophysiology; vasospasm, increased vascular permeability and a systemic inflammatory response are all attributable to widespread vascular endothelial dysfunction. In some women, severe pre-eclampsia is accompanied by headache, visual disturbance, epigastric/upper abdominal pain, progressive oedema or nausea/vomiting. Women may also present with complications of pre-eclampsia, such as pulmonary oedema or eclampsia.

Management

Women should be managed in a consultant-led unit and admission to hospital is recommended for all women with pre-eclampsia (NICE, 2010).

BP Monitoring and Control

The latest Confidential Enquiry into Maternal Deaths and Morbidity (2009–14) emphasised the importance of urgently reducing BP <150/100 mmHg in women with severe hypertension in order to reduce maternal mortality due to intracerebral haemorrhage, the commonest cause of death attributable to pre-eclampsia.

BP should be monitored at least four times a day. Current NICE recommendations are to commence antihypertensive medication for moderate hypertension, with a target BP of <150/80–100 mmHg (NICE,

2010). In the acute situation blood pressure should be measured every 15 minutes and a reduction in blood pressure should be evident within 30–60 minutes. In the absence of a response to first-line therapy, a second antihypertensive agent should be used.

Fetal Well-being

At the time of diagnosis, fetal well-being should be established. Depending on the gestation, a CTG should be performed. When it is appropriate, an ultrasound scan should be performed for fetal growth, liquor volume, dopplers and if necessary, presentation. If the findings are normal a repeat ultrasound should be performed fortnightly (NICE, 2010).

Management of Severe Pre-eclampsia

Local protocols for the management of SPE should be up to date and easily accessible in an acute situation. Most units will have a clearly designated 'eclampsia trolley' (or equivalent) containing required equipment and drugs. Ensuring that all team members are aware of the existence and location of these is an important component of induction and training. Multidisciplinary management with early involvement of experienced clinicians and ensuring rapid maternal stabilisation before contemplating delivery are cornerstones of good management. Women with SPE needing IV therapy require Level 2 care.

Management of severe pre-eclampsia involves:

- Close monitoring of BP and managing acute hypertension to maintain systolic blood pressure $\leq$ 150 mmHg.
- Prevention of eclampsia with magnesium sulphate (see discussion in Chapter 17).
- Fluid restriction and strict monitoring of fluid balance.
- Consideration of timing of delivery.

BP Monitoring and Treatment

The response of maternal BP to each administered dose of an antihypertensive must be checked and documented. If BP remains above target (150/80–100 mmHg), further doses of the same or other agents will be required.

Many units will use continuous intra-arterial BP monitoring in severe pre-eclampsia to allow titration of antihypertensive therapy, particularly if intravenous infusions of antihypertensive agents are required.

Fluid Management

The incidence of maternal deaths due to pulmonary oedema in the UK has fallen following the 1994–1996 Confidential Enquiry into Maternal Deaths due to widespread adoption of more stringent fluid management practices in pre-eclampsia.

Fluid input should be restricted to 80 ml/h for women with SPE (including PO and IV fluids and drugs). A concentrated regime of syntocinon may be used in pre-eclampsia, according to local protocol. In addition to maintenance of 80 ml/h, fluid losses due to haemorrhage (e.g. related to abruption or delivery) require replacement. These regimes require accurate, contemporaneous documentation of fluid balance.

Timing of Delivery

Delivery is the only definitive treatment for severe pre-eclampsia. Timing delivery is a balance between avoiding maternal complications and risks of preterm delivery for the fetus. When expectant management is appropriate, close surveillance of maternal and fetal well-being is necessary.

Beyond 37 weeks delivery is indicated. A multicentre randomised controlled trial compared expectant management and induction of labour (IOL) in a cohort of 756 women with gestational hypertension or mild PE between 36 and 41 weeks gestation. IOL was associated with improvement in maternal outcomes (RR 0.71) (Koopmans et al., 2009).

Prior to 34 weeks expectant management is suggested. Delivery prior to 34 weeks for severe PE reduces the risk of abruption (RR 0.43). However, this puts the neonate at risk of complications (Wang et al., 2017).

It is uncertain whether delivery or expectant management is best for women between 34 and 37 weeks. Planned early delivery appears to reduce the risk of adverse maternal outcomes such as: thromboembolic disease, pulmonary oedema, eclampsia, HELLP syndrome, placental abruption, or maternal death (RR 0.36). However, this comes at the cost of increased neonatal respiratory distress (RR 3.3) (Broekhuijsen et al., 2015). This area of clinical practice is likely to evolve in coming years with the advent of multicentre, randomised clinical trials designed to address these uncertainties.

Complications

Pre-eclampsia is associated with significant maternal and fetal morbidity and mortality.

In the UK, maternal deaths due to pre-eclampsia are at historical lows, occurring in less than one per million live births. This is due in large part to the implementation of local protocols for the management of severe pre-eclampsia to ensure timely application of core interventions to reduce complications (Knight et al., 2016).

Acute maternal complications include:

- Placental abruption
- Disseminated intravascular coagulation (DIC)
- HELLP syndrome
- Pulmonary oedema
- Acute renal failure
- Eclampsia
- Liver failure
- Stroke
- Thromboembolism
- Posterior reversible encephalopathy syndrome (PRES).

Long-term maternal complications include:

- Chronic hypertension
- Coronary artery disease
- Cerebrovascular disease
- Peripheral vascular disease
- Diabetes
- Risk of chronic renal failure.

Fetal complications include:

- Prematurity
- Fetal growth restriction (FGR)
- Hypoxic–ischaemic encephalopathy (HIE)
- Perinatal death
- Long-term cardiovascular morbidity (Sibai et al., 2005).

HELLP Syndrome

Definition/Classification

HELLP is characterised by **H**aemolyisis, **E**levated **L**iver enzymes and **L**ow **P**latelets. Two classification systems have been described: the Tennessee (Sibai et al., 1986) and the Mississippi (Martin et al., 2006). The Tennessee classification defines 'true' HELLP as requiring all three components:

1. Platelets $\leq 100,000 \times 10^9/l$
2. AST ≥ 70 IU/l
3. LDH ≥ 600 IU/l

The Mississippi classification is stratified according to the platelet count:

- Class 1: Platelets $\leq 50,000 \times 10^9$/l, AST/ALT ≥ 70 IU/l and LDH ≥ 600 IU/l
- Class 2: Platelets $50,000–100,000 \times 10^9$/l, AST/ALT ≥ 70 IU/l and LDH ≥ 600 IU/l
- Class 3: Platelets $100,000–150,000 \times 10^9$/l, AST/ALT ≥ 40 IU/l and LDH ≥ 600 IU/l

Incidence

HELLP syndrome occurs in 10–20% of pregnancies that are complicated with severe pre-eclampsia.

Risk Factors

- Multiparity
- Caucasian
- Previous pre-eclampsia/HELLP
- Age > 25 years
- Raised BMI > 30
- Chronic hypertension.

Clinical Presentation

Seventy percent of cases are diagnosed antenatally with peak frequency between 27 and 37 weeks gestation (Sibai et al., 1993). When it occurs postpartum, this is usually within 48 hours of delivery.

Symptoms usually develop over a short period of time and women typically present with:

- Right upper quadrant pain or epigastric pain (90%)
- Malaise (90%)
- Nausea or vomiting (50%) (Sibai, 1990).

Management

Delivery is advised after 34 weeks if multisystem disease is present. A small case-control study found similar outcomes in women who had delivery delayed by up to 48 hours compared to women who had immediate delivery (Fitzpatrick et al., 2014). In cases of prematurity it may be appropriate to delay the delivery until corticosteroids have been administered for fetal lung maturation. Prior to 27 weeks conservative management (of at least 48–72 hours) may be considered. However, the potential short-term gain must be weighed against the increased risk of maternal and fetal complications developing which could result in an emergency caesarean section being required.

Mode of delivery should be determined taking into account maternal history and clinical status as well as fetal gestation and well-being.

Management of the mother is supportive. As with pre-eclampsia, BP control should be maintained and magnesium sulphate should be considered. To date there is no evidence to support the use of corticosteroids in the treatment of HELLP (Woudstra et al., 2009).

Complications

A rare but life-threatening complication is spontaneous rupture of a subcapsular liver haematoma.

More common complications include placental abruption, DIC and postpartum haemorrhage. Perinatal mortality and morbidity is higher than maternal and can be attributed to the gestational age at disease onset, FGR and fetal distress (Aslan et al., 2004).

Anaesthetic Considerations in Severe Pre-eclampsia

Good labour analgesia is important for the woman with severe pre-eclampsia in order to reduce the surges in BP seen with contraction pain. Regional analgesia can be considered in the absence of contraindications. Due to the associated risk of thrombocytopaenia, a recent platelet count should be reviewed prior to regional analgesia. A platelet count of $>100,000 \times 10^9$/l in the 6 hours prior to insertion of neuraxial block is not thought to present any increased risk of vertebral canal haematoma. There is no absolute platelet count below which a central neuraxial block should not be performed; it is a continuum of risk and the decision should be made by a consultant anaesthetist, taking into account the individual circumstances. If the platelet count is $<100 \times 10^9$/l, then a coagulation screen should also be checked. If this is normal, it would be reasonable to perform a central neuraxial block down to a platelet count of 75×10^9/l, depending on the rate of decrease in platelet count (Association of Anaesthetists of Great Britain and Ireland et al., 2013).

For operative delivery, in the absence of contraindications, regional anaesthesia is the preferred method of anaesthesia in severe pre-eclampsia in terms of control of hypertension and avoiding managing a potentially difficult airway. The haemodynamic stability of spinal and epidural anaesthesia is comparable (Visalyaputra et al., 2005). Spinal hypotension is known to be less severe in pre-eclampsia and vasopressor requirements are reduced.

General anaesthesia may be indicated, for example, in the presence of severe thrombocytopenia or developing DIC. In pre-eclamptic women, difficult intubation due to pharyngolaryngeal oedema should be anticipated.

Laryngoscopy and intubation cause a rise in blood pressure and heart rate. With pre-eclampsia, the hypertensive response to intubation is exaggerated. This rise in BP can cause cerebral haemorrhage, cerebral oedema or pulmonary oedema; therefore, the anaesthetic technique for general anaesthesia in a pre-eclamptic woman must be adapted to attenuate the pressor response to laryngoscopy and intubation.

Many drugs have been used to attenuate the haemodynamic response to airway manipulation under general anaesthesia and a useful 2014 review (Pant et al., 2014) looked at the evidence for many of these drugs in the setting of general anaesthesia in patients with severe pre-eclampsia. Some options are outlined in Table 18.1.

Table 18.1 Drugs used to attenuate the haemodynamic response to laryngoscopy and intubation in women with pre-eclampsia.

Drug	Mode of action	Dose studied in pre-eclampsia	Effective at attenuating response to laryngoscopy and intubation?	Onset time	Notes
Esmolol	Selective β-1 antagonist	2 mg/kg or 1 mg/kg in combination with 1.5 mg/kg of lidocaine	Yes	1.5–3 min	May cause transient maternal bradycardia or heart block
Labetalol	Mixed β-1 and β-2 antagonist with some α-antagonist activity (1:7 α:β)	20 mg titrated up to 1 mg/kg	Yes	2–5 min	
Alfentanil	Opioid receptor agonist	10 µg/kg	Yes – when lidocaine 1 mg/kg also given*	1–2 min	Inform neonatal team that opioids have been given
Fentanyl	Opioid receptor agonist	2.5 µg/kg	Yes – when lidocaine 1 mg/kg also given*	3–5 min	
Remifentanil	Opioid receptor agonist	Bolus of 0.5 µg/kg	Yes – 1 µg/kg also studied but resulted in more post-intubation hypotension	< 60 s	
GTN	Direct-acting smooth muscle relaxant via the nitric oxide/cyclic GMP pathway	1.5–2.5 µg/kg bolus (in non-pregnant population) or IV infusion (5 µg/min or titrated to response)	Yes	< 30 s	Can cause short-lived maternal tachycardia and hypotension
Hydralazine	Direct-acting vasodilator	5–10 mg	No	5–20 min	Onset time and long duration of action (1–4 h) make it unsuitable
Lidocaine	Central sodium blockade	1.5 mg/kg	Not when used alone – but can be effective used in combination with other agents	1–2 min	
Magnesium sulphate	Direct-acting vasodilator, α-adrenergic antagonist and inhibits the release of catecholamines	40 mg/kg or 30 mg/kg given with alfentanil 7.5 µg/kg	Yes	< 30 s if given by bolus	Potentiates non-depolarising neuromuscular agents

*Note that lidocaine 1 mg/kg and etomidate 0.3 mg/kg were also given at induction in this small study of pre-eclamptic women. In another study looking at alfentanil 10 µg/kg given with thiopentone and suxamethonium at induction in women with pre-eclampsia, there was a failure to control systolic blood pressure to 180 mmHg or less at laryngoscopy and intubation and for 4 minutes after intubation in 25% of mothers in the alfentanil group, despite satisfactory overall mean values for the change in systolic BP (Allen et al., 1991).
In the non-pregnant population, alfentanil 10–30 µg/kg and fentanyl 2–8 µg/kg have been shown to be effective at attenuating the haemodynamic response to laryngoscopy and intubation.

Bibliography

Allen, R. W., James, M. F. and Uys, P. C. (1991). Attenuation of the pressor response to tracheal intubation in hypertensive proteinuric pregnant patients by lignocaine, alfentanil and magnesium sulphate. *British Journal of Anaesthesia*, 66, 216–223.

Aslan, H., Gul, A. and Cebeci, A. (2004). Neonatal outcome in pregnancies after preterm delivery for HELLP syndrome. *Gynecologic and Obstetric Investigations*, 58(2), 96–99.

Association of Anaesthetists of Great Britain and Ireland, Obstetric Anaesthetists' Association and Regional Anaesthesia UK. (2013). Regional anaesthesia and patients with abnormalities of coagulation. *Anaesthesia*, 68, 966–972.

Broekhuijsen, K., Van Baaren, G. J., Van Pampus, M. G., et al. (2015). Immediate delivery versus expectant monitoring for hypertensive disorders of pregnancy between 34 and 37 weeks of gestation (HYPITAT-II): an open-label, randomised controlled trial. *Lancet*, 385(9986), 2492–2501.

Duckitt, K. and Harrington, D. (2005). Risk factors for pre-eclampsia at antenatal booking: systematic review of controlled studies. *British Medical Journal*, 330(7491), 565.

Duley, L. (2009). The global impact of pre-eclampsia and eclampsia. *Seminars in Perinatology*, 33, 130–137.

Fitzpatrick, K. E., Hinshaw, K., Kurinczuk, J. J. and Knight, M. (2014). Risk factors, management, and outcomes of hemolysis, elevated liver enzymes, and low platelets syndrome and elevated liver enzymes, low platelets syndrome. *Obstetrics and Gynecology*, 123(3), 618–627.

Knight, M., Nair, M., Tuffnell, D., et al. (2016). *Saving Lives, Improving Mothers' Care – surveillance of maternal deaths in the UK 2012–14 and lessons learned to inform maternity care from the UK and Ireland Confidential Enquiries into Maternal Deaths and Morbidity 2009–2014.* Available from: www.npeu.ox.ac.uk/mbrrace-uk

Koopmans, C. M., Bijlenga, D., Groen, H., et al. (2009). Induction of labour versus expectant monitoring for gestational hypertension or mild pre-eclampsia after 36 weeks' gestation (HYPITAT): a multicentre, open-label randomised controlled trial. *Lancet*, 374(9694), 979–988.

Martin, J. N., Rose, C. H. and Briery, C. M. (2006). Understanding and managing HELLP syndrome: The integral role of aggressive glucocorticoids for mother and child. *American Journal of Obstetrics and Gynecology*, 195, 914–934.

Ness, R. B. and Roberts, J. M. (1996). Heterogeneous causes constituting the single syndrome of preeclampsia: a hypothesis and its implications. *American Journal of Obstetrics and Gynecology*, 175(5), 1365–1370.

NICE. (2010). *CG107 Hypertension in Pregnancy: NICE Guideline.* Manchester: NICE. Available from: http://guidance.nice.org.uk/CG107/NICEGuidance/pdf/English (accessed February 17, 2014).

Pant, M., Fong, R. and Scavone, B. (2014). Prevention of peri-induction hypertension in preeclamptic patients: a focused review. *Anesthesia Analgesia*, 119, 1350–1356.

Redman, C. W. G. (1991). Current topic: Pre-eclampsia placenta and the placenta. *Placenta*, 12(4), 301–308.

Redman, C. W. G. and Sargent, I. L. (2004). Preeclampsia and the systemic inflammatory response. *Seminars in Nephrology*, 24, 565–570.

Sibai, B. M. (1990). The HELLP syndrome (hemolysis, elevated liver enzymes, and low platelets): much ado about nothing? *American Journal of Obstetrics and Gynecology*, 162(2), 311–316.

Sibai, B. M., Taslimi, M. M., El-Nazer, A., Amon, E., Mabie, B. C. and Ryan, G. M. (1986). Maternal–perinatal outcome associated with the syndrome of hemolysis, elevated liver enzymes, and low platelets in severe preeclampsia-eclampsia. *American Journal of Obstetrics and Gynecology*, 155(3), 501–507.

Sibai, B. M., Ramadan, M. K., Usta, I., Salama, M., Mercer, B. M. and Friedman, S. A. (1993). Maternal morbidity and mortality in 442 pregnancies with hemolysis, elevated liver enzymes, and low platelets (HELLP syndrome). *American Journal of Obstetrics and Gynecology*, 169(4), 1000–1006.

Sibai, B., Dekker, G. and Kupferminc, M. (2005). Pre-eclampsia. *Lancet*, 365(9461), 785–799.

Tranquilli, A. L., Dekker, G., Magee, L., et al. (2014). The classification, diagnosis and management of the hypertensive disorders of pregnancy: a revised statement from the ISSHP. *Pregnancy and Hypertension*, 4(2), 97–104.

Visalyaputra, S., Rodanant, O., Somboonviboon, W., Tantivitayatan, K., Thienthong, S. and Saengchote, W. (2005). Spinal versus epidural anesthesia for cesarean delivery in severe preeclampsia: a prospective randomized, multicenter study. *Anesthesia Analgesia*, 101(3), 862–888.

Wang, Y., Hao, M., Sampson, S. and Xia, J. (2017). Elective delivery versus expectant management for pre-eclampsia: a meta-analysis of RCTs. *Archives of Gynecology and Obstetrics*, 295(3), 607–622. Available from: www.ncbi.nlm.nih.gov/pubmed/28150165%0Ahttp://link.springer.com/10.1007/s00404-016-4281-9

Woudstra, D. M., Chandra, S. and Hofmeyr, G. J. (2009). Corticosteroids for HELLP (hemolysis, elevated liver enzymes, low platelets) syndrome in pregnancy. *Cochrane Database of Systematic Reviews*, (9), CD008148.

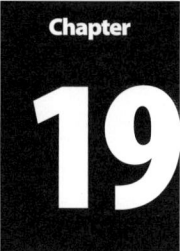

Chapter

19

Microangiopathic Haemolytic Anaemia (MAHA) in Pregnancy Presenting in A&E

Louise Simcox and Jo Gillham

Scenario in a Nutshell

Patient presents with hypertension, proteinuria, headache and confusion. MAHA on blood results. Has seizure. Probable thrombotic thrombocytopenic purpura (TTP).

Stage 1: Initial assessment and management by the emergency department team of a hypertensive, proteinuric, pregnant patient with history of abdominal pain, headache and confusion.

Stage 2: Assessment of patient by obstetrician and anaesthetist. Fetal death in utero (FDIU) diagnosed. MAHA on blood results. Patient becoming increasingly agitated.

Stage 3: Patient deteriorates and has tonic–clonic seizure on critical care. Further multidisciplinary input regarding likely diagnosis of TTP and management.

Target Learner Groups

A+E staff, obstetricians, anaesthetists, critical care doctors and nurses.

Specific learning opportunities
Effective team management of obstetric emergency – MAHA
Exploration of differential diagnosis: TTP/atypical haemolytic uraemic syndrome (HUS)/acute fatty liver/HELLP
Demonstrate appropriate leadership and communication with other specialities
Appropriate use/interpretation of investigations

Suggested learners (to represent their normal roles)	In the room from the start	Available when requested
Emergency department (ED) Registrar	√	
Emergency department (ED) Nurse	√	
Obstetric ST3+		√

Suggested learners (to represent their normal roles)	In the room from the start	Available when requested
Anaesthetic ST3+		√
Critical care ST3+		√
Critical care nurse		√
Suggested facilitators		
Faculty to play role of patient's partner	√	
Haematology ST7		√ in critical care at end of scenario

Details for Facilitators

Patient Demographics

Name: Clare

Age: 32

Gestation: 25+4

Booking weight: 81 kg

Parity: P0

Scenario Summary for Facilitators

32-year-old 25+4/40 gestation primigravida attended emergency department (ED) with headache, abdominal pain and reported confusion.
Seen by ED team in Majors – hypertension with proteinuria, confused and agitated. Transferred to Resuscitation bay.
Seen by Obstetric Team – identify FDIU.
Abnormal blood results – explore differential diagnosis of MAHA.
CT head and liver USS.
Transfer to Critical Care Unit.
Seizure on critical care.
Confirm likely diagnosis of TTP – management plan for plasma exchange and delivery.

Set-up Overview for Facilitators

Clinical setting	On a trolley in Emergency Department Majors
Patient position	Semi-recumbent
Initial monitoring in place	Pulse oximeter NIBP cuff ECG
Other equipment	Nil
Useful manikin functions	Seizures

Medical Equipment

For core equipment checklist, see Chapter 9 including advanced airway equipment.

Additional equipment specific to scenario		
Doppler fetal monitor	Ultrasound machine	Magnesium Sulphate (MgSO$_4$)
Labetalol PO/IV, hydralazine or other antihypertensives as per local severe pre-eclampsia protocol	Pen torch	Tendon hammer
Arterial line	Benzodiazepines	

Information Given to the Learners

Information given to ED nurse and ED registrar who are taking over care at start of their shift

Time: 08:00

This handover is given by a facilitator playing the role of the ED nurse from the night shift who is now going home.

The SBAR handover is as follows:

Situation: This is Clare. She has just come around from the waiting room with a bad headache, abdominal pain and a history of being confused a bit earlier.

Background: 32 years old, previously fit and well primip who is 25+4 weeks pregnant. She has no allergies and is on no regular medication. History from partner – unwell for 4–5 days with abdominal pain, headache for past 2 days and intermittently confused over last 24 hours. Noted blood in urine today. Referred following telephone consultation with GP.

Assessment: I have done her first set of observations.

Recommendation: Are you two OK to take over her care?

Scenario Schedule

Stage 1: Initial assessment and management by the emergency department team of a hypertensive, proteinuric, pregnant patient with history of abdominal pain, headache and confusion.

Information given	Expected actions
Patient is intermittently confused and complaining of abdominal pain. Concerned about her baby	
Patient is usually well, no significant past medical history	Elicit history from patient/husband while performing a set of observations
Started with abdominal pain 4-5 days ago. She has had a headache for the last 2 days. No visual symptoms. No nausea and vomiting. No diarrhoea.	
Odd behaviour intermittently over last 24 hrs. Partner reports confused speech –eg: She was talking about one of her work colleagues being in their kitchen but Clare and her partner were at home alone.	
She noticed some blood in her urine this morning and when husband rang the GP, she told them to come to A+E	

Observations	
A	Clear
B	RR 14/min SpO$_2$ 97% on air
C	HR 77bpm BP 162/110 CRT 2s
D	**A**VPU
E	Temp 36.7°C

Information given	Expected actions
On examination, patient noted to have facial oedema and jaundiced sclera. Some petechiae noted on lower legs.	Commence systematic ABCDE approach
Patient talking	Assess airway and apply O_2 if required to maintain $SpO_2 \geq 94\%$
Chest clear, no added sounds	
Abdomen is soft and non-tender	
Neurological examination: Difficult as patient struggling to perform the tasks requested and then getting upset Brisk reflexes at ankle and knee, right more than left 3 beats clonus Pupils equal and reactive to light GCS 14-15, some confused speech intermittently –saying she doesn't have enough money and wants to leave	
	Secure IV access and take blood for FBC, U+E, LFT, CRP, Coagulation including fibrinogen and G+S
CBG 6.6 mmol/L	Check CBG
Urine noted to have 2+ protein and 4+blood	Dipstick urine and send urine for uPCR (urinary protein:creatinine ratio)
ABG if requested: (on air) pH 7.4 pO2 13.1 kPa pCO2 4.0 kPa Hb 90 g/L BE -2mmol/L HCO3- 20 mmol/L Lactate 1.8 mmol/L	Consider ABG
	Contact Obstetric on-call team to urgently review
	Recognise and treat hypertension: eg. PO labetalol 200mg /IV bolus 50mg labetalol slowly over 5-10mins or nifedipine PO 10mg (or as per local guidance)
	Start IV bolus of 4g MgSO4 as per local guidance
Becoming agitated and upset – doesn't want any more tests done. Trying to get off trolley and leave.	Book urgent CT head in view of recent onset confusion and headache
	Transfer to resus

Proceed to stage 2 once initial assessment complete and treatment for hypertension commenced.

Stage 2: Assessment of patient by obstetrician and anaesthetist. Fetal death in utero (FDIU) diagnosed. Microangiopathic haemolytic anaemia (MAHA) on blood results. Patient becoming increasingly agitated

Observations	
A	Clear
B	RR 22/min SpO$_2$ 98% on air
C	HR 89bpm BP 168/112 CRT 2s
D	**A**VPU
E	Temp 36.8°C

Information given	Expected actions
Patient now in resus	
Obstetric registrar and anaesthetic registrar arrive	SBAR from emergency department (ED) registrar
	Recheck observations
Unable to find fetal heart (FH) on auscultation	Listen in to fetal heart (FH)
USS confirms FDIU. Obstetrician informs Clare and husband	Scan for FH
	If history or examination incomplete from ED registrar, complete now
Husband worried, patient obviously confused now, getting very agitated, trying to remove ECG stickers and pulse oximeter.	
	Consultant obstetrician, consultant anaesthetist and ED consultant called
	Commence loading dose of 4g magnesium sulphate if not done already, made up and infused according to local protocol
	Then maintenance dose of magnesium sulphate: 1g/hr.
	BP control as per local severe pre-eclampsia guidelines Local example: • Labetolol 50mg IV bolus slowly repeat after 10 mins (up to dose 200mg) +/- Infusion of neat labetalol (5mg/ml): 20mg /hr double every 30 mins to maximum up to 160mg/hr • Hydralazine 2.5mg IV slowly. Repeat at 20 min intervals if necessary up to max of 20mg. Infusion if required: hydralazine 1mg/ml at rate of 1-5ml/hr
	Insert urinary catheter and urometer for hourly urine output, fluid restrict to 80 mls/hr

Information given	Expected actions
Blood results are back from lab: **FBC:** WCC 21.8 X 10 9/L Hb 88 g/L PLTs 27 X 10 9/L Lab have performed peripheral blood film in view of thrombocytopenia and anaemia: increased reticulocyte count (7.92%), red blood cell fragments	Diagnose MAHA from blood results
	Discussion with team regarding differential diagnosis of MAHA in this scenario: • HELLP syndrome • Acute fatty liver of pregnancy • Atypical haemolytic uraemic syndrome (HUS) • Thromotic thrombocytopenic purpura (TTP) (see discussion)
U+Es: Na+ 135 mmol/L K+ 5.2 mmol/L Urea 24.6 mmol/L Creat 244 µmol/L	
LFTs: ALP 95 I.U/L ALT 22 I.U/L Bilirubin 49 µmol/L LDH 1546 I.U/L (<450 I.U/L)	
Coagulation screen: PT 12.6 s APTT 33.6 s Fib 5.1 g/L FDP 1985 mg/L	
	Appropriate discussion with relevant specialties - haematology/renal
Critical care accept patient	Recognise that ongoing care of this patient needs to be in a critical care setting – discuss with critical care team
	Consider specific investigations to aid diagnosis: • liver ultrasound scan • expedite CT head • ADAMTS 13

Information given	Expected actions
HIV negative	Check HIV status in notes (association with TTP)
ABG if done: pH 7.38 pO2 13.1 kPa pCO2 3.8 kPa Hb 87 g/L HCO3- 19 mmol/L BE -3mmol/L Lactate 2.2 mmol/L	Anaesthetist inserts arterial line

Proceed to stage 3 once differential diagnosis has been considered, further investigations planned and transfer to critical care planned

Stage 3: Patient deteriorates and has tonic-clonic seizure on critical care. Further multidisciplinary input regarding likely diagnosis of TTP and management

Information given	Expected actions
Patient has been for a CT head and liver USS and transferred to the critical care unit. Obstetric registrar is on the critical care unit. Also present is anaesthetic ST3+ or critical care ST3+	
CT head scan suggests a left parietal lobe infarct	Recognise this picture is more typical of TTP/HUS and re-contact haematology for advice
Liver ultrasound scan results normal	
Patient is now oliguric 5ml/hr Reflexes still present	Recognise poor urine output Check reflexes Send serum Mg2+ levels and decrease/stop MgSO$_4$ infusion according to local protocol
Patient less responsive GCS now 10: E =2, V=3, M=5	Recognise that patient continues to deteriorate Repeat observations
	Assess airway
	Give 15L/min of oxygen via non re-breathing facemask
	Critical care ST/anaesthetic ST prepare for intubation in case GCS continues to deteriorate Consider repeat CT head with fall in GCS
Whilst awaiting response from haematology: Patient becomes less responsive and then starts to fit	Call for help

Observations	
A	Clear
B	RR 24/min SpO$_2$ 100% on 15L/min O$_2$
C	HR 92 bpm BP 139/90 CRT 2s
D	AV**P**U
E	Temp 36.7°C

Information given	Expected actions
	Keep patient safe
Obstructed, noisy breathing until airway-opening manoeuvres performed	Perform airway assessment and airway-opening manoeuvres Continue 15L/min of oxygen via non re-breathing facemask
	Left lateral position
	Reasonable to consider 2nd loading dose of magnesium- 2g IV over 10 mins but clinical picture more in keeping with TTP/HUS
Seizure self-terminates after 2 minutes	Prepare to give benzodiazepine but seizure terminates
GCS improving post-seizure. Drowsy but says a few words	Keep in left lateral position until GCS improves post-seizure
	Titrate O_2 to SpO2 to SpO2 $\geq$94%
Haematology ST7 arrives to review the patient (faculty): They feel TTP more likely diagnosis at this point – generally, in aHUS PLTs are >50X10 9/l at presentation and aHUS more commonly occurs in postpartum period. Also renal impairment less severe than commonly seen with HUS. They recommend: • Octaplas • Methylprednisolone 1g IV • Plasma exchange – the Haematology team will arrange: (patient will need urgent transfer to a specialist centre if plasma exchange service not available locally as ideally it should be commenced within 4-8 hours – give steroid and octaplas infusion in meantime) • This initial treatment will be appropriate for both TTP and aHUS until further results are available.	
	Multidisciplinary discussion with team regarding management of FDIU: aim for induction of labour (IOL) with mifepristone/misoprostol (vaginal delivery) with blood product cover (but note contraindication to PLT transfusion (unless advised by an expert Haematologist from a TTP centre – see discussion)

Information given	Expected actions
	Optimal timing of IOL to be discussed with Haematologist/Critical Care consultant/Obstetrician/obstetric anaesthetist Plasma exchange should be first priority

Scenario ends when haematologist has assessed patient and made plan

Suggested Topics for Debrief Discussion

- Did ED team recognise severe hypertension in a pregnant patient and treat it while waiting for obstetricians to arrive?
- Were there any problems obtaining appropriate antihypertensives/MgSO$_4$ in ED?
- Were the team confident with the differential diagnosis of MAHA in pregnancy?
- Were consultants in obstetrics and anaesthetics contacted early and multidisciplinary help from haematology/renal/medicine/critical care sought early?

Discussion

Definition

Microangiopathic haemolytic anaemia (MAHA) is the collective term for a group of haemolytic anaemias where red blood cells are destroyed due to factors in small blood vessels. MAHA is characteristic of a number of conditions known as thrombotic microangiopathies (TMAs), and is characterised by the presence of anaemia and schistocytes (red cell fragments) on blood film examination. TMAs, although diverse, are all similar in the presence of endothelial injury or change that results in microthrombus formation. The resultant shear forces on circulating red cells result in damage to the red cell membrane (hence the anaemia and red cell fragmentation), with the microthrombus formation leading to small-vessel ischaemia and end-organ damage.

Differential Diagnosis of MAHA in Pregnancy and Clinical Presentation

The differential diagnosis of severe MAHA in pregnancy includes:

- Pre-eclampsia/HELLP syndrome
- Thrombotic thrombocytopenic purpura (TTP)
- Acute fatty liver of pregnancy (AFLP)
- Complement-mediated thrombotic microangiopathy (C-TMA; also referred to as atypical haemolytic uraemic syndrome (aHUS))
- HUS (also known as STEC-HUS).

Trying to distinguish between these different pathologies is often difficult because they share similar clinical features. Unlike pre-eclampsia, both TTP and HUS/aHUS are rare during pregnancy and the puerperium. TTP or HUS/aHUS can present with central nervous system involvement and patients often have confusion, irritability and/or seizures. Hypertension is a predominant feature in pre-eclampsia/HELLP and although sometimes present, is not common in TTP or AFLP. The presentation of AFLP is somewhat different, with severe abdominal pain, vomiting, abnormal liver function tests, profound hypoglycaemia and a consumptive coagulopathy. Although thrombocytopaenia may be present in all of the syndromes, coagulopathy is not a feature of TTP or HUS/aHUS. The features of the TMAs in pregnancy are compared in the Table 19.1. PET, HELLP and AFLP characteristically improve following delivery of the fetus, with such spontaneous improvement not usually seen in the other MAHAs.

The approach to a patient presenting with a MAHA is to ensure the complete differential diagnosis is considered. As such, the clinical assessment and investigations should be directed to elicit the key distinguishing features of these conditions, which have different management strategies. The history should determine if there is a history of diarrhoea (as in HUS) or abdominal symptoms (such as in HELLP and AFLP). The presence of neurological symptoms would be more suggestive of a diagnosis of pre-eclampsia, TTP or HUS/aHUS. Investigations should first be directed at confirming the presence of a MAHA (anaemia, thrombocytopenia, red cell fragmentation with markers of haemolysis such as an elevated LDH, low haptoglobin and elevated bilirubin). The direct antiglobulin test is negative in contrast with autoimmune haemolytic

Table 19.1 Typical features in pregnancy-associated microangiopathies (Scully et al., 2012).

	MAHA	Thrombocy-topenia	Coagulopathy	Hypertension	Abdominal symptoms	Renal impairment	Neurological symptoms
PET	+	+	±	+++	±	±	++
HELLP	+	++	±	+	+++	+	±
TTP	++	+++	-	±	+	++	+++
HUS	+	++	±	++	+	+++	±
AFLP	±	+	++++	+	+++	++	+
SLE	+	+	±	+	±	++	+
APLS	+	++	±	±	±	±	±

PET, Pre-eclampsia; HELLP, haemolysis, elevated liver enzymes and low platelets; TTP, thrombotic thrombocytopenic purpura; HUS, haemolytic uraemic syndrome; AFLP, acute fatty liver of pregnancy; SLE, systemic lupus erythematosus; APLS, antiphospholipid syndrome (catastrophic); MAHA, microangiopathic haemolytic anaemia.

anaemia. Further investigations should attempt to differentiate between the different possible diagnoses.

Thrombotic Thrombocytopenic Purpura (TTP)

TTP is a rare disorder, which, without appropriate treatment, is invariably fatal. It is caused by a deficiency of the von Willebrand factor cleaving enzyme ADAMTS13, where the presence of ultralong (uncleaved) von Willebrand multimers and the resultant platelet aggregation results in microthrombi. The deficiency of ADAMTS13 is usually caused by the presence of an acquired autoantibody directed against ADAMTS13, although congenital forms (with a persistent low level of the enzyme throughout life) are seen, often presenting during pregnancy due to the physiological reduction in ADAMTS13 activity in pregnancy and the peripartum period. Reduced ADAMTS13 activity (<10%) is seen in TTP; however, treatment should not be withheld pending such specialist investigations – it is suggested that any MAHA with low platelets and no clear cause should be treated as TTP pending confirmation due to its high untreated mortality.

The first-line therapy for TTP is plasma exchange (to remove the offending autoantibody and replace with plasma containing ADAMTS13), with concomitant immunosuppression to inhibit antibody formation. Supportive management should be provided for end-organ damage, such as cerebral involvement and renal impairment. Platelet transfusion is usually contraindicated in TTP (unless advised by an expert Haematologist from a TTP centre) due to concerns about accelerating microthrombus formation.

Troponin should be checked as it is a prognostic indicator in TTP (it indicates microvascular cardiac involvement).

Haemolytic Uraemic Syndrome

HUS is characterised by MAHA, thrombocytopenia and acute kidney injury. *Shigella*-like toxin-producing *E. coli* (STEC)-HUS is the commonest form (although far more common in children than adults), usually presenting with a prodrome of (bloody) diarrhoea. *Escherichia coli* 0157 is the commonest serotype of these bacteria. The binding of the *Shigella* toxin to the endothelium results in cell damage and leukocyte adhesion. The endothelium becomes thrombogenic, with the binding action of the *Shigella* toxin inactivating ADAMTS-13 – as such, TTP and STEC-HUS are considered part of the same spectrum of disease. The management of STEC-HUS is largely supportive, again with platelet transfusion being generally contraindicated.

Atypical HUS (aHUS), although presenting in the same way as STEC-HUS, apart from the associated diarrhoea, has a different underlying pathology with chronic, uncontrolled activation of complement leading to platelet activation, endothelial damage and an uncontrolled systemic TMA with a renal preponderance. Pregnancy can be the trigger for aHUS(p-aHUS: pregnancy-associated atypical HUS) affecting ~1 in 25,000 pregnancies. The urgent exclusion of TTP (through demonstration of normal ADAMTS13 activity) is vital in the diagnosis of aHUS. The only therapy directed against aHUS is eculizumab, a monoclonal antibody directed against C5, blocking part of the compliment pathway. aHUS more commonly occurs in the postpartum period.

Acute Fatty Liver of Pregnancy (AFLP)

AFLP typically presents in the third trimester of pregnancy with nausea/vomiting, right upper quadrant or epigastric pain, headache and fatigue. The patient is often jaundiced and may have coexisting features of pre-eclampsia/HELLP, but often in a milder form.

A subgroup of women with AFLP and HELLP are heterozygous for LCHAD (3-hydroxy-acyl-coenzyme A dehydrogenase) deficiency. If the fetus is homozygous for this defect, it results in accumulation of fetal fatty acids which return to the mother's circulation. The mother cannot metabolise these extra fatty acids, leading to fat deposition in the hepatocytes and impaired liver function.

Features of AFLP that help to differentiate it from HELLP include profound hypoglycaemia and coagulopathy often in the absence of thrombocytopenia. The mainstay of management is to expedite delivery and to treat the associated coagulopathy, hypoglycaemia and hypertension if present. Severely ill patients can develop hepatic failure and encephalopathy and require management in a critical care setting with early involvement of the regional liver unit.

The neonate should be tested for disorders of fatty acid oxidation.

HELLP Syndrome

See discussion in Chapter 18. If PET or HELLP don't improve within 48 hours of delivery, then TTP should be considered.

Summary

Diagnosis in a woman presenting with a MAHA in pregnancy can be very challenging due to the overlap of several conditions in their clinical presentation and initial laboratory testing as outlined above. TTP and HUS, although rare, should be considered in the pregnant patient presenting with MAHA as early, expert haematological input and urgent plasma exchange may be life-saving.

Bibliography

George, J. N., Nester, C. M. and McIntosh, J. J. (2015). Syndromes of thrombotic microangiopathy associated with pregnancy. *Hematology American Society of Hematology Education Program*, 2015, 644–648.

Liu, J., Ghaziani, T. T. and Wolf, J. L. (2017). Acute fatty liver disease of pregnancy: updates in pathogenesis, diagnosis and management. *American Journal of Gastroenterology*, 112, 838–846.

Scully, M., Hunt, B. J., Benjamin, S., et al. (2012). Guidelines on the diagnosis and management of thrombotic thrombocytopenic purpura and other thrombotic microangiopathies. *British Journal of Haematology*, 158, 323–335.

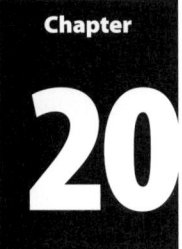

Chapter

20

Subdural Block in Labour

Kathryn Wood and Lorna Howie

Scenario in a Nutshell

Subdural catheter in labour.
 Stage 1: Assessment and management of inadequate epidural.
 Stage 2: Horner's syndrome and high patchy sensory block develops following epidural bolus.

Target Learner Groups

Anaesthetists and midwifery staff. Useful scenario for anaesthetists new to obstetrics.

Specific learning opportunities
Demonstrate sensory and motor assessment following insertion of labour epidural
Recognise features of a potential subdural catheter
Demonstrate appropriate management of a suspected subdural catheter and its complications

Suggested learners (to represent their normal roles)	In the room from the start	Available when requested
Anaesthetic CT2 or ST3+	√	
Midwife caring for patient	√	
Suggested facilitators		
Faculty to play role of husband	√	
Faculty to play role of daytime anaesthetist finishing shift, handing over the case to the night team	√	

Details for Facilitators

Patient Demographics

Name: Hannah

Age: 32

Gestation: Term + 10

Booking weight: 78 kg

Parity: P0

Scenario Summary for Facilitators

Patient is on delivery suite having an induction of labour, on IV syntocinon, for post maturity. She had an epidural sited (for labour analgesia) at the level L2–3 by the daytime team. The procedure was difficult, with bony obstruction on multiple attempts. 5 cm of catheter have been left in the space.

45 minutes following an initial 15 ml bolus of 0.1% bupivacaine with 2 µg/ml fentanyl, the patient is still complaining of pain.

On assessment, she has a sensory block to cold to T11 on the right and L1 on the left, with bilateral Bromage score of 0.

Patient very keen for further epidural top-up.

On administration of a further epidural bolus, the patient complains of ongoing labour pains and a strange sensation in her face.

She has a subdural catheter with a high patchy sensory block to T2 right, T4 left and right-sided Horner's syndrome.

The scenario ends with the description of subsequent management of the patient.

Set-up Overview for Facilitators

Clinical setting	In a delivery room, on a delivery bed
Patient position	Semi-recumbent
Initial monitoring in place	Pulse oximeter NIBP cuff CTG
Other equipment	16G cannula dorsum left hand attached to 1 litre Hartmann's solution at 80 ml/h and 10 IU syntocinon in 500 ml normal saline running at 48 ml/h Epidural catheter secured to back and attached to an epidural pump
Useful manikin functions	Pupillary accommodation

143

Medical Equipment

For core equipment checklist, see Chapter 9.

Additional equipment specific to scenario		
Epidural pump and epidural catheter	Local anaesthetics as per local epidural policy with syringes and drawing-up needles	Syntocinon infusion with infusion pump and giving set
Ethyl chloride spray		Pen torch

Information Given to the Learners

Information given to the anaesthetic trainee and midwife caring for the patient by the daytime anaesthetist finishing shift (played by a facilitator).

SBAR handover is as follows:

Situation: This is Hannah. She has ongoing pain from labour despite me siting an epidural.

Background: 32 years old, fit and well primip having IOL for post maturity, 6 cm dilated, on IV syntocinon with normal CTG.

Epidural was very difficult to site, multiple bony obstructions but I managed to get it in at L2–3, 5 cm catheter left in space. I administered a total of 15 ml 0.1% bupivacaine with 2 µg/ml fentanyl (or local anaesthetic as per local guidance) 40 min ago and commenced the pump at the standard labour patient-controlled epidural analgesia (PCEA) settings.

Assessment: She still has pain 40 min after her loading dose.

Recommendation: Are you able to review her epidural?

Scenario Schedule

Observations	
A	Clear
B	RR 20/min SpO$_2$ 97% on air
C	HR 112bpm BP 135 / 90
D	**A**VPU
E	Nil to note
CTG:	Normal

Stage 1. Assessment and management of inadequate epidural	
Information given	Expected actions
Patient remains in significant pain with very little improvement since the epidural was sited. Pain worse on the left.	Assess pain
Block height to cold up to and including T11 on the right and L1 on the left. Lower level to L4 on right and L5 on left.	Assess sensory level of epidural block
Bromage score 0 bilaterally (free movement of legs and feet)	Assess motor block
Patient very keen not to have epidural removed, wants every effort made to make this epidural work	Consider options for rescuing the epidural
	Top up epidural whilst patient on left side
No CSF on aspiration	Aspirate catheter before and during injection of local anaesthetic
	May consider withdrawing catheter slightly– would usually try top-up first

Progress to stage 2 once epidural top up administered

Stage 2: Horner's syndrome and high, patchy, sensory block develops after epidural bolus

Information given	Expected actions
Midwife requests that you return to the room 25 minutes after epidural top up given. Patient still complaining of pain and face feels funny.	
On arrival, the husband is panicking because his wife's face looks abnormal. He is asking why her right eyelid is drooping.	
Patient says the pain is no better. Her husband says her right eyelid definitely looks different.	Take a history from the patient and husband regarding block and facial symptoms
	Check observations
	Sit patient upright
	Apply Oxygen via non-rebreathing mask at 15 L/min whilst stabilising the patient (then titrate oxygen to SpO$_2$ 94-98%)
Bilaterally patchy sensory block: upper block height to cold up to and including T2 on right and T4 on left with patchy dermatomal sensory block below this to L5 No sensory block below L5 Bromage score 0	Reassess sensory and motor block
Upper limbs: power is normal, if checks, altered sensation to cold in T2 distribution: medial upper arm, on the right	
Faculty to describe the features of right sided Horner's syndrome: Right-sided pupil constricted and partial ptosis, left-sided pupil normal	Recognise the facial features of Horner's Syndrome
No headache, no history of migraine No ipsilateral head, neck or facial pain	Recognise that epidural most likely cause but seeks to rule out other causes of acute Horner's syndrome, eg: Migraine Carotid artery dissection
Patient upset, asking for further top-up	Doesn't administer further local anaesthetic
	Anaesthetist explains to patient and husband what they think has happened and proposes a plan.
	Plan to take out epidural and offer re-site of epidural or alternative analgesia- discuss with anaesthetic consultant

Observations	
A	Clear
B	RR 25/min SpO$_2$ 97% on air
C	HR 110bpm BP 108/68
D	**A**VPU
E	Nil to note
CTG:	Normal

Scenario ends when plan made to take out epidural catheter and offer re-site or alternative analgesia.

Suggested Topics for Debrief Discussion

- Where do you think the epidural catheter was?
- What made you think that?

Discussion

Anatomy of the Subdural Space

Subdural blocks are a rare complication and are caused by the injection of local anaesthetic into the subdural space. They can occur as an unintended complication of both epidurals and spinals. In spinals, the needle is thought to breach the dura and the arachnoid mater and some local anaesthetic is injected into each.

The subdural space (Figure 20.1) is thought of as a potential space. It is filled with a small amount of serous fluid and lies between the dura and arachnoid mater. The space extends from the second sacral vertebra into the cranial cavity contrasting with the epidural space which ends at the foramen magnum (Ajar et al., 2002). The subdural space is larger both laterally and dorsally (Agarwal et al., 2010). It extends over the dorsal nerve roots and the dorsal root ganglion but is attached to the ventral nerve roots, which explains why the anterior nerve roots (motor and sympathetic nerve fibres) are spared (see clinical features below) (Agarwal et al., 2010).

More recently, it has been proposed that rather than there being an existing potential space, the subdural space is actually created by trauma and tissue damage between the layers of dura and arachnoid mater (Collier, 2004). However, it may be that anatomical differences exist between patients causing variability in the existence of this space: the injection of fluoroscopic fluid into the subdural space has been demonstrated to vary from being extremely easy in some patients to near impossible in others (Blomberg, 1987).

Incidence

The exact incidence of unintended subdural blocks from epidurals is unknown and is probably underestimated due to anaesthetists not recognising the potential for a poorly working epidural to be a subdural catheter placement. The incidence is generally quoted as less than 1%. A prospective study by Jenkins (2005) suggests that the incidence is 1 in 4200 patients (0.024%). Other journals suggest higher rates of up to 7%. Inadvertent subdural injection of local anaesthetic during a subarachnoid block may occur in up to 13% (Agarwal et al., 2010). Most of the cases reported in the literature relate

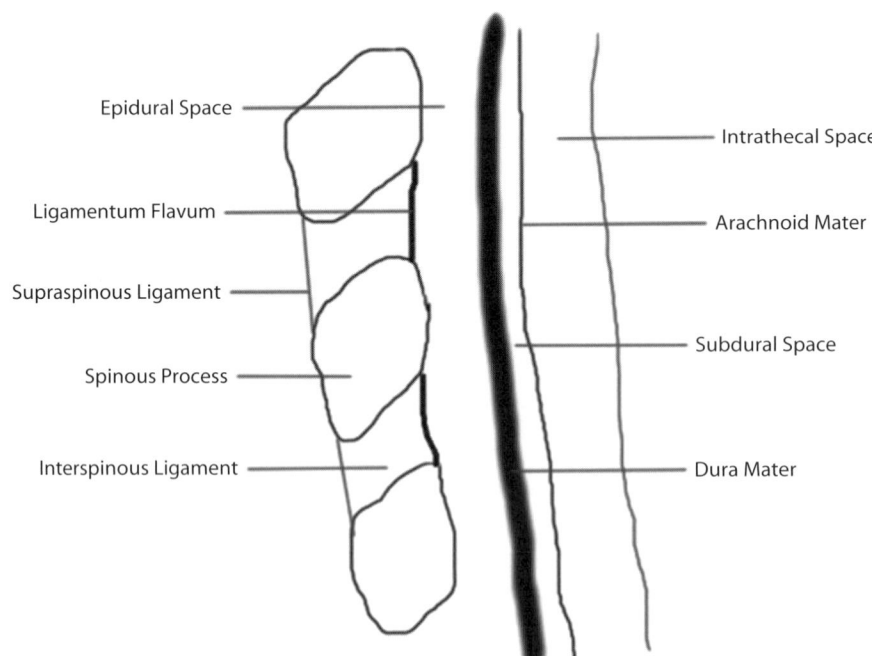

Epidural Space

Ligamentum Flavum

Supraspinous Ligament

Spinous Process

Interspinous Ligament

Intrathecal Space

Arachnoid Mater

Subdural Space

Dura Mater

Figure 20.1 Anatomy of the subdural space.

to epidurals for labour analgesia with very few from the non-obstetric population (Collier, 2004).

Risk Factors

Several risk factors for the accidental insertion of a subdural catheter have been proposed (see below); however, Hoftman and Ferrante (2009) found that these were absent in the majority of cases with radiologically proven subdural catheters.

Risk factors:

- Difficult epidural insertion.
- Previous back surgery.
- Recent lumbar puncture.
- Rotating the Tuohy epidural needle in the epidural space (Lubenow et al., 1988).

Operator experience is not believed to affect the incidence of subdural blocks (Agarwal et al., 2010).

Clinical Features of a Subdural Block

Inadvertent subdural injection of local anaesthetic was first described as a 'massive epidural' with a delayed onset and a high, widespread sensory block, which was out of proportion to the amount of local anaesthetic that had been administered (Lubenow et al., 1988).

In reality, it is now felt that there is a wide variability in the presentation of a subdural block, but the most common feature appears to be a patchy block. It may also be associated with any of the following symptoms:

- Unilateral block.
- Slow onset.
- High sensory block with sacral sparing.
- Minimal/moderate hypotension.
- Motor sparing.
- Unconsciousness.
- Horner's syndrome.
- Trigeminal nerve palsy.
- Frontal headache at the time of drug injection (signifying the displacement of the CSF).
- Respiratory symptoms – progressive respiratory incoordination rather than sudden apnoea.

The features of a subdural block in terms of degree of motor block and incidence of hypotension generally fall in the middle of a continuum with spinal at one end of the spectrum and epidural at the other.

A subdural block is typically suspected when an epidural is slow in onset. However, case reports have also suggested that the onset may be rapid. Duration may also be varied (Agarwal et al., 2010).

Although the volume of local anaesthetic injected has been proposed to be related to the extent of the symptoms, a clear link has not been demonstrated. It has been proposed that this may be more related to anatomical variations in the space between patients (Hoftman and Ferrante, 2009).

As the subdural space extends laterally, the dorsal root ganglions are exposed to more local anaesthetic than the anterior nerve roots which explains the potential sparing of both motor and sympathetic nerve fibres (Ajar et al., 2002). There have, however, been reported cases of subdural catheters with both motor weakness as well as pronounced hypotension (Agarwal et al., 2010).

With the subdural space extending intracranially, there is the potential for the local anaesthetic to affect the brainstem, resulting in bradycardia and respiratory depression and apnoea (Kalil, 2006). However, effects are less sudden than a high intrathecal block – progressive respiratory depression and incoordination tend to be seen rather than sudden apnoea.

The literature contains several descriptions of patients with a subdural catheter developing Horner's syndrome and less commonly trigeminal nerve palsy. Horner's syndrome (miosis, ptosis and anhydrosis) appears to develop over a period of around 30 minutes and can last as long as several hours. The development of Horner's syndrome is usually associated with a high sensory block (Rodriguez et al., 2005).

There is a huge variation in the presentation of a subdural block, but the most common presentation appears to be one which fails to provide adequate analgesia (Hoftman and Ferrante, 2009) and does not fit the normal expected clinical picture of an epidural (Kalil, 2006).

Another factor increasing the difficulty in interpreting the clinical signs of an unusually behaving neuraxial block is that the block may be multicompartment with the end hole and side holes of the catheter in different spaces: subarachnoid, subdural or epidural. At low pressures seen with continuous infusions, the local anaesthetic will be delivered preferentially via the side holes of the catheter, but with the higher pressures seen with a bolus, the drug will be delivered via the end hole as well as the side holes.

Diagnosis

There have been several proposed diagnostic criteria for subdural blocks, although given the variability in the presentation as described above, it is clear that specific and reliable criteria can be difficult to produce. Many of the older criteria have needed to be reviewed due to the increasing number of atypical presentations arising in the literature (Hoftman and Ferrante, 2009).

In 2009, Hoftman and Ferrante developed a four-step algorithm for the diagnosis of a subdural catheter:

Step 1: Identify whether the catheter is intrathecal or epidural: from the tactile feel of the operator and presence or absence of CSF.

Step 2: Is the extent of the block excessive or restrictive or neither?

Step 3: Were any minor criteria present:

Onset of the block > 20 min?

Was there cardiovascular stability?

Motor sparing and a patchy spread?

Respiratory failure or cranial nerve involvement?

Step 4: Confirm the site of the catheter with: X-ray, CT or MRI.

In a presumed epidural catheter (no CSF aspirated) when the block was excessive, with one of the minor criteria (onset of > 20 min, cardiovascular instability, motor sparing, patchy/asymmetrical spread, respiratory failure, facial or head involvement), the sensitivity in identifying a subdural block was 93%. In a restrictive block with either an onset of > 20 min or motor sparing, the sensitivity was 100%. However, the sample size from which the sensitivities were derived was very small. Regardless, the common themes of patchy blocks with motor sparing remain.

Lateral X-ray, CT and MRI imaging with the injection of contrast through the epidural catheter can definitively identify the location of the catheter.

Complications

Use of a recognised subdural catheter for labour or caesarean section has been described in the literature, but continued use of the subdural catheter may risk:

- Inadequate, patchy block.
- High sensory block ± cardiorespiratory compromise.
- Subsequent intrathecal block with potential for a high/total spinal due to:
  - migration of the catheter from the subdural to the subarachnoid space: the soft epidural catheters used in the UK are unable to

puncture the dura in cadavers, but it is possible for them to spontaneously migrate through the arachnoid membrane. Therefore, continued use of a subdural catheter comes with a risk of catheter migration into the intrathecal space (Reynolds and Speedy, 1990),
  - rupture of the arachnoid membrane, particularly with a large bolus.
- Nerve damage: compression of nerves and the accompanying radicular arteries with the infusion of a large volume of local anaesthetic into the relatively confined subdural space (Reynolds and Speedy, 1990). Although this serious complication is rare, a case was reported in 2017 where a patient developed permanent paraplegia after an accidental subdural infusion of 0.1% levobupivacaine after a combined spinal–epidural (Chen et al., 2017).

Management

In view of the potential risks outlined above in continuing to use the subdural catheter, the most appropriate management would be to remove the catheter and either re-site the epidural at a different level or offer alternative analgesia.

If a subsequent subarachnoid block is performed, enhanced cephalad spread of local anaesthetic should be anticipated, because of the potential compression of the subarachnoid space by the subdural injection.

Conclusion

Inadvertent subdural blocks remain a poorly recognised complication of epidural analgesia, primarily due to the variability in presentation. A high level of suspicion is required when an intended epidural or intrathecal block presents itself in a way that is unexpected.

Bibliography

Agarwal, D., Mohta, M., Tyagi, A. and Seth, A. K. (2010). Subdural block and the anaesthetist. *Anaesthesia and Intensive Care*, 38(1), 20–26.

Ajar, A. H., Rathmell, J. P. and Mukherji, S. K. (2002). The subdural compartment. *Regional Anaesthesia and Pain Medicine*, 27(1), 72–76.

Blomberg, R. G. (1987). The lumbar subdural extraarachnoid space of humans: an anatomical study using spinaloscopy in autopsy cases. *Anesthesia and Analgesia*, 66(2), 177–180.

Chen, J., Hu, Y. and Lv, L. (2017). Paraplegia after accidental continuous subdural analgesia. *International Journal of Obstetric Anesthesia*, 30, 61–64.

Collier, C. B. (2004). Accidental subdural injection. *Regional Anaesthesia and Pain Medicine*, 29(1), 47–51.

Hoftman, N. N. and Ferrante, F. M. (2009). Diagnosis of unintentional subdural anaesthesia/analgesia: analysing radiographically proven cases to define the clinical entity and to develop a diagnostic algorithm. *Regional Anaesthesia and Pain Medicine*, 34(1), 12–16.

Jenkins, J. G. (2005). Some immediate serious complications of obstetric epidural analgesia and anaesthesia: a prospective study of 145,550 epidurals. *International Journal of Obstetric Anaesthesia*, 14, 37–42.

Kalil, A. (2006). Unintended subdural injection: a complication of epidural anaesthesia – a case report. *Journal of the American Association of Nurse Anaesthetists*, 74(3), 207–211.

Lubenow, T., Keh-Wong, E., Kristof, K., Ivankovich, O. and Ivankovich, A. D. (1988). Inadvertent subdural injection: a complication of an epidural block. *Anaesthesia and Analgesia*, 67, 175–179.

Reynolds, F. and Speedy, H. M. (1990). The subdural space: the third space to go astray. *Anaesthesia*, 45, 120–123.

Rodriguez, J., Barcena, M. and Taboada-Muniz, J. (2005). Horner syndrome after unintended subdural block: a report of 2 cases. *Journal of Clinical Anaesthesia*, 17, 473–477.

Chapter
21

Total Spinal Anaesthesia in Labour

Katie Gott and Sophie Kimber-Craig

Scenario in a Nutshell

Total spinal develops after epidural top-up for caesarean section administered in the delivery unit room.
  Stage 1: Developing symptoms and signs of high spinal. Recognition and initial management.
  Stage 2: Total spinal develops. Cardiovascular support, intubation and ventilation, and delivery.

Target Learner Groups

Anaesthetists, midwives, obstetricians and operating department practitioners (ODPs)/anaesthetic nurses and theatre team.

Specific learning opportunities
Demonstrate safe planning of transfer to theatre after an epidural top-up
Recognition of symptoms and signs of high/total spinal
Demonstrate safe management of a high/total spinal

Suggested learners (to represent their normal roles)	In the room from the start	Available when requested
Anaesthetic CT2	√	
Operating department practitioner/anaesthetic nurse		√
Midwife Coordinator		√
Midwife in room	√	
Obstetric ST3+	√	
Suggested facilitators		
Faculty to play role of night midwife finishing shift (can be played by facilitator running scenario)	√	
Faculty to play role of patient's partner	√	

Details for Facilitators

Patient Demographics

Name: Amelia	
Age: 31	
Gestation: 38+2	
Booking weight: 85 kg	
Parity: P0	

Scenario Summary for Facilitators

A 31-year-old, 38-week pregnant primigravida who is being induced for obstetric cholestasis.
She received an epidural for labour analgesia 7 hours ago.
On siting the epidural, three attempts were required at two different levels as the patient was very needle-phobic and unable to sit still. When the catheter was threaded, the patient reported some right leg paraesthesia and jumped in response. The catheter threaded easily and had a meniscal drop and negative aspiration.
Loading dose resulted in good analgesia and also a degree of weakness in the legs, particularly at the ankle joint. BP remained stable. Patient was monitored and given the PCEA once her pain returned. The epidural has worked well since.
CTG becomes pathological and the departing night anaesthetist administers epidural top-up in the room for category 1 caesarean section.
Patient develops symptoms and signs of a high spinal that develops into a total spinal.
Fetal bradycardia develops.
Patient requires emergency treatment of hypotension and bradycardia, intubation and ventilation followed by urgent caesarean delivery.

Set-up Overview for Facilitators

Clinical setting	In a delivery room, on a delivery bed
Patient position	Semi-recumbent
Initial monitoring in place	Pulse oximeter NIBP cuff CTG
Other equipment	16G cannula dorsum left hand attached to 1 litre Hartmann's solution at 80 ml/h and 10 IU syntocinon in 500 ml normal saline running at 48 ml/h Epidural catheter secured to back
Useful manikin functions	Intubation Pupillary accommodation

Medical Equipment

For core equipment checklist, see Chapter 9 including advanced airway equipment.

Additional equipment required for this scenario		
Epidural catheter (taped over shoulder) with epidural pump attached	Syntocinon infusion/ infusion pump	High/total spinal block emergency checklist (if locally available
Vomit bowl	Ethyl chloride spray	
Arterial line	Cardiovascular drugs: Phenylephrine Atropine Ephedrine Adrenaline	Induction agents (thiopentone or propofol), neuromuscular blockers (suxamethonium or rocuronium)

Scenario Schedule

Observations	
A	Clear
B	RR 16/min SpO$_2$ 98% on air
C	HR 85bpm BP 112/62
D	**A**VPU
E	Nil to note
CTG:	Baseline 140 bpm, baseline variability <5bpm, deep late decelerations

Information Given to the Learners

Information given to CT2 anaesthetic trainee, midwife and obstetric ST3+ by the anaesthetic ST3 finishing their shift.

Time: 20:00

SBAR handover:

Situation: We are just going for a category 1 caesarean section for a pathological CTG.

Background: Amelia is a 31-year-old primigravida. She is 38 weeks pregnant and being induced for obstetric cholestasis.

She has raised bile acids (22 µmol/l). ALT 42 IU/l, FBC and coagulation screen are normal.

She is on a syntocinon infusion and I sited an epidural 7 hours ago. Epidural insertion was difficult as Amelia is very needle-phobic and she found it very difficult to sit still. When I threaded the catheter, she reported some right leg paraesthesia and jumped in response. The catheter threaded easily and had a meniscal drop and negative aspiration. I spoke to the consultant after the first dose because she got some weakness in her legs, particularly dorsi-flexing her feet. Her blood pressure never dropped. We have kept a close eye on it and it has been absolutely fine ever since. I have just completed the top-up with 15 ml of 0.5% bupivacaine.

Assessment: All her observations have been fine.

Recommendation: Theatre team are ready whenever you are. All her paperwork is done.

Stage 1: Developing symptoms and signs of high spinal. Recognition and initial management.

Information given	Expected actions
Patient is comfortable	Staff prepare to move patient to theatre
	Anaesthetist should: • Stay with patient • Monitor HR, BP, SpO$_2$ during transfer • Have vasopressors available for transfer
Vasopressors and transfer monitor not available in the room – will need to send someone to theatre	Continue to monitor patient in room while member of staff sent for vasopressors and transfer monitor
If wants to start transfer of patient to theatre, allow. *In which case, symptoms develop as below on the way to theatre and next set of observations once arrive in theatre are as per start of stage 2*	

Observations	
A	Clear
B	RR 22/min SpO$_2$ 96% on air
C	HR 122bpm BP 83/48
D	**A**VPU
E	nil to note
CTG:	Baseline 140 bpm, baseline variability <5bpm, deep late decelerations

Information given	Expected actions
Patient starts to feel unwell – starts vomiting	
Still talking – feels awful, light-headed	ABCDE assessment of patient with repeat set of observations
No perioral numbness, no tinnitus, no metallic taste. Pulse looks regular on SpO$_2$ monitor.	Consider differential diagnosis with high suspicion of epidural complication:
Can't move legs and arms starting to feel tingly and heavy	High spinal/ local anaesthetic toxicity
No chest pain, not short of breath at this point	
Vasopressors only available once staff member returns from theatre	Hypotension noted Rapid IV fluid bolus
If sit patient upright she complains of feeling more light-headed, thinks she might faint	Activate emergency buzzer
	Apply Oxygen via non-rebreathing mask at 15 L/min whilst stabilising the patient (then titrate oxygen to Sp0$_2$ 94-98%)
Midwife co-ordinator and further midwives (if available) respond to emergency buzzer	State the emergency to team: high spinal
	Locate emergency checklist for high/total spinal and allocates scribe
	Anaesthetist communicating with patient and partner– reassuring them that they know what is happening, they will treat the problem and keep her safe
	Ensure uterine displacement
Bromage 3 bilaterally. Block to cold to C5 and rising.	Checks sensorimotor block
	Urgently call second anaesthetist, ODP/ anaesthetic nurse
	Ask team member to get cardiac arrest trolley
	Call anaesthetic consultant in from home
	Urgently call neonatal team
Over next few minutes develops: tingling in jaw rapid, shallow breathing voice barely audible becoming very drowsy	Repeat observations

Observations	
A	Clear
B	RR 30/min SpO$_2$ 91% on O$_2$
C	HR 64bpm BP 74/35
D	A**V**PU
E	Nil to note
CTG	Baseline 140 bpm, baseline variability <5bpm, deep late decelerations

Observations	
A	Clear
B	RR 30/min SpO$_2$ 84% on O$_2$
C	HR 43bpm BP 62/30
D	AVP**U**
E	Nil to note
CTG	fetal bradycardia, 84bpm

Information given	Expected actions
If anaesthetist commenced transfer at start of scenario, now arrive in theatre	

Progress to stage 2 once high spinal diagnosed, help called for and initial emergency management commenced.

Stage 2: Total spinal develops. Cardiovascular support, intubation, ventilation and delivery

Information given	Expected actions
Patient unrousable now	Recognise total spinal
	Team note fetal bradycardia but realise first priority is to secure airway and ventilation and commence cardiovascular support for mother
	Repeat observations and commence ABCDE approach to assessment and management: Anaesthetist assists ventilation with BVM and cricoid pressure as soon as equipment available
Not speaking Very shallow breathing	
Observations improve according to dose and drug given If give metaraminol/phenylephrine alone, becomes more bradycardic	As soon as drugs arrive in delivery unit room/patient arrives in theatre, anaesthetist gives appropriate dose of vasopressor and anticholinergic: titrate atropine 0.5mg boluses and vasopressor of choice
If check pupils, dilated and non-reactive	
	Prepare drugs and equipment for GA
	Discuss airway plan with ODP/anaesthetic nurse
Grade 1 laryngoscopy	Induction and intubation (care with dose of induction agent)
	Continue to administer vasopressors as required
	If still in delivery room, moves to theatre now
Fetal bradycardia now for 3 minutes	Proceed with caesarean section

Information given	Expected actions
	Insert arterial line
	Continues to administer vasopressors as required – may need CVP insertion for vasopressor infusion
	Inform critical care team of need for transfer
	Maintain sedation once caesarean section complete and prepare for transfer
Can aspirate clear fluid back from epidural catheter if attempts to at any point	

Scenario ends once plan for ongoing care on critical care is planned

Suggested Topics for Debrief Discussion

- How could the departing anaesthetist have made the epidural top-up safer?
- Are you happy with the point at which you moved to theatre or would you do it differently on reflection?

Discussion

Detecting Inadvertent Intrathecal or Intravascular Placement

Visible CSF

When the dura has been breached by a Tuohy needle a visible jet of CSF is often evident. This is more pronounced in the upright position when the CSF pressure is above 40 cmH$_2$O (compared with 5–15 cmH$_2$O when supine) (Turnbull and Sheperd, 2003).

If the dura has been damaged but not fully breached by the Tuohy needle at the time of insertion, then the epidural catheter can penetrate the intrathecal space without the initial gush of CSF, resulting in an inadvertent spinal catheter. CSF may be aspirated freely from the catheter but not always, hence the importance of using a test dose routinely in epidural management.

If, at the time of aspiration, fluid is present but it is not clear whether this is CSF or residual saline used for insertion, then it can be tested using urinalysis dipsticks with the following results.

- The pH of CSF would be 7.5–8.5 compared to 5–7.5 for 0.9% saline.

- CSF would have at least a trace of glucose and protein compared to 0.9% saline, which would be negative for both.
- The temperature of CSF would be warm compared to 0.9% saline.

Falling (and Rising) Meniscus in Epidural Catheter

The meniscus test has previously been reported to have a 95.5% sensitivity, 63.6% specificity and 98.5% positive predictive value of confirming correct epidural placement in non-obstetric patients (Trojanowski and Murray, 1995). However, a cohort study has since shown that the meniscus test does not improve diagnostic accuracy of aspiration in detecting intravascular catheters (Servin et al., 2009).

Negative Aspiration of Blood or CSF

Most intravascular catheters will be detected by a positive aspiration test (Norris et al., 1999).

Epidural Test Dose

Ideally, an epidural test dose will ensure that the catheter is neither intrathecal nor intravascular.

Detecting Intravascular Placement

Adrenaline has been used to identify intravascular placement of an epidural catheter, as it can cause a detectable rise in heart rate, but this is not reliable in pregnant, labouring women (Norris et al., 1999).

Lidocaine 100 mg IV produces tinnitus and metallic taste in labouring parturients (Colonna-Romano et al., 1993), but 100 mg is in excess of a usual lidocaine epidural test dose and would be a dangerous dose if placed intrathecally (see below). Michels et al. (1995) found that at least 1 mg/kg of lidocaine would be required to reliably produce subjective symptoms after IV injection of lidocaine (in non-pregnant women).

Detecting Intrathecal Placement

Lidocaine has been used as a test dose due to its fast onset and short duration of action, but doses in the range commonly used as an epidural test dose (≥45 mg) may have the potential to cause a dangerously high block if injected into the intrathecal space (Palkar et al., 1992; Richardson et al., 1996). If lidocaine is to be used as a test dose for intrathecal placement, 20 mg is a more appropriate dose (Camorcia and Capogna, 2004).

Low-dose bupivacaine and fentanyl is recommended in the UK as an epidural test dose in obstetrics (NICE, 2014). This will reliably detect intrathecal placement, but not intravascular; 10 mg bupivacaine and 20 μg fentanyl intrathecally was 100% sensitive and specific for intrathecal placement by 6 minutes (dense motor block – no or minimal movement at ankle). Warm feet were also a good differentiating sign between epidural and spinal at 4 minutes (Dalal et al., 2003). A test dose of 10 mg bupivacaine and 20 μg fentanyl inadvertently placed intrathecally will also produce rapid analgesia.

High/Total Neuraxial Anaesthesia
Definition

Definitions vary, but a high neuraxial block may be defined as a sensorimotor block above that which is required for the surgery and which is associated with significant cardiovascular/respiratory compromise, sometimes culminating in cardiorespiratory arrest.

Total spinal involves anaesthesia of at least part of the brainstem.

Incidence

The incidence of high neuraxial block is largely unknown, but a retrospective study from the USA suggested an incidence of high neuraxial block necessitating intubation of 1:4336 obstetric regional anaesthetics (D'Angelo et al., 2014). Loss of consciousness as a complication of

epidural is very rare, with an incidence quoted by the Obstetric Anaesthetists' Association of around 1:100,000.

The UK Obstetric Surveillance System (UKOSS) Cardiac Arrest in Pregnancy study (Beckett et al., 2017) identified anaesthetic causes, including high neuraxial block, as the leading cause of maternal cardiac arrest in the UK, with 25% of maternal cardiac arrests being due to anaesthetic causes. UKOSS are now leading a study investigating high neuraxial block in obstetrics.

Aetiology

High/total spinal can occur in the following situations.

- A large volume local anaesthetic top-up given down a previously undetected intrathecal catheter.
- A spinal anaesthetic performed in a patient who recently received an epidural top-up.
- A spinal anaesthetic performed using an inappropriately large dose of local anaesthetic.
- A top-up given down an epidural catheter that has migrated into the intrathecal space (soft epidural catheters were unable to puncture the dura in a cadaver study (Hardy et al., 1986) but it is possible that the physical characteristics of dura in a live patient may be different to that of a cadaver.).

Clinical Effects

The clinical effects of a high regional block depend on the level of the spinal roots affected. Knowledge of the signs and symptoms allows the detection and diagnosis of an ascending block to be made quickly as shown in Table 21.1.

Management

Early recognition of an ascending high regional block is vital and instigation of prompt and appropriate management is imperative to prevent harm to mother and baby. A systematic ABCDE approach should be used (see Figure 21.1). With prompt recognition of high neuraxial block and support of ventilation and the cardiovascular system, there should be no long-term sequelae.

Severe respiratory compromise may occur without loss of consciousness and the decision on whether to intubate and ventilate will be determined by the clinical state of the patient and the progression of the block. If the decision is made to induce general anaesthesia then psychological reassurance and explanation should be

Table 21.1 Clinical manifestations of a high neuraxial block (Poole, 2009).

Root level	System affected	Clinical signs and symptoms
T1–T4	Cardiac sympathetic fibres Intercostal nerves	Bradycardia Hypotension compounded by vasodilation Weakness of respiratory accessory muscles
C6–C8	Arms and hands	Paraesthesia Weakness
C3–C5	Respiratory	Diaphragmatic paralysis
Intracranial spread		Paraesthesia of face and jaw Weakness/hoarseness of voice Sedation Loss of consciousness

---

Emergency management of high neuraxial block

- Turn off epidural if running
- Call for HELP involving anaesthetic and obstetric teams
- Uterine displacement
- Commence full monitoring (SpO$_2$, BP, ECG)
- Explain to patient and partner
- Head up/reverse Trendelenburg position if BP OK
- AIRWAY
    - Apply 15 l O$_2$ via non-rebreathing mask
    - Assess airway patency
    - Intubation may be required
- BREATHING
    - Assess ventilation adequacy
    - Assist ventilation if required and prepare for intubation and ventilation if consciousness level is impaired or ventilation inadequate
- CIRCULATION
    - Uterine displacement if not already applied
    - Assess maternal BP and pulse
    - Treat hypotension with:
        - IV fluids
        - Intravenous vasoconstrictors/ionotropes such as:
            - Phenylephrine IV 100 µg boluses
            - Metaraminol IV 0.5 mg boluses
            - Ephedrine IV 6 –12 mg boluses
        - Consider adrenaline IV 50–100 µg boluses if resistant hypotension
    - Treat maternal bradycardia with atropine IV 0.5 mg boluses
    - In the event of cardiac arrest commence CPR as per ALS guidelines
- Check fetal heart rate/CTG and consider the need to expedite delivery with obstetric team

Figure 21.1 Emergency management of high neuraxial block.

given to the patient and her partner prior to doing so to minimise any further anxiety.

Deciding whether to expedite delivery or not will largely depend on the well-being of the baby. With profound hypotension ± maternal hypoxia, it is highly likely that urgent delivery of the fetus will be needed. If the CTG is normal once emergency treatment of the mother has been undertaken, then vaginal delivery, once the block has receded and the mother has been extubated, is an option. This, however, will be a decision involving both senior obstetricians and anaesthetists.

Bibliography

Beckett, V. A., Knight, M. and Sharpe, P. (2017). The CAPS Study: incidence, management and outcomes of cardiac arrest in pregnancy in the UK: a prospective, descriptive study. *British Journal of Obstetrics and Gynaecology*, 124, 1374–1381.

Camorcia, M. and Capogna, G. (2004). Standard lidocaine epidural test dose: isn't it too much? *European Journal of Anaesthesiology*, 21, 154–155.

Colonna-Romano, P., Lingaraju, N. and Braitman, L. E. (1993). Epidural test dose: lidocaine 100 mg, not chloroprocaine, is a symptomatic marker of i.v. injection in labouring parturients. *Canadian Journal of Anaesthesia*, 40(8), 714–717.

Dalal, P., Reynolds, F., Gertenbach, C., Harker, H. and O'Sullivan, G. (2003). Assessing bupivacaine 10 mg/fentanyl 20 mcg as an intrathecal test dose. *International Journal of Obstetric Anaesthesia*, 12, 250–255.

D'Angelo, R., Smiley, R. M., Riley, E. T. and Segal, S. (2014). Serious complications related to obstetric anesthesia: the serious complication repository project of the Society for Obstetric Anesthesia and Perinatology. *Anesthesiology*, 120, 1505–1505.

Hardy, P. A. (1986). Can epidural catheters penetrate dura mater? An anatomical study. *Anaesthesia*, 41, 1146–1147.

Kar, G. S. and Jenkins, J. G. (2000). High spinal anaesthesia: a survey of 81322 obstetric epidurals. *International Journal of Obstetric Anaesthesia*, 10, 172–176.

Michels, M. J., Lyons, G. and Hopkins, P. M. (1995). Lignocaine test dose to detect intravenous injection. *Anaesthesia*, 50, 211–213.

NICE (2014). *NICE Guidelines CG190: Intrapartum Care: Care of Healthy Women and Their Babies During Childbirth*. Manchester: NICE.

Norris, M. C., Ferrenbach, D., Dalman, H., et al. (1999). Does epinephrine improve the diagnostic accuracy of aspiration during labor epidural analgesia? *Anesthesia & Analgesia*, 88(5), 1073–1076.

Palkar, N. V., Boudreaux, R. C. and Mankad, A. V. (1992). Accidental total spinal block: a complication of an epidural test dose. *Canadian Journal of Anaesthesia*, 39, 1058–1060.

Poole, M. (2009). Management of high regional block in obstetrics. Update in Anaesthesia. www.esafe-anaesthesia.org/e.../High_regional_block_in_obstetrics_Update_2009.pdf

Richardson, M. G., Lee, A. C. and Wissler, R. N. (1996). High spinal anaesthesia after epidural test dose in five obstetric patients. *Regional Anesthesia*, 21, 119–123.

Servin, M. N., Mhyre, J. M., Greenfield, M. V. and Polley, L. S. (2009). An observational cohort study of the meniscus test to detect intravascular epidural catheters in pregnant women. *International Journal of Obstetric Anaesthesia*, 18, 215–220.

Trojanowski, A. and Murray, W. B. (1995). A test to prevent subarachnoid and intravascular injections during epidural analgesia. *South African Medical Journal*, 85, 531–534.

Turnbull, D. K. and Shepherd, D. B. (2003). Post-dural puncture headache: pathogenesis, prevention and treatment. *British Journal of Anaesthesia*, 91, 718–729.

Chapter

22

Severe Local Anaesthetic Toxicity in Labour

Charlotte Ash and Suna Monaghan

Scenario in a Nutshell

Local anaesthetic toxicity with seizure then pulseless ventricular tachycardia (VT) requiring perimortem caesarean section in delivery room.

Stage 1: Patient dizzy and unwell after epidural top-up.

Stage 2: Patient suffers tonic–clonic seizure.

Stage 3: Cardiovascular collapse with pulseless VT.

Stage 4: Return of spontaneous circulation.

Target Learner Groups

All members of the multidisciplinary obstetric team: anaesthetists, midwives, obstetricians, operating department practitioners/anaesthetic nurses and emergency response teams.

Specific learning opportunities
Knowledge of differential diagnosis of acute deterioration following epidural top-up
Recognise symptoms and signs of local anaesthetic toxicity
Knowledge of Association of Anaesthetists of Great Britain and Ireland (AAGBI) local anaesthetic toxicity guidelines and their location
Knowledge of location of intralipid on delivery unit
Demonstrate fast and accurate delivery of intralipid
Demonstrate safe and effective cardio-pulmonary resuscitation (CPR) and defibrillation
Demonstrate timely decision-making to perform perimortem caesarean section
Demonstrate good team communication, leadership and decision-making

Suggested learners (to represent their normal roles)	In the room from the start	Available when requested
Anaesthetic CT2	√	
Anaesthetic ST3+		√

Suggested learners (to represent their normal roles)	In the room from the start	Available when requested
Obstetric ST3+		√
Midwife Coordinator		√
Midwife in room	√	
Operating Department Practitioner (ODP)/ anaesthetic nurse		√
Suggested facilitators		
Faculty to play role of night anaesthetist finishing shift (can be played by facilitator running scenario)	√	
Faculty to play role of patient's partner	√	

Details for Facilitators

Patient Demographics

Name: Trisha

Age: 22

Gestation: 38+4

Booking weight: 56 kg

Parity: P0

Scenario Summary for Facilitators

Patient had an epidural sited (for labour analgesia) with difficulty during the night shift. Three attempts were made. On the last attempt, there was blood in the catheter which then cleared on withdrawing 1 cm. Epidural was working well initially but required top-up within last hour.

Patient now requires Category 2 caesarean section for failure to progress.

The night-time anaesthetist who sited the epidural (faculty) administers epidural top-up for theatre,

20 ml 0.5% bupivacaine with 100 μg fentanyl. He hands over to the daytime team – midwife and CT2 anaesthetist – and then goes home.

Patient becomes unwell in labour room. Differential diagnosis of her symptoms of dizziness to be explored.

Patient goes on to experience seizures.

Diagnosis of local anaesthetic toxicity and appropriate management.

Ultimately develops pulseless VT and requires perimortem caesarean section.

Return of spontaneous circulation occurs after second bolus of intralipid and defibrillation.

Set-up Overview for Facilitators

Clinical setting	In a delivery room, on a delivery bed
Patient position	Semi-recumbent
Initial monitoring in place	Pulse oximeter NIBP cuff CTG
Other equipment	16G cannula dorsum left hand attached to 1 litre Hartmann's solution at 80 ml/h and 10 IU syntocinon in 500 ml normal saline running at 48 ml/h
	Epidural catheter secured to back
Useful manikin functions	Seizures Defibrillation

Medical Equipment

For core equipment checklist, see Chapter 9, including advanced airway equipment.

Additional equipment specific to scenario		
Defibrillator and external pads	Epidural catheter (taped over shoulder) with epidural pump attached	Syntocinon infusion with giving set and infusion pump
	Ethyl chloride spray	Perimortem caesarean section pack or scalpel/swabs/cord clamp

Additional equipment specific to scenario			
Arterial line	CVP line		Severe local anaesthetic toxicity guidelines + local emergency checklist for local anaesthetic toxicity if available
Intralipid 20% emulsion with giving set and infusion pump	Induction/sedative agents (thiopentone, propofol, benzodiazepine)	Neuromuscular blockers (depolarising and non-depolarising)	Cardiovascular drugs: adrenaline 1 mg, amiodarone 300 mg

Information Given to the Learners

Information given to CT2 anaesthetic trainee and midwife who are taking over care at start of their shift.

Time: 08:00

This handover is given by a facilitator playing the role of the night anaesthetist who is now going home. Night anaesthetist is just completing epidural top-up as midwife and CT2 anaesthetics come in for handover.

The SBAR handover is as follows:

Situation: This is an epidural top-up for a category 2 section.

Background: Trisha is a 22-year-old, previously fit and well primip who is 38+4 weeks pregnant with no allergies. She had an induction for prolonged rupture of membranes and has failed to progress. She had an epidural sited 2 hours ago. I had multiple attempts at siting it. On my third attempt there was blood in the catheter, but I flushed it, pulled it back 1 cm and it worked well initially. She has had one midwife top-up when the block had regressed a little 40 min ago.

Assessment: Observations were all normal. I have got monitoring on ready for transfer and I have just finished giving an epidural top-up of 20 ml 0.5% bupivacaine with 100 μg fentanyl.

Recommendation: Are you happy to take over? Theatres said they will be ready for you in about 5 minutes.

Brief information given to obstetric team and midwifery coordinator who will respond to the emergency when called. You have arrived on shift and have been told there is a category 2 section for failure to progress being brought around to theatre shortly.

Scenario Schedule

Stage 1 – Patient dizzy and unwell after epidural top-up	
Information given	**Expected actions**
Night shift anaesthetist has delivered epidural top-up bolus and leaves the room	
Following the epidural bolus, Trisha starts to feel unwell. She states: 'I do not feel quite right, I feel very dizzy'.	
	Perform all observations and commence ABCDE approach
Patient talking	Assess airway
	Apply oxygen via non-rebreathing mask at 15 L/min whilst stabilising the patient (then titrate oxygen to SpO$_2$ 94-98%)
Chest clear, good air entry bilaterally, no added sounds	Examine repiratory and cardiovascular system
Good volume, regular peripheral pulse, heart sounds normal, no peripheral oedema	
Give information below if asked: Felt completely well up until a few minutes ago No other symptoms: no chest pain, no shortness of breath, no wheeze, no palpitations, no metallic taste, no peri-oral tingling or tinnitus. Legs or arms don't feel weak. No other recent medications administered No known allergies No rash No history of cardiac problems Vials of local anaesthetic checked and confirmed to be 20ml 0.5% bupivacaine with 100mcg fentanyl No obvious blood loss If checks block: upper sensory level up to and including T12 to cold bilaterally, free movement of legs (Bromage 0 bilaterally)	Consider the broad differential diagnosis, to include: • vasovagal episode • high epidural/intrathecal/subdural block • local anaesthetic toxicity • anaphylaxis • haemorrhage • cardiac event • drug error • ammniotic fluid embolism (AFE)
Patient getting increasingly agitated	Repeat observations as patient getting more agitated
CBG 5.8 mmol/L	Check CBG
Progress to stage 2 once differential diagnosis considered	

Observations

A	Clear
B	RR 18/min SpO$_2$ 97% on air
C	HR 99bpm BP 121/70
D	**A**VPU
E	Temp 36.8°C
CTG:	Normal

Observations

A	Clear
B	RR 28/min SpO$_2$ 99% on O$_2$
C	HR 130bpm BP 125/82
D	**A**VPU
E	Temp 36.9°C
CTG	Normal

Stage 2: Patient suffers tonic-clonic seizure

Information given	Expected actions
Tonic-clonic seizure	Pull emergency buzzer
	Keep patient safe
	Oxygen 15L/min administered via non-rebreathing mask if not done so already
Noisy breathing until airway opening manoeuvres performed	Perform airway assessment and airway-opening manoeuvres
Obstetric ST3 and midwife co-ordinator enter room	State the emergency: tonic-clonic seizure after epidural top-up – likely local anaesthetic toxicity
	Left lateral position
Palpable central pulse	Attempt observations but very difficult while fitting
	Consultant anaesthetist and consultant obstetrician asked to attend if not already done so
	Urgently call ODP/anaesthetic nurse
	Alert the neonatal team
	Request intravenous lipid emulsion 20% and local anaesthetic toxicity guidelines/emergency checklist
(Remember it is difficult to analyse blood samples after intralipid has commenced- but do not let this delay treatment)	Site second IV access, and send blood for FBC, U+Es, LFTs, coagulation screen, G+S
CBG 6.5 mmol/l	Check CBG if not done in stage 1
	Commence rapid IV Hartmann's
	Control seizures: give a benzodiazepine, thiopental or propofol in small incremental doses
	Although temporally related to the epidural top-up - consider eclampsia as a potential cause of the seizure. Team may consider $MgSO_4$ 4g IV over 5-10 mins or according to local guidelines
BP has been normal throughout labour	Administer lipid emulsion in the appropriate dose: An initial bolus of (56kg x 1.5mls/kg = 84mls IV)
	After bolus given, start the infusion of lipid emulsion (15ml x 56kg/hr =) 840mls/hour

Progress to stage 3 once initial bolus of intralipid has being administered and infusion commenced

Observations

A	Noisy, obstructed
B	RR 35/min SpO_2 not reading
C	HR 137bpm BP unable to record
D	AVP**U**
E	Nil to note
CTG:	Unable to record during seizure. Fetal bradycardia FHR 76bpm once seizure stopped.

Stage 3: Cardiovascular collapse with pulseless VT

Information given	Expected actions
Inform team that seizure has stopped	
ECG monitor change: now shows a broad complex tachycardia at 190bpm	Team recognise the change in rhythm and commence advanced life support (ALS) algorithm
No breath sounds, no palpable central pulse	Look, listen and feel for breath sounds and central pulse for 10 seconds
	Obstetric cardiac arrest call made (urgent call to neonatal emergency team at the same time)
	Ask staff member to bring cardiac arrest trolley
	Promptly commence cardiopulmonary resuscitation with chest compressions and ventilation (30:2)
	Perform airway opening manoeuvres +/- airway adjuncts as appropriate (caution with nasopharyngeal airway as bleeding risk)
	Manual bag-valve-mask(BVM) ventilation with 100% oxygen and cricoid pressure
	Attention to good manual left uterine displacement
	Identification of team leader / role allocation including scribe
Patient still in ventricular tachycardia with no palpable central pulse	Attach defibrillation pads and briefly pause chest compressions to analyse cardiac rhythm
	Identify shockable rhythm and perform safe defibrillation
	Recommence chest compressions / ventilations immediately after defibrillation
Grade 2a laryngoscopy	Early intubation
Attenuated ETCO2 trace present	Attach capnograph and confirm trace
	Deliver uninterrupted chest compressions and continuous ventilations at ~10/min
	Early discussion and decision for peri-mortem caesarean section with senior obstetrician
	Perform perimortem caesarean section in the delivery room (commence by 4 minutes and deliver baby by 5 minutes)

Observations	
A	Intubated
B	RR as per anaesthetist SpO2 not reading ETCO$_2$ 1.9kPa
C	HR 190bpm, broad complex No palpable central pulse except with chest compressions
D	AVP**U**
E	Nil to note

Information given	Expected actions
Remains in pulseless VT until delivery at peri-mortem section	Give adrenaline 1mg and amiodarone 300mg before 3rd shock (if get to this point prior to delivery)
	Give 2nd bolus of intralipid (84ml) 5 minutes after initial bolus and increase infusion to 1680ml/hr
Once baby delivered, patient reverts to sinus rhythm (although in debrief need to remind learners that this could take up to an hour)	
Palpable central pulse	Team recognise change to sinus rhythm at next rhythm check and check for central pulse

Progress to Stage 4 once baby delivered and return of spontaneous circulation

Stage 4: Return of spontaneous circulation

Information given	Expected actions
	Repeat all observations
If no sedation commenced patient starts coughing	Maintain general anaesthesia with IV agent
	Transfer to theatre, when appropriate, for wound closure
	Site invasive monitoring including arterial line & central venous catheter
	Refer to critical care
	Site urinary catheter
	Debrief with team
	Critical incident report

Scenario ends when post-return of spontaneous circulation care discussed

Observations	
A	Intubated
B	RR as per anaesthetist SpO$_2$ 95%, FiO$_2$ 0.7 ETCO$_2$ 6.0kPa
C	HR 118bpm, SR BP 89/52
D	AVP**U**
E	Temp 35.6°C

Suggested Topics for Debrief Discussion

- Was the Intralipid administered in the most efficient way?
- Were there limitations of equipment, e.g. maximum infusion rates on pumps?
- Consideration of maximum doses of intralipid (max cumulative dose of 12 ml/kg)
- Did the team share their mental model for the cause of the collapse?

Discussion

Local Anaesthetic Systemic Toxicity (LAST)

Incidence

In his review, Mulroy (2002) reported a rate of LAST for epidural anaesthesia in the general population of 1.2–11 per 10,000 epidural anaesthetics.

Aetiology

Wrong-Route Errors

The Third National Audit Project (NAP 3) in 2009 by the Royal College of Anaesthetists (RCoA)

163

addressed Major Complications of Central Neuraxial Block (CNB) in the UK. Wrong-route errors were identified as the third most commonly occurring complication after abscess and nerve injury (Cook, 2009).

Nine cases of genuine wrong-route drug errors were described. Six of these nine reports involved misconnection and administration of an epidural infusion (all containing low-dose 0.1% bupivacaine with opioid) intravenously. Five of these six events occurred in obstetric patients during labour. The other three cases involved the administration of vasopressors via the epidural route. Two cases of migration of an epidural catheter tip into a vessel were also noted (Cook, 2009).

One fatality was reported in a non-obstetric patient when a large volume of bupivacaine (250–300 ml) was given intravenously. Fortunately, none of the five obstetric patients came to harm despite an infusion of local anaesthetic (LA) running intravenously for over 3 hours in one case. Further fatalities were avoided by the use of low doses over long time periods in some cases and in others by the prompt recognition and management of the wrong-route errors. The report concluded that measures should be taken to prevent wrong-route errors occurring; for example, separate storage of intravenous and epidural infusions. Introduction of non-Luer devices for neuraxial techniques should reduce the risk of near-patient misconnection.

In the event of a wrong-route error, the impact must be minimised and systemic toxicity must be treated promptly and aggressively.

Factors Predisposing to LAST

A number of factors, pertaining to both the patient and the drug, are known to increase the risk of accumulation of local anaesthetic resulting in LAST.

Patient Factors

*   Distension of epidural veins in the parturient is known to occur, which increases the risk of intravascular epidural catheter tip migration (Bern and Weinberg, 2011). Increased reabsorption of local anaesthetic from the epidural space occurs, and can result in potentially toxic plasma levels of local anaesthetic. Migration of an epidural catheter can be difficult to detect: indicators include failure of an epidural to provide a sensory block

or adequate pain relief, or aspiration of blood from a catheter, which may not have been present at insertion. Failure of an epidural block may not be attributable to intravascular catheter tip placement and the patient may progress to showing signs and symptoms consistent with LA toxicity before recognition occurs.

*   Decrease in protein binding in pregnancy increasing the free fraction of the local anaesthetic drug available.
*   The direct effect of pregnancy hormones on cardiac myocytes increases their arrythmogenic potential. Similarly, an increase in neuronal sensitivity to local anaesthetic results in a reduced seizure threshold (Bern and Weinberg, 2011).
*   Increasingly parturients are older and present with comorbidities. Pre-existing renal and hepatic disease can decrease the elimination of local anaesthetic. Those with pre-existing cardiac disease such as heart failure are also more susceptible.
*   Acidosis and hypoxaemia potentiate LA toxicity (Rajan, 2009).

Drug Factors

*   Dose: the lowest effective dose of LA should always be used. The Society for Obesity and Bariatric Anaesthesia suggest lean body weight (which plateaus at 70 kg for women) is used for calculating bupivacaine-dosing regimes (Nightingale et al., 2015).
*   Mode of administration: signs of toxicity are usually apparent shortly after an intravascular injection of LA. However, symptoms and signs may be delayed if the rate of administration or is slow, e.g. by continuous infusion.
*   Site of administration: risk of LAST with nerve block is affected by the site or administration with rapid, system absorption of LA occuring in highly vascular tissues.
*   The choice of LA solution used is a factor in LA toxicity. Levobupivacaine, containing only the S-enantiomer, has a more desirable safety profile compared to bupivacaine (a mixture of S- and R-enantiomers), requiring higher doses to induce cardiac effects in animal models (Mazoit et al., 1993) and resulting in fewer seizures when used in similar doses to bupivacaine (Huang et al., 1998). Vasoconstriction seen with levobupivacaine may

be beneficial in comparison to the vasodilatory effect seen with bupivacaine, reducing its systemic absorption while still offering a prolonged block.

- Additives: addition of adrenaline to a test/loading dose is known to decrease the peak plasma LA concentration (Rajan, 2009) and can be a marker of intravascular placement should a tachycardia or hypertension occur post injection. However, in a review of epidural test doses in 2006, the injection of epidural adrenaline in pregnant patients had a poor positive predictive value in detecting intravascular catheter placement, may be associated with side effects and was not recommended (Guay, 2006).

Clinical Features of LAST

Systemic toxicity attributed to local anaesthetic has a varied presentation and includes both cardiac and neurological effects. The more common symptoms include the following:

- Conduction abnormalities particularly resulting in prolonged PR & QRS intervals; arrhythmias including bradycardia and AV node dissociation (Rajan, 2009); myocardial depression and ultimately ventricular tachycardia or asystolic cardiac arrest.
- Neurologically, patients may experience dizziness, metallic taste, agitation, visual and auditory disturbances (e.g. tinnitus) in addition to seizures and coma. Not all patients will experience the peri-oral tingling so often described.

The onset of any such cardiac or neurological symptoms in a patient with a neuraxial block for analgesia or anaesthesia should always alert the anaesthetist to the possibility of LA toxicity.

Management

The Association of Anaesthetists of Great Britain and Ireland (AAGBI) have produced guidelines on the Management of Severe Local Anaesthetic Toxicity (AAGBI Working Party, 2010). See Figure 22.1.

The first action in any such scenario should always incorporate ceasing any injection or infusion of local anaesthetic. All other drug/fluid infusions should be reviewed in order to rule out direct wrong-route administration. The use of low-dose continuous local anaesthetic infusions as opposed to single-dose techniques poses a risk of delayed toxicity.

Airway management is critical to prevent hypoxia and acidosis and hence the potentiation of LAST. Should intubation be required, thiopentone or propofol can be used. Propofol may be more easily available although thiopentone may offer more effective seizure control. However, both will cause a myocardial depressant effect and should be used with caution. The lipid content of propofol is too low to be beneficial and it is not an appropriate substitute for Intralipid®.

Intravenous lipid emulsion was first used in the treatment of LAST in the late 1990s. The mechanism of action of lipid emulsion appears to be multifaceted, with effects thought to include:

- intravascular effects such as the well-documented 'lipid sink hypothesis', whereby the drug is retained bound in the plasma to the large lipid load having moved down a gradient from toxic target sites such as the heart;
- intracellular metabolic effects, including increased fatty acid uptake by mitochondria for use as a substrate for metabolism in the heart, and activation of a protein kinase resulting in cytoprotective pathways and ultimately cell survival;
- membrane effects including reduction in the local anaesthetic-induced inhibition of the sodium channel (Weinberg, 2012).

Safety in pregnancy is still to be fully determined. A systematic review of adverse events reported after use of IV lipid emulsion highlighted that many adverse effects appeared to be proportional to rate of infusion and total dose administered (Hayes et al., 2016). Consequently, users should take care to adhere to national protocols when using such drugs and not give over the maximum recommended dose of Intralipid of 12 ml/kg.

Summary

It is important to remain vigilant when siting any neuraxial blocks, connecting epidural infusions and administering any epidural bolus doses. Block failure should alert the anaesthetist to the possibility of epidural catheter tip migration and ultimately the risk of LAST. LAST has a varied presentation incorporating both cardiac and neurological effects. Clear guidance is available from the AAGBI regarding the management of systemic LA toxicity and the use of lipid emulsion.

AAGBI Safety Guideline

Management of Severe Local Anaesthetic Toxicity

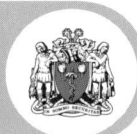

1 **Recognition**	**Signs of severe toxicity:** • Sudden alteration in mental status, severe agitation or loss of consciousness, with or without tonic-clonic convulsions • Cardiovascular collapse: sinus bradycardia, conduction blocks, asystole and ventricular tachyarrhythmias may all occur • Local anaesthetic (LA) toxicity may occur some time after an initial injection	
2 **Immediate management**	• Stop injecting the LA • Call for help • Maintain the airway and, if necessary, secure it with a tracheal tube • Give 100% oxygen and ensure adequate lung ventilation (hyperventilation may help by increasing plasma pH in the presence of metabolic acidosis) • Confirm or establish intravenous access • Control seizures: give a benzodiazepine, thiopental or propofol in small incremental doses • Assess cardiovascular status throughout • Consider drawing blood for analysis, but do not delay definitive treatment to do this	
3 **Treatment**	**IN CIRCULATORY ARREST** • Start cardiopulmonary resuscitation (CPR) using standard protocols • Manage arrhythmias using the same protocols, recognising that arrhythmias may be very refractory to treatment • Consider the use of cardiopulmonary bypass if available **GIVE INTRAVENOUS LIPID EMULSION** (following the regimen overleaf) • Continue CPR throughout treatment with lipid emulsion • Recovery from LA-included cardiac arrest may take >1 h • Propofol is not a suitable substitute for lipid emulsion • Lidocaine should not be used as an anti-arrhythmic therapy	**WITHOUT CIRCULATORY ARREST** Use conventional therapies to treat: • hypotension, • bradycardia, • tachyarrhythmia **CONSIDER INTRAVENOUS LIPID EMULSION** (following the regimen overleaf) • Propofol is not a suitable substitute for lipid emulsion • Lidocaine should not be used as an anti-arrhythmic therapy

4 **Follow-up**	• Arrange safe transfer to a clinical area with appropriate equipment and suitable staff until sustained recovery is achieved
	• Exclude pancreatitis by regular clinical review, including daily amylase or lipase assays for two days
	• Report cases as follows:
	   in the United Kingdom to the National Patient Safety Agency
	   (via www.npsa.nhs.uk)
	   in the Republic of Ireland to the Irish Medicines Board (via **www.imb.ie**)
	If Lipid has been given, please also report its use to the international registry at **www.lipidregistry.org**. Details may also be posted at **www.lipidrescue.org**	

Your nearest bag of Lipid Emulsion is kept..

This guideline is not a standard of medical care. The ultimate judgement with regard to a particular clinical procedure or treatment plan must be made by the clinician in the light of the clinical date presented and the diagnostic and treatment options available.

© The Association of Anaesthetists of Great Britain & Ireland 2010

Figure 22.1 AAGBI safety guideline on the management of severe local anaesthetic toxicity (reproduced with the kind permission of The Association of Anaesthetists of Great Britain and Ireland).

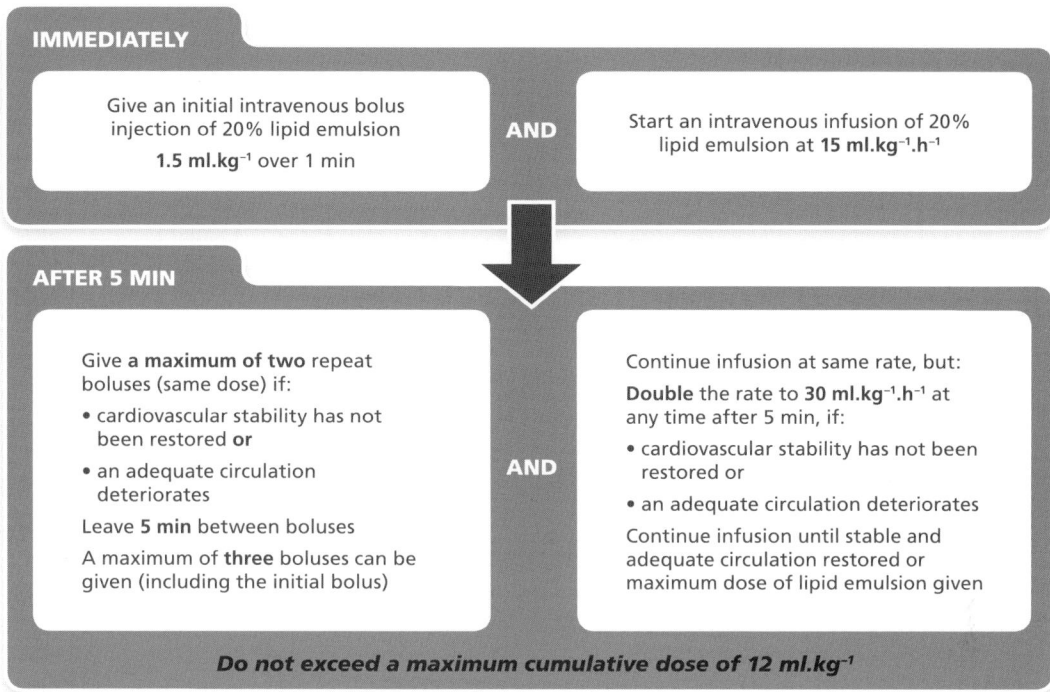

IMMEDIATELY

Give an initial intravenous bolus injection of 20% lipid emulsion **1.5 ml.kg⁻¹** over 1 min

AND

Start an intravenous infusion of 20% lipid emulsion at **15 ml.kg⁻¹.h⁻¹**

AFTER 5 MIN

Give **a maximum of two** repeat boluses (same dose) if:
• cardiovascular stability has not been restored **or**
• an adequate circulation deteriorates
Leave **5 min** between boluses
A maximum of **three** boluses can be given (including the initial bolus)

AND

Continue infusion at same rate, but:
Double the rate to **30 ml.kg⁻¹.h⁻¹** at any time after 5 min, if:
• cardiovascular stability has not been restored or
• an adequate circulation deteriorates
Continue infusion until stable and adequate circulation restored or maximum dose of lipid emulsion given

Do not exceed a maximum cumulative dose of 12 ml.kg⁻¹

An approximate dose regimen for a 70-kg patient would be as follows:

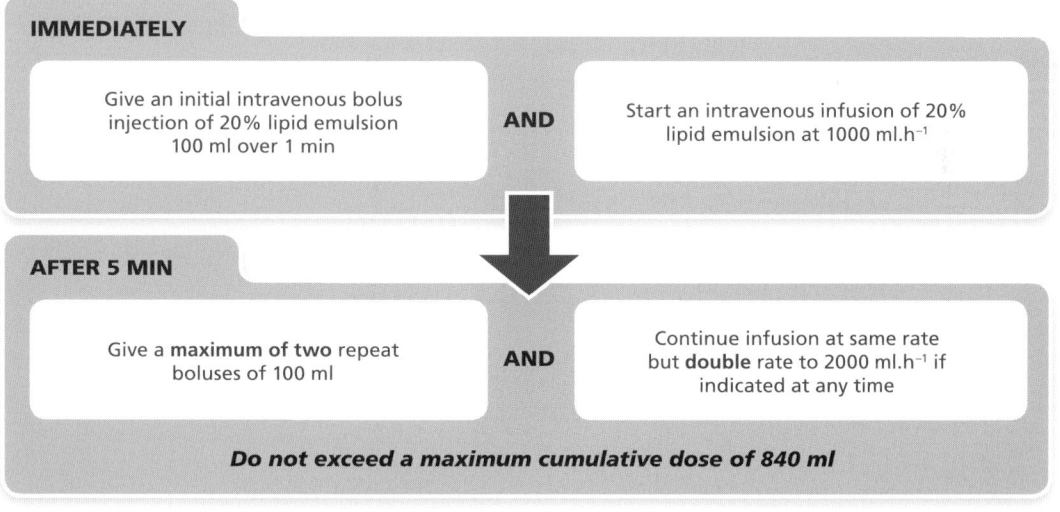

IMMEDIATELY

Give an initial intravenous bolus injection of 20% lipid emulsion 100 ml over 1 min

AND

Start an intravenous infusion of 20% lipid emulsion at 1000 ml.h⁻¹

AFTER 5 MIN

Give a **maximum of two** repeat boluses of 100 ml

AND

Continue infusion at same rate but **double** rate to 2000 ml.h⁻¹ if indicated at any time

Do not exceed a maximum cumulative dose of 840 ml

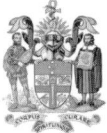

This AAGBI Safety Guideline was produced by a Working Party that comprised:
Grant Cave, Will Harrop-Griffiths (Chair), Martyn Harvey, Tim Meek, John Picard, Tim Short and Guy Weinberg.
This Safety Guideline is endorsed by the Australian and New Zealand College of Anaesthetists (ANZCA).

Figure 22.1 (Continued)

Further Reading

www.lipidrescue.org for up-to-date reviews and articles on the use of lipid emulsion.

Bibliography

AAGBI Working Party. (2010). *Guidelines for the Management of Severe Local Anaesthetic Toxicity*. London: AAGBI. Available from: www.aagbi.org/sites/default/files/la_toxicity_2010_0.pdf (accessed March 16, 2017).

Bern, S. and Weinberg, G. (2011). Local anesthetic toxicity and lipid resuscitation in pregnancy. *Current Opinion in Anesthesiology*, 24, 262–267.

Cook, T. (2009). The 3rd National Audit of The Royal College of Anaesthetists: Major Complications of Central Neuraxial Block in the United Kingdom. Available from: www.rcoa.ac.uk/nap3 (accessed March 16, 2017).

Guay, J. (2006). The epidural test dose: a review. *Anaesthesia and Analgesia*, 102, 921–929.

Hayes, B. D., Gosselin, S., Calello, D. P., et al. (2016). Lipid Emulsion Workgroup. Systematic review of clinical adverse events reported after acute intravenous lipid emulsion administration. *Clinical Toxicology (Philadelphia)*, 54(5), 365–404.

Huang, Y., Pryor, M., Mather, L., et al. (1998). Cardiovascular and central nervous system effects of intravenous levobupivacaine and bupivacaine in sheep. *Anesthesia and Analgesia*, 86, 797–804.

Levine, M., Hoffman, R. S., Lavergne, V., et al. (2016). Lipid Emulsion Workgroup. Systematic review of the effect of intravenous lipid emulsion therapy for non-local anesthetics toxicity. *Clinical Toxicology (Philadelphia)*, 54(3), 194–221.

Mazoit, J., Boico, O. and Samii, K. (1993). Myocardial uptake of bupivacaine: II. Pharmacokinetics and pharmacodynamics of bupivacaine enantiomers in the isolated perfused rabbit heart. *Anesthesia and Analgesia*, 77, 477–482.

Mulroy, M. F. (2002). Systemic toxicity and cardiotoxicity from local anesthetics: incidence and preventive measures. *Regional Anesthesia and Pain Medicine*, 27, 556–561.

Nightingale, C., Margarson, M. P., Shearer, E., et al. (2015). *Peri-operative Management of the Obese Surgical Patient*. London: AAGBI: Society for Obesity and Bariatric Anaesthesia. Available from: www.aagbi.org/sites/default/files/Peri_operative_management_obese_patientWEB.pdf (accessed March 29, 2017).

Rajan, N. (2009). Management of severe local anaesthetic toxicity. *Updates in Anaesthesia*. Available from: www.anaesthesiologists.org (accessed March 16, 2017).

Weinberg, G. (2012). Lipid emulsion infusion: resuscitation for local anesthetic and other drug overdose. *Anesthesiology*, 117(1): 180–187.

23

Respiratory Arrest in a Woman Using Remifentanil PCA for Labour

Michael McGinlay and Susan Davies

Scenario in a Nutshell

Respiratory arrest in a woman using remifentanil patient-controlled analgesia (PCA) for labour with a fetal death in utero (FDIU).

    Stage 1: Assessment and immediate management of collapsed patient in labour.

    Stage 2: Management of respiratory arrest and consideration of differential diagnosis.

Target Learner Groups

Midwives and anaesthetists. For remifentanil to be used safely on a delivery unit, staff must have a robust training programme and be confident in recognising and managing serious complications such as severe respiratory depression or arrest. This scenario would fit well with a midwifery staff training programme for remifentanil PCA.

Specific learning opportunities
Demonstrate rapid assessment and resuscitation of respiratory arrest in labour
Identify the key safety concerns surrounding the use of remifentanil on the labour ward and steps that should be taken to minimise this risk
Demonstrate effective communication, appropriate leadership and team-working

Suggested learners (to represent their normal roles)	In the room from the start	Available when requested
Anaesthetic CT2/ST3		√
Midwife Coordinator		√
Midwife in room	√	
Operating Department Practitioner (ODP)/ anaesthetic nurse		√
Obstetric ST3+		√

Suggested learners (to represent their normal roles)	In the room from the start	Available when requested
Suggested facilitators		
Faculty to play role of patient's partner	√	

Details for Facilitators

Patient Demographics

Name: Cheryl

Age: 24

Gestation: 31+4

Booking weight: 51 kg

Parity: P0

Scenario Summary for Facilitators

A 24-year-old, primiparous woman is admitted to the labour ward at 31 weeks gestation for induction of labour after an unexplained fetal intrauterine death. Otherwise uneventful pregnancy to date.

No significant medical history. No regular medications or known drug allergies.

Given oral mifepristone one day previously.

A dose of IM diamorphine was administered at 11:00 a.m. She became increasingly distressed and was requesting further analgesia by 3 p.m. She did not want an epidural.

Anaesthetist set up a remifentanil PCA 30 minutes ago. The PCA pump was programmed as per local protocol to deliver a bolus of 40 μg with a 2-min lockout and no background infusion (*can be adapted to adhere to local protocol*).

Supplemental oxygen was given via nasal cannula at 2 l/min (*or as per local protocol*). Patient was observed by anaesthetist for six boluses with no evidence of desaturation or apnoea.

Midwife left room briefly approximately 30 minutes later. Partner noted patient to be unresponsive and shouted for help in the corridor. Midwife assesses the collapsed patient, calls for help and initiates basic life support.

Emergency team attends immediately. On arrival, patient unresponsive and deeply cyanosed. Respiratory arrest with low blood pressure.

With adequate and prompt resuscitatory efforts, the patient's oxygen saturations improve along with the return of spontaneous respiratory effort.

If the respiratory arrest is not effectively managed the scenario will end with maternal cardiorespiratory arrest.

Set-up Overview for Facilitators

Clinical setting	In a delivery room, on a delivery bed
Patient position	Semi-recumbent
Initial monitoring in place	Pulse oximeter
Other equipment	16G cannula dorsum left hand attached to 10 IU syntocinon in 500 ml normal saline running at 12 ml/h
	20G cannula dorsum right hand attached to remifentanil PCA pump O_2 at 2 l/min via nasal cannulae (if this is local policy)
Useful manikin functions	Pupillary accommodation Intubation

Medical Equipment

For core equipment checklist, see Chapter 9, including advanced airway equipment.

Scenario Schedule

Additional equipment required for this scenario

Remifentanil pump with syringe/bag of remifentanil and giving set	Syntocinon infusion with infusion pump and giving set	Naloxone (keep naloxone in usual place on delivery unit)
Perimortem caesarean section pack	External defibrillator pads	Pen torch
Cardiovascular drugs: e.g. metaraminol, phenylephrine, atropine, adrenaline	Sedative drugs: benzodiazapines, propofol	

Information Given to the Learners

Information given to midwife who is taking over care at start of their shift

Time: 19.50

This handover is given by a facilitator:

Situation: This is Cheryl. She is having an IOL for FDIU.

Background: She has been admitted for induction of labour at 31 weeks gestation with a confirmed fetal intrauterine death. She is on an oxytocin infusion. A remifentanil PCA was started 30 min ago and has been working very well for her.

Assessment: She is currently 3–4 cm dilated. HR and BP are fine. She is so much more comfortable with the remifentanil. SpO_2 drop a little when she dozes but come straight back up again when she wakes.

Recommendation: Are you OK to take over her care?

To anaesthetist: You received the same information at your handover.

To midwife: You have had to briefly leave the room to get some ranitidine that the anaesthetist had prescribed. As you return to the room, the woman's partner rushes into the corridor, looking very worried and shouting for help.

Stage 1: Assessment and immediate management of collapsed patient	
Information given	**Expected actions**
Midwife enters the room with partner(played by facilitator), who is frantic	
Woman is slumped unconscious on the bed, cyanosed	Midwife activates emergency buzzer
Facilitator playing patient's partner: 'I was trying to just let her sleep – she hasn't slept properly for days but I can't wake her, her colour looks wrong, do something!'	
No response	Check responsiveness: shake and shout

Information given	Expected actions
No breath sounds	Look, listen and feel for breath sounds +/- central pulse for 10 seconds
Midwife unsure - doesn't think there is a central pulse	
Cyanosed	
Anaesthetic CT2, Obstetric ST3+ and midwife delivery unit co-ordinator enter room	State the emergency: cardiorespiratory arrest in a labouring, previously well woman using a remifentanil PCA
	Put out cardiac arrest call for obstetric and neonatal cardiac arrest teams

Proceed to stage 2 once cardiorespiratory arrest diagnosed and cardiac arrest call made

Stage 2: Management of respiratory arrest and consideration of differential diagnosis

Information given	Expected actions
	Send one of team for cardiac arrest trolley
If midwife asks anaesthetist to confirm, they can feel weak palpable central pulse – proceed as respiratory arrest as below. If chest compressions already commenced, don't stop to check pulse until ready to analyse cardiac rhythm and a rhythm compatible with a pulse has been found	Promptly commence life support as per advanced life support (ALS) algorithms 30 chest compressions:2 ventilations
	Perform airway opening manoeuvres+/- airway adjuncts as appropriate (caution with nasopharyngeal airway as bleeding risk)
	Manual bag-valve-mask(BVM) ventilation with 100% oxygen and cricoid pressure
	Manual left uterine displacement in supine position
	Identification of team leader / role allocation including scribe and staff member to support distressed partner
	Call for senior anaesthetic and obstetric help
	Contact ODP/anaesthetic nurse urgently if they have not responded to emergency buzzer
Sinus bradycardia	Attach defibrillation pads and briefly pause chest compressions to analyse cardiac rhythm

171

Observations	
A	Clear
B	RR as per BVM ventilation SpO$_2$ 88%
C	HR 48 bpm BP 70/42
D	AVP**U**
E	Nil to note

Information given	Expected actions
Confirmation of palpable pulse with ongoing respiratory arrest	Anaesthetist checks central pulse
	Check BP once central pulse noted
Alter observations according to drug and dose given	Administer dose of vasopressor +/- anticholinergic
	Continue mask ventilation, stop cardiac compressions
	Identify and treat potential causes of respiratory arrest:
Pupils equal and pin-point	High index of suspicion for remifentanil toxicity: Check pupils Consider naloxone: 400 micrograms IV; if no response after 1 minute, give 800 micrograms IV
No history of asthma, no cardiac history If partner asked for more details about event: Sudden deterioration - was completely well on admission. No preceding headache, neurological symptoms or cardiorespiratory symptoms. No anxiety or increasing agitation prior to event. After commencing remifentanil PCA, partner reports that she was falling asleep between contractions. He then noticed she had slumped a bit to one side and went to try and help her get more comfortable but she didnt respond to him at all.	Opioid overdose most likely cause for respiratory arrest but also consider and try to rule out a primary respiratory, cardiovascular or neurological event: Pulmonary embolism Amniotic fluid embolism Pulmonary oedema Aspiration Asthma exacerbation Community-acquired pneumonia Intracranial haemorrhage Primary cardiac event Anaphylaxis
Respiratory examination: trachea central, good air entry bilaterally with BVM ventilation, no added sounds HS 1+2+0 No PV bleeding No rash	Examine patient
	Insert second large-bore IV access and take bloods for FBC, U+Es, LFTs, coagulation screen, troponins, tryptase
CBG 6.9mmol/l	Check capillary blood glucose
	Consider need for early peri-mortem caesarean section if no rapid improvement or deteriorates to cardiorespiratory arrest
	Prepare equipment and staff for tracheal intubation

Information given	Expected actions
	If proceed to perimortem Caesarean Section, anaesthetist must be anticipating potential for recovery from remifentanil and have IV anaesthetic agent/sedatives ready to administer
Patient starts to make respiratory efforts within 1 minute of naloxone administration or 2 minutes of effective BVM ventilation if naloxone not given. Then starts to groan and regain consciousness	Assist ventilation until patient has regular breathing pattern with good tidal volumes
If delay in initiating BVM ventilation or inadequate ventilation established, patient deteriorates to PEA cardiopulmonary arrest	

Observations	
A	Clear
B	RR 14/min, SpO$_2$ 94%
C	HR 59bpm BP 84/48
D	A**V**PU
E	Nil to note

Scenario ends once spontaneous breathing returns and patient starts to regain consciousness

Suggested Topics for Debrief Discussion

- Do you think this patient was at an increased risk of adverse respiratory effects with a remifentanil PCA?
- Was it easy to locate naloxone?

Discussion

Remifentanil is a potent opioid with unique pharmacological properties that are desirable for labour analgesia. Over the last 15 years it has increasingly been used as a primary mode of labour analgesia in many centres across the UK and Europe.

Pharmacological Properties of Remifentanil

Remifentanil is a synthetic, ultra-short-acting, pure mu opioid receptor agonist characterised by rapid onset and offset of action. The effect-site concentration peaks at 1–2 minutes following intravenous administration.

It is then rapidly hydrolysed to non-active metabolites by non-specific esterases, independent of organ metabolism, and is completely eliminated by 10 minutes. As a result, it does not accumulate even after prolonged use.

Theoretically, its pharmacological profile makes remifentanil well-suited for labour analgesia, especially if its peak effect is matched with uterine contraction. However, it is important to remember that most pharmacokinetic models are based on non-pregnant individuals and evidence suggests that there is a large patient variability in the pregnant population.

Clinical Efficacy

Remifentanil PCA lowers pain scores more effectively than Entonox (Volmanen et al., 2005) or intramuscular pethidine (Van de Velde and Carvelho, 2016), but not to the same degree as epidural analgesia. Despite this, maternal satisfaction scores with remifentanil are high and comparable to satisfaction scores with epidurals (Stocki et al., 2014). Conversion rates to epidurals are approximately 10%.

Protocol for Remifentanil PCA for Labour

A variety of protocols for remifentanil administration in labour have been described. The commonest used within the UK is a bolus of 20–40 µg with a lockout time of 2–5 min and no background infusion.

It has been accepted that the use of a fixed-dose regimen is not ideal because there is a risk of both underdosing for some patients leading to inadequate analgesia and excessive dosing for others, leading to unwanted adverse effects.

Remifentanil PCA must be administered via a dedicated cannula. Only the patient is permitted to use the PCA at all times. BP should be measured on the opposite arm to the cannula and staff should be vigilant to avoid obstruction of the cannula, e.g. due to

173

positioning of wrist. Specific giving sets incorporating a non-return and anti-syphon valve must be used.

Contraindications

Most clinical trials investigating the efficacy and safety of remifentanil include healthy women with no comorbidities at term pregnancy. The use in pre-term labour has not been evaluated and as such the use of remifentanil in parturients less than 36 weeks gestation is relatively contraindicated.

The absolute and relative contraindications vary between different institutions although generally include those summarised in Box 23.1. It is prudent to exclude any of these when assessing a patient for remifentanil. If a relative contraindication is present, then this should be clearly explained to the patient along with the increased risk of adverse maternal and fetal effects.

In the case of FDIU, altered fetal–placental circulation may contribute to the increased maternal side effects. The lack of need for fetal monitoring and potential for less-stringent maternal monitoring during labour may also place patients at an increased risk of unrecognised respiratory depression. Extra vigilance should be taken in such cases. Some institutions opt to use an alternative opioid PCA instead.

Side Effects

Fetal

Remifentanil crosses the placenta to a significant degree (umbilical vein:maternal artery ratio of 0.88), but the mean umbilical vein:umbilical artery ratio of 0.29 suggests rapid metabolism and rapid redistribution of remifentanil in the fetus.

Reduced fetal heart rate variability has been observed with remifentanil *infusions*; however, overall the effects of remifentanil PCA on the fetus appear to be less than with other parental opioids (Van de Velde and Carvelho, 2016).

Maternal

Sedation, dizziness, nausea, vomiting and pruritus are all reported with remifentanil PCA. Maternal respiratory depression and desaturation remain the most concerning risks associated with remifentanil use in labour, with evidence suggesting an incidence of some degree of respiratory depression in up to 20–30% (Van de Velde and Carvelho, 2016). One study evaluating the respiratory effects of remifentanil noted that maternal apnoea (defined as > 20 seconds of respiratory arrest) occurred in 26% of patients within the first hour of administration (Stocki et al., 2014), but bolus doses up to 60 µg with a lockout interval of 1–2 min were used in this study.

An important risk factor includes preceding opioid administration and therefore remifentanil is contraindicated in a patient who has received parenteral opioids within the previous 4 hours.

Significant safety concerns remain around its use in labour, with several published case reports of significant maternal respiratory depression and cardiorespiratory arrest over the last few years. These case reports implicated medication errors and non-adherence to remifentanil PCA protocol, particularly the need for non-interrupted one-to-one midwifery care (Bonner and McClymont, 2012; Marr et al., 2013).

Monitoring

It is mandatory that patients are continuously monitored for signs of respiratory depression throughout use. One-to-one uninterrupted midwifery care and continuous pulse oximetry are mandatory. See Box 23.2.

It has recently been suggested that an additional form of ventilatory monitoring, such as capnography, should also be used, with pulse oximetry alone being inadequate as an early alert to apnoea (Van de Velde and Carvelho, 2016).

Summary

Remifentanil PCA is a useful analgesic for labour, but for it to be used safely there must be:

- one-to-one uninterrupted midwifery care;
- continuous monitoring of oxygenation and, ideally, ventilation;
- strict adherence to local protocols for its use; and
- ongoing education for staff including recognition of severe respiratory depression and respiratory arrest and confidence in its emergency management as practised in the above scenario.

Bibliography

Bonner, J. C. and McClymont, W. (2012). Respiratory arrest in an obstetric patient using remifentanil patient controlled analgesia. *Anaesthesia*, 67, 538–540.

Hill, D. (2001). Remifentanil patient controlled analgesia should be routinely available for use in labour. *International Journal of Anaesthesia*, 87, 415–420.

Kinney, M. A. O., Rose, C. H., Traynor, K. D., et al. (2012). Emergency bedside cesarean delivery: lessons learned in teamwork and patient safety. *BMC Research Notes*, 5, 412.

Marr, R., Hyams, J. and Bythell, V. (2013). Cardiac arrest in an obstetric patient using remifentanil patient-controlled analgesia. *Anaesthesia*, 68, 283–287.

Stocki, D., Matot, I., Einav, S., Eventov-Friedman, S., Ginosar, Y. and Weiniger, C. F. (2014). A randomized control trial of the efficacy and respiratory effects of patient-controlled intravenous remifentanil analgesia and patient controlled epidural analgesia in labouring women. *Anaesthesia and Analgesia*, 118, 589–597.

Van de Velde, M. and Carvelho, B. (2016). Remifentanil for labour analgesia: an evidence-based narrative review. *International Journal of Obstetric Anaesthesia*, 25, 66–74.

Volmanen, P., Akural, E., Raudaskoski, T., Ohtonen, P. and Alahuhta, S. (2005). Comparison of remifentanil and nitrous oxide in labour analgesia. *Acta Anaesthesiologica Scandinavica*, 49, 453–458.

General Anaesthesia and Failed Intubation in a Category 1 Caesarean Section

Richard McGuire and Sharon Smith

This chapter contains two scenarios relating to general anaesthesia for a category 1 caesarean section.

The first scenario takes the anaesthetist through a straightforward category 1 caesarean section requiring general anaesthesia. This may be used to assess conduct of general anaesthesia for caesarean section as per requirement for the Royal College of Anaesthetists (RCOA) initial assessment of competence in obstetric anaesthesia.

The second scenario is a failed intubation. This is appropriate for all grades of anaesthetists and should be practised with the whole theatre team including obstetricians and midwives.

Suggested learners (to represent their normal roles)	In theatre from the start	Available when requested
Anaesthetic CT2	√	
Obstetric ST3+	√	
Midwife	√	
Operating Department Practitioner (ODP)/ anaesthetic nurse	√	
Theatre team – scrub nurse	√	
Theatre team – runner	√	
Suggested facilitators		
Faculty to play role of midwife finishing shift (can be played by facilitator running scenario)	√	

Scenario 1

Scenario in a Nutshell

General anaesthesia for a category 1 caesarean section.
    Stage 1: Preparation for a GA category 1 caesarean section.
    Stage 2: Induction and maintenance of anaesthesia.
    Stage 3: Waking and extubation.

Target Learner Groups

Anaesthetists, midwives, operating department practitioners/anaesthetic nurses, theatre scrub team, obstetricians.

Specific learning opportunities

Demonstrate competencies around general anaesthesia for caesarean section as described in RCOA 2010 Curriculum – Annex B

Effective preparation for and management of induction of general anaesthesia for category 1 caesarean section

Demonstrate clear communication in the team, particularly the verbalising of Plan A, B and C of the airway strategy, how to contact emergency anaesthetic assistance in case of difficult airway and whether planning to continue surgery using a supraglottic airway or wake the patient up in the event of a failed intubation

Details for Facilitators

Patient Demographics

Name: Freya

Age: 29

Gestation: 38+4

Booking weight: 78 kg

Parity: P0

Scenario Summary

29-year-old primiparous woman at 38+4 weeks gestation.
Labouring on Delivery Suite following induction of labour for reduced fetal movements.
Has progressed slowly to 6 cm dilated using entonox for analgesia.
Developed sustained fetal bradycardia resulting in decision for category 1 caesarean section for fetal distress.

Set-up Overview for Facilitators

Clinical setting	Obstetric theatre
Patient position	Just arrived in theatre, being positioned on operating table
Initial monitoring in place	None
Other equipment	16G cannula dorsum left hand
Useful manikin functions	Intubation

Medical Equipment

For core equipment checklist, see Chapter 9, including advanced airway equipment.

Additional equipment specific to scenario		
Premedication: Ranitidine (IV if not had PO) Sodium citrate	**Induction drugs:** Induction agents – thiopentone, propofol Opioids – alfentanil, fentanyl, morphine Muscle relaxants – suxamethonium, rocuronium, atracurium	**Other drugs:** Oxytocin Anti-emetics Reversal agents: neostigmine, sugammadex Paracetamol Diclofenac
Quantitative peripheral nerve stimulator	Contact details for emergency anaesthetic assistance	WHO checklist/time out

Information Given to the Learners

Information given to anaesthetic trainee and obstetric trainee before they enter theatre

You have both just arrived to start your night shift on delivery unit. As you arrive, you are told that a woman has just been rushed through to theatre for a category 1 caesarean section for a fetal bradycardia.

Information given in theatre to anaesthetic trainee, obstetric trainee, theatre team, midwife and obstetrician from midwife who has just transferred the patient to theatre

Time: 20:30

The SBAR handover from the transferring midwife is as follows:

Situation: This is Freya, who is having a fetal bradycardia.

Background: 29-year-old, fit and well primip, BMI 27, who is 38 weeks pregnant with no allergies. She was induced for reduced fetal movements and laboured uneventfully to 6 cm dilatation, then had a fetal bradycardia. She was using entonox for analgesia.

Assessment: Observations were all normal.

Recommendation: She needs a category 1 caesarean section.

Scenario Schedule

Observations	
A	Clear
B	RR 20/min SpO$_2$ 98%
C	HR 125bpm BP 125/75
D	**A**VPU
E	Nil to note
CTG: baseline FHR 80bpm	

Stage 1: Preparation for a GA category 1 Caesarean Section	
Information given	**Expected actions**
Patient is on operating table, clearly anxious	Ensure correct positioning – 15° left lateral tilt, head-up for preoxygenation and position optimised for intubation
	Start O$_2$ at 15L/min via nasal cannulae
	Apply monitoring (NIBP, ECG, SpO$_2$, quantitative peripheral nerve stimulator)
Fit and well. BMI 27. No regular meds. No allergies. Previous uneventful GA for tonsillectomy. No problems with this pregnancy. Last meal: 08:00 (>12 hours ago), drinking water since	Anaesthetist takes a focussed history
Difficult as lying down but mouth opening looks OK and Calder A	Perform airway assessment

Information given	Expected actions
	Brief explanation of procedure including cricoid pressure and consent for GA including mention of risk of awareness
	Check OK for Diclofenac suppositories
	Check patency of IV cannula and ensure fluid attached and running
If asked: she has been prescribed 6 hourly oral ranitidine, but has not had the dose she was due at 20:00.	Antacid prophylaxis: Sodium citrate 30mls and IV ranitidine 50mg
	Give antibiotic prophylaxis as per local guidance
	Prepare drugs for induction of anaesthesia – have 2 syringes of induction agent available
	Check suction available and switched on
	Once history taken, commence preoxygenation with facemask in addition to nasal cannulae for 2-3 mins or $ETO_2 \geq 0.9$.
	Meanwhile, scrub team, obstetrican and midwife are preparing for caesarean section: • Theatre team scrubbed • Abdomen prepared • Bladder catheterised
	Neonatal team called to attend
Plan to continue/wake up may vary but should show consideration of factors in Figure 24.2 (OAA DAS guidelines)	WHO checklist undertaken as per local guidance. As part of this, the anaesthetist should clearly verbalise: • Plan A, B and C of their airway strategy • Who their emergency anaesthetic assistance is and how they can be contacted in case of difficult airway • Plan made to either continue surgery using a supraglottic airway or wake the patient up in the event of a failed intubation

Proceed to stage 2 once all preparations for GA have been made

Observations	
A	Clear
B	As per BVM ventilation
C	HR and BP to reflect the doses of induction agent/ analgesia given
D	Anaesthetised
E	Nil to note

Observations	
A	ETT
B	RR as per ventilator SpO$_2$ 98% ETCO$_2$ 5.4kPa
C	HR and BP to reflect the doses of induction agent/ analgesia given
D	Anaesthetised
E	Temp 36.8^{0}C

Stage 2: Induction and maintenance of anaesthesia

Information given	Expected actions
	Application of cricoid pressure
	Induction of anaesthesia with appropriate agents and dose: • Thiopentone 5-7mg/kg or propofol 2-2.5mg/kg (induction agent titrated to response) with second syringe of induction agent available • Suxamethonium 1-1.5mg or rocuronium 1-1.2mg/kg • Consider opioid: eg alfentanil 500-1000mcg
	Anaesthetist may gently bag/valve/mask(BVM) ventilate, maintaining peak airway pressures <20 cmH20, or if not, should maintain airway patency to facilitate apnoeic oxygenation
Grade 2a laryngoscopy	Intubation with size 7.0 endotracheal tube(ETT) and ETT secured
	ETT position checked with ETCO$_2$ and auscultation
	Commence volatile agent and oxygen/nitrous oxide mix (33%/66%) at appropriate fresh gas flows (see discussion)
	Anaesthetist instructs ODP/anaesthetic nurse to release cricoid pressure once happy that ETT in correct position and cuff inflated adequately to create seal
	Obstetrician should check with anaesthetist prior to commencing surgery
	Monitor patient temperature and initiate active warming measures
Delivery of the infant in good condition	At delivery candidate should administer oxytocin as a slow bolus
	Anaesthetist should administer: • Analgesia and antiemetics in accordance with local policies • Consideration of further dose of non-depolarising muscle relaxant if suxamethonium given at induction

Proceed to stage 3 once analgesia and antiemetic given and surgery complete

Stage 3: Waking and extubation

Information given	Expected actions
Surgery finished	Anaesthetist assesses for residual neuromuscular block using a quantitative peripheral nerve stimulator and reverses with appropriate reversal agent and dose at end of surgery
	Don't proceed to wake up patient if train-of-four (TOF) ratio <0.9
	Check temperature
	Suction oropharynx
	Position appropriately for extubation and turn off volatile anaesthetic – switch to 100% oxygen.
	Extubate fully awake
Scenario ends when patient is extubated and breathing spontaneously on facemask O$_2$	

Observations	
A	ETT
B	RR 20/min
SpO$_2$ 98%
ETCO$_2$ 4.9kPa
C	HR 110bpm
BP 140/85
D	A**V**PU
E	Temp 36.9°C

Suggested Topics for Debrief Discussion

- **To anaesthetist:** did you feel that you prioritised tasks appropriately and got everything prepared in a timely way prior to induction of anaesthesia?
- Would you change any aspects of how you did this for your next GA category 1 caesarean section?
- How was communication within the theatre team: in particular, prior to induction, did the anaesthetist clearly verbalise:
  · Plan A, B and C of their airway strategy?
  · Who their emergency anaesthetic assistance is and how they could be contacted in case of difficult airway?
  · Plan made to either continue surgery using a supraglottic airway or wake the patient up in the event of a failed intubation?

Scenario 2
Scenario in a Nutshell

Caesarean section under general anaesthesia with failed intubation.
   Stage 1: Preparation for a GA category 1 caesarean section.
   Stage 2: Induction of anaesthesia and failed intubation.
   Stage 3: Difficult mask ventilation, airway rescue with supraglottic airway device, decision to proceed/wake patient.

Target Learner Groups

Anaesthetists, midwives, operating department practitioners/anaesthetic nurses, theatre scrub team, obstetricians.

Specific learning opportunities
Demonstrate competencies around general anaesthesia for caesarean section as described in RCOA 2010 Curriculum – Annex B
Effective preparation for and management of induction of general anaesthesia for category 1 caesarean section
Demonstrate clear communication in the team, particularly the verbalising of Plan A, B and C of the airway strategy, how to contact emergency anaesthetic assistance in case of difficult airway and whether planning to continue surgery using a supraglottic airway or wake the patient up in the event of a failed intubation
Knowledge of and timely progression through the DAS/OAA failed intubation in obstetrics algorithm

Suggested learners (to represent their normal roles)	In theatre from the start	Available when requested
Anaesthetic CT2	√	
Anaesthetic ST3+		√
Obstetric ST3+	√	
Midwife	√	
Operating Department Practitioner (ODP)/anaesthetic nurse	√	
Theatre team – scrub nurse	√	
Theatre team – runner	√	

Suggested learners (to represent their normal roles)	In theatre from the start	Available when requested
Suggested facilitators		
Faculty to play role of midwife transferring patient to theatre (can be played by facilitator running scenario)	√	

Details for Facilitators
Patient Demographics

Name: Felicity

Age: 32

Gestation: 39+5

Booking weight: 90 kg

Parity: P0

Scenario Summary for Facilitators

32-year-old, 39+5 weeks gestation primiparous woman.
Labouring spontaneously on Delivery Suite.
Has progressed slowly to 5 cm dilated using entonox for analgesia.
Developed sustained fetal bradycardia resulting in decision for category 1 caesarean section for fetal distress.
Requires a general anaesthetic.
Failed intubation occurs.
Able to ventilate with a supraglottic airway.
Decision to wake patient or proceed with caesarean section.

Set-up Overview for Facilitators

Clinical setting	Obstetric theatre
Patient position	Just arrived in theatre, being positioned on operating table
Initial monitoring in place	None
Other equipment	16G cannula dorsum left hand
Useful manikin functions	Intubation

Medical Equipment

For core equipment checklist, see Chapter 9, including advanced airway equipment.

Additional equipment specific to scenario		
Premedication:	**Induction drugs:**	**Other drugs:**
Ranitidine (IV if not had PO)
Sodium citrate	Thiopentone, propofol
Opioids – alfentanil, fentanyl, morphine
Muscle relaxants – suxamethonium, rocuronium, atracurium	Reversal agents: neostigmine, sugammadex
Quantitative peripheral nerve stimulator	Contact details for emergency anaesthetic assistance	WHO checklist/ timeout

Information Given to the Learners

Information given to anaesthetic trainee before they enter theatre
The midwife coordinator comes in to say there is a category 1 section for a prolonged fetal bradycardia. As you go to assess her, the team are wheeling her into theatre.

Information given in theatre to anaesthetic trainee, obstetric trainee, theatre team, midwife and obstetrician from midwife who has just transferred the patient to theatre (faculty)
Time: 10:00 Sunday
The SBAR handover is as follows:
Situation: This is Felicity, who is having a fetal bradycardia.
Background: 32-year-old, fit and well primip, BMI 31, who is 39+5 weeks pregnant with no allergies. She presented in spontaneous labour and progressed to 5 cm dilatation, then has just had a fetal bradycardia. She has had diamorphine and entonox for analgesia.
Assessment: We have come straight through from the room. She has signed her consent form.
Recommendation: She needs a category 1 caesarean section.

Scenario Schedule

Stage 1: Preparation for GA category 1 caesarean section	
Information given	**Expected actions**
Patient has just been moved onto operating table	Ensure correct positioning – 15° left lateral tilt, head-up position for pre-oxygenation
	Start O_2 via nasal cannulae at 15L/min
	Consider ramped position/positioning aids eg: Oxford HELP® pillow
If asked: Usually fit and well. BMI 31. No antenatal problems. No previous general anaesthetic or family history of problems with general anaesthesia. No regular medications or drug allergies. Last drank 30 minutes ago – water. Last ate 10 hours ago. Had PO ranitidine 150mg 2 hours ago.	Focussed history taken by anaesthetist
No dental problems Mallampati 2, average mouth opening, Calder B	Perform airway assessment
	Brief explanation of procedure including cricoid pressure and consent for GA including mention of risk of awareness
	Monitoring applied (NIBP, ECG, SpO_2, quantitative peripheral nerve stimulator)
	Check patency of IV cannula and ensure fluid attached and running
	Antacid prophylaxis: Sodium citrate 30mls
	Check suction available and switched on
	Commence facemask preoxygenation in addition to nasal cannulae for 2-3mins or until $ETO_2 \geq 0.9$
	Meanwhile, scrub team, obstetrican and midwife are preparing for caesarean section: • Theatre team scrubbed • Abdomen prepared • Bladder catheterised
	Neonatal team called to attend

Observations	
A	Clear
B	RR 20/min SpO_2 98%
C	HR 102bpm BP 135/75
D	**A**VPU
E	Nil to note
CTG	Baseline FHR 80bpm

Information given	Expected actions
	WHO checklist undertaken as per local guidance. As part of this, the anaesthetist should clearly verbalise: • Plan A, B and C of their airway strategy • Who their emergency anaesthetic assistance is and how they can be contacted in case of difficult airway
Plan to continue/wake up may vary but should show consideration of factors in Figure 24.2 (OAA DAS guidelines)	• Plan made to either continue surgery using a supraglottic airway or wake the patient up in the event of a failed intubation

Proceed to stage 2 once all preparations for GA have been made.

Stage 2: Induction of anaesthesia and failed intubation

Information given	Expected actions
	Application of cricoid pressure Induction of anaesthesia with appropriate agents and dose: • Thiopentone 5-7mg/kg or propofol 2-2.5mg/kg (induction agent titrated to response) with second syringe of induction agent available • Suxamethonium 1-1.5mg or rocuronium 1-1.2mg/kg • Consider opioid eg alfentanil 500-1000mcg
	Candidate may gently bag/valve/mask(BVM) ventilate, maintaining peak airway pressures <20 cmH20, or if not, should maintain airway patency to facilitate apnoeic oxygenation
1st laryngoscopy attempt: Grade 4 view	Laryngoscopy attempted
	Anaesthetist should: • Optimise positioning • Apply/ask ODP/anaesthetic nurse to apply BURP(backwards/upwards/right pressure) • Ease/remove cricoid pressure

Observations

A	Clear
B	RR as per BVM ventilation SpO$_2$ 97%
C	Alter HR and BP as appropriate for doses of induction drugs given
D	Anaesthetised
E	Nil to note

Stage 2: Induction of anaesthesia and failed intubation

Information given	Expected actions
2nd laryngoscopy attempt: difficult grade 3 view – tip of epiglottis seen	2nd attempt at laryngoscopy – use alternative laryngoscope
No ETCO$_2$ seen once ETT railroaded over bougie	Anaesthetist may attempt to place bougie
	Remove ETT and revert to BVM ventilation via facemask
	No more than 3 attempts at laryngoscopy in total (Limit to 2 by same anaesthetist, if 3rd attempted should be by experienced colleague)
	Anaesthetist makes clear statement of emergency to the team: failed intubation

Progress to stage 3 once failed intubation recognised and clearly stated

Observations

A	Obstructed
B	RR as per BVM ventilation SpO$_2$ 92% and falling
C	HR 132bpm BP 150/80
D	Anaesthetised
E	Nil to note

Stage 3: Difficult mask ventilation, airway rescue with supraglottic airway device. Decision to proceed/wake patient.

Information given	Expected actions
	Anaesthetist calls for anaesthetic assistance stating clearly who they require
Mask ventilation difficult with minimal chest movement	Reverts to BVM ventilation +/- oropharyngeal airway and 2-handed technique
	Consider further boluses of induction agent
Able to ventilate with SAD – SpO$_2$ slowly improves	Insertion of 2nd generation supraglottic airway device (SAD) – no more than 2 attempts, with relaxation of cricoid during insertion
	2nd anaesthetist arrives: SBAR from 1st anaesthetist No further attempts at intubation at this stage as able to ventilate via SAD, particularly if patient has had suxamethonium (may be wearing off) or had 3 attempts at intubation already
	Decision on whether to proceed with surgery with SAD and cricoid pressure or wake patient - refer to earlier decision and verbalise with team if any changes have occurred that alter decision

Observations

A	Obstructed
B	RR as per BVM ventilation SpO$_2$ 85%
C	HR 112bpm BP 110/75
D	Anaesthetised
E	Nil to note

Observations

A	SAD
B	RR as per anaesthetist SpO$_2$ 94%
C	HR 110bpm BP 108/68
D	Anaesthetised
E	Nil to note
CTG	Baseline FHR 150bpm, variability <5bpm and late decelerations

Information given	Expected actions
	Considerations if proceeding with caesarean section with SAD in situ:
	• Most senior obstetrician available to complete LSCS to minimise length of procedure
	• Consider paralysis with rocuronium to facilitate surgery and ventilation if sugammadex available
	• If not paralysed, deep inhalational anaesthesia
	• Minimise aspiration risk:
	• Maintain cricoid pressure until delivery if ventilation not compromised
	• Head-up position
	• Empty stomach with gastric drain if 2nd generation SAD used (if paralysed)
	• Minimise fundal pressure
	• If not had ranitidine (or similar) administer IV dose
	Considerations if decide to wake patient:
	• Maintain cricoid pressure if ventilation not compromised
	• Maintain head-up position or turn left-lateral recumbent
	• If rocuronium used, reverse with sugammadex
	• Monitor neuromuscular block, manage awareness if paralysis prolonged
	• If not had ranitidine (or similar) administer IV dose
	Inform neonatal team of failed intubation
	The scenario could be modified by failure of a SAD to rescue the airway, forcing the candidate down the OAA/DAS 2015 failed intubation/failed ventilation algorithm with a resultant cricothyroidotomy

Scenario ends once decision to proceed on SAD or wake the patient is agreed

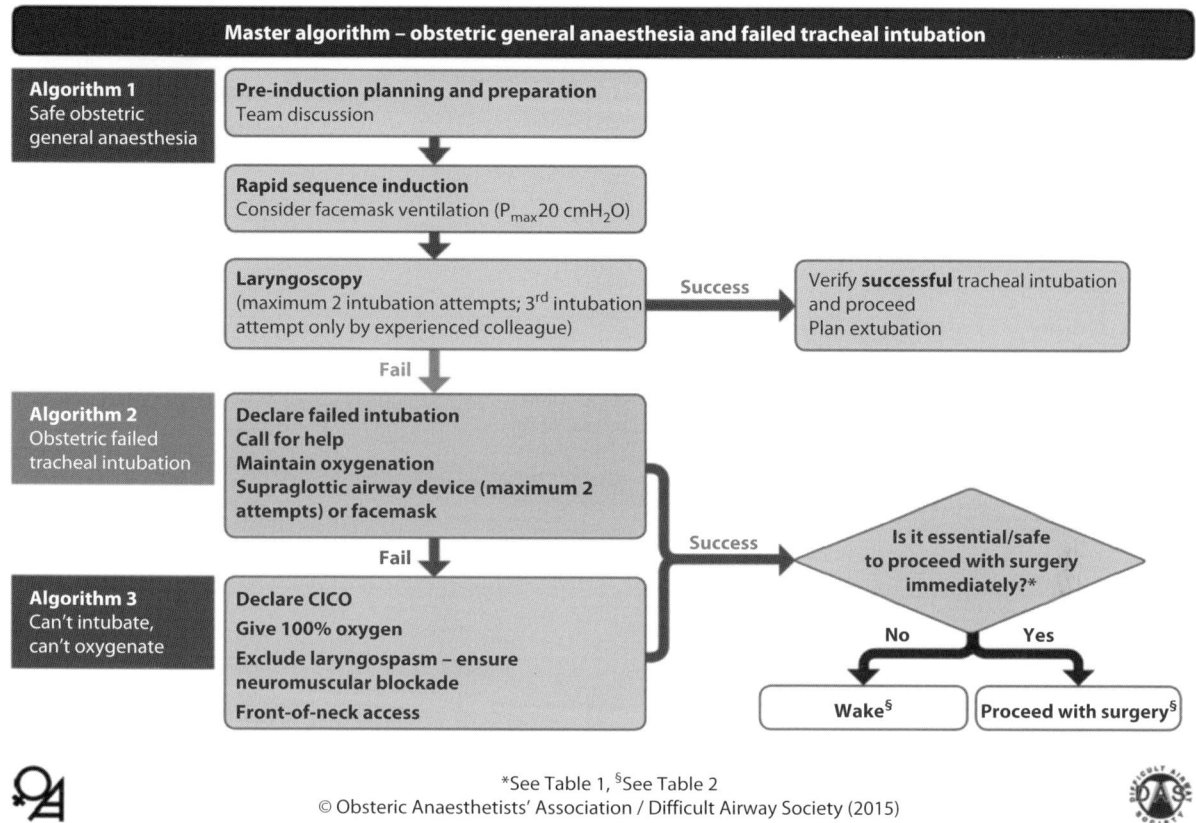

Figure 24.1 Obstetric Anaesthetists' Association and Difficult Airway Society guidelines for the management of difficult and failed tracheal intubation in obstetrics.

Reproduced from Mushambi, M. C., Kinsella, S. M., Popat, M., Swales, H., Ramaswamy, K. K., Winton, A. L. Quinn, A. C. Anaesthesia 2015, 70, 1286–1306, and with permission from Obstetric Anaesthetists' Association/Difficult Airway Society.

Suggested Topics for Debrief Discussion

- Was all the airway equipment available that was requested?
- Did everyone know where to find the failed intubation trolley, including obstetric/midwifery staff?
- Were the team clear regarding who to call for emergency assistance in failed intubation?
- Did the obstetric/midwifery/theatre team recognise the significance when 'failed intubation' stated and understand their role in the emergency?
- Did the theatre team/obstetricians/midwife understand the relevance of the team discussion at WHO checklist regarding proceeding or waking in the event of failed intubation (show the group the DAS/OAA, Figure 24.2).

Discussion

The technique of choice for many anaesthetists providing anaesthesia for caesarean section remains a 'classical' rapid sequence induction (RSI), comprising thiopentone, suxamethonium, volatile anaesthetic agent and cricoid pressure. In this regard, the technique remains unchanged from that used in 1970 (Lucas and Yentis, 2015).

The provision of anaesthesia for such cases can be a source of anxiety, particularly among inexperienced trainees, due to perceptions around the risks associated with such cases; namely, the increased risk of difficulty in managing the airway (incidence of failed intubation in obstetric general anaesthetics is 1 in 390: Kinsella et al., 2015), risk of accidental awareness under general anaesthesia (AAGA) and concerns regarding the well-being of both mother and fetus.

Table 1 – proceed with surgery?				
Factors to consider	**WAKE** ⟵⟶			**PROCEED**
Before induction — Maternal condition	• No compromise	• Mild acute compromise	• Haemorrhage responsive to resuscitation	• Hypovolaemia requiring corrective surgery • Critical cardiac or respiratory compromise, cardiac arrest
Fetal condition	• No compromise	• Compromise corrected with intrauterine resuscitation, pH < 7.2 but > 7.15	• Continuing fetal heart rate abnormality despite intrauterine resuscitation, pH < 7.15	• Sustained bradycardia • Fetal haemorrhage • Suspected uterine rupture
Anaesthetist	• Novice	• Junior trainee	• Senior trainee	• Consultant / specialist
Obesity	• Supermorbid	• Morbid	• Obese	• Normal
Surgical factors	• Complex surgery or major haemorrhage anticipated	• Multiple uterine scars • Some surgical difficulties expected	• Single uterine scar	• No risk factors
Aspiration risk	• Recent food	• No recent food • In labour • Opioids given • Antacids not given	• No recent food • In labour • Opioids not given • Antacids given	• Fasted • Not in labour • Antacids given
Alternative anaesthesia • regional • securing airway awake	• No anticipated difficulty	• Predicted difficulty	• Relatively contraindicated	• Absolutely contraindicated or has failed • Surgery started
After failed intubation — Airway device/ventilation	• Difficult facemask ventilation • Front-of-neck	• Adequate facemask ventilation	• First generation supraglottic airway device	• Second generation supraglottic airway device
Airway hazards	• Laryngeal oedema • Stridor	• Bleeding • Trauma	• Secretions	• None evident

 Criteria to be used in the decision to wake or proceed following failed tracheal intubation. In any individual patient, some factors may suggest waking and others proceeding. The final decision will depend on the anaesthetist's clinical judgement.
© Obstetric Anaesthetists Association / Difficult Airway Society (2015)

Figure 24.2 Obstetric Anaesthetists' Association and Difficult Airway Society guidelines for the management of difficult and failed tracheal intubation in obstetrics.
Reproduced from Mushambi, M. C., Kinsella, S. M., Popat, M., Swales, H., Ramaswamy, K. K., Winton, A. L. and Quinn, A. C. Anaesthesia 2015, 70, 1286–1306, with permission from Obstetric Anaesthetists' Association/Difficult Airway Society.

Anaesthetic Considerations of the Anatomical and Physiological Changes of Pregnancy

The anatomical and physiological changes associated with pregnancy are key to the challenges posed when delivering general anaesthesia to the obstetric population.

Changes to the Airway

• Engorgement of capillary beds in the airway soft tissues results in swelling and friability of nasal and oropharyngeal mucosae, meaning these areas can be easily traumatised during airway instrumentation, with the risk of bleeding and airway compromise.

• This swelling, combined with an increase in size of the breasts and the increasing incidence of obstetric obesity, means that there may be difficulty in laryngoscopy.

Respiratory Changes

• Reduction in functional residual capacity (FRC): the expanding uterus causes compression of intra-abdominal organs with reduction (up to 30% when supine at term) in diaphragmatic excursion during ventilation and reduced efficacy of pre-oxygenation.

• Increased oxygen requirements: maternal oxygen requirements and carbon dioxide production increase up to 60% due to increased metabolic demand.

The combination of these factors results in the potential for rapid desaturation following induction of anaesthesia, particularly if difficultly in managing the airway is experienced.

Cardiovascular Changes

- Aortocaval compression: after 20 weeks gestation, the increasing mass of the gravid uterus causes compression of the aorta and inferior vena cava, particularly when supine, resulting in a reduction in venous return and thus cardiac output. This may compromise maternal blood pressure and consequently end-organ perfusion and, as there is no uteroplacental autoregulation, placental blood flow. This is compensated for with an increase in sympathetic tone resulting in vasoconstriction and increased maternal heart rate, a response that may be obtunded by induction of anaesthesia.
- Increased cardiac output: There is an increase in both stroke volume and heart rate with a resultant increase in cardiac output. This has implications for the risk of accidental awareness, as the increased cardiac output reduces the duration of action of an induction bolus of intravenous anaesthetic agent, while increasing the time to attain an effective partial pressure of volatile agent, potentially giving rise to a 'gap' in anaesthesia.

Central Nervous System

- In a pregnant woman, the central nervous system is theoretically more sensitive to anaesthetic agents, traditionally necessitating a reduction in MAC of volatile agents of up to 30%. However, the findings of NAP 5 counter this (Pandit et al., 2014), and the high risk of AAGA in obstetric anaesthesia means low end-tidal concentrations of volatile agents are not recommended.

Gastrointestinal

- The stomach is displaced upwards during pregnancy causing an increase in intragastric pressure. In association with a reduction in gastro-oesophageal sphincter tone, this gives rise to the characteristic symptoms of acid reflux experienced by many pregnant women.
- The pain and anxiety of labour, as well as the use of opioid analgesia, can cause a reduction in gastric

emptying in women presenting for emergency caesarean section.

There is thus an increased risk of regurgitation and aspiration during obstetric general anaesthesia.

Organisational Factors in Obstetric General Anaesthesia

Caesarean section under general anaesthesia is increasingly uncommon, as the majority of obstetric cases are performed under regional anaesthesia. Only 25% of category 1 and 2 caesarean sections are undertaken with a consultant anaesthetist present (Pandit et al., 2014). Therefore, these cases are most commonly managed by (potentially inexperienced) trainees, often outside normal working hours and in sites remote from the main theatre complex.

The most common choice of induction drug for caesarean section remains thiopentone, the use of which is dwindling rapidly in non-obstetric practice, resulting in trainees potentially using an induction technique in obstetrics that they would otherwise use rarely, if ever (Murdoch et al., 2013).

These factors, along with anaesthetising in a noisy theatre rife with distractions as it is prepared for urgent surgery, result in an environment that is less than ideal for the delivery of safe anaesthesia.

Current Areas of Interest in General Anaesthesia for Obstetrics

A number of recent publications (including NAP 4 and 5, MBRRACE (Knight et al., 2014) and the 2015 joint guidelines from the Difficult Airway Society and the Obstetric Anaesthetists' Association) have prompted us to reflect on our current practice of general anaesthesia in obstetrics. In particular, the problems with airway difficulty (Cook et al., 2011) and the disproportionately high incidence of reported awareness under anaesthesia in the obstetric population, with their associated morbidity, have obliged anaesthetists to examine carefully our existing technique for GA caesarean section.

Because of these concerns, various components of the process involved in delivering general anaesthesia have been debated in the literature.

Consent

Given the high incidence of AAGA, with obstetric cases over-represented in NAP 5 by a factor of more than 10, some discussion around the potential for awareness is advised. However, given the time-critical nature of many cases, a detailed discussion is not feasible. It is suggested that along with a brief explanation of cricoid pressure, the woman should be warned that she might be aware of some sensations as the ETT is introduced and removed at the end of the procedure (Bogod and Plaat, 2015).

Positioning

All patients should be positioned with at least 15° of left lateral tilt to obviate aorto-caval compression. In addition, positioning in the ramped position (in which the external auditory meatus is in line with the suprasternal notch) may have multiple benefits, including improving the efficacy of pre-oxygenation by increasing FRC, reducing the risk of aspiration of gastric contents, allowing easier access and improving the view at laryngoscopy and facilitating ventilation. In obese patients, consideration should be given to using positioning aids such as the Oxford HELP® pillow.

Pre-oxygenation

Women at term are at high risk of rapid desaturation following induction of anaesthesia due to a reduction in FRC and increased metabolic demand for oxygen. Rigorous pre-oxygenation is essential in order to decrease the time to hypoxaemia in case of airway difficulty.

Pre-oxygenation using a tight-fitting face mask and 100% inspired oxygen to achieve an end-tidal O_2 (ETO_2) in excess of 0.9 is common practice. This can be augmented with 5–15 l/min of oxygen via nasal cannulae, continued after induction with maintenance of the airway to both increase oxygen delivery during pre-oxygenation and provide a degree of apnoeic oxygenation after induction.

Consideration should be given to gentle mask ventilation (maintaining peak airway pressures below 20 cmH_2O) to prevent desaturation (Mushambi et al., 2015).

Some units are beginning to use high-flow humidified nasal oxygen delivery systems for pre-oxygenation and prolongation of apnoea time, currently used in head and neck anaesthesia and critical care. The application of these systems in obstetric practice is intriguing, but further research is needed in this patient population.

Induction Drugs

Thiopentone has a long-established record in obstetric anaesthesia. It remains the drug of choice for general anaesthesia in obstetrics for the majority of anaesthetists (Murdoch et al., 2013). Recently, numerous high-profile publications have expressed concerns regarding the use of thiopentone in obstetrics. NAP 5 involved thiopentone as one of the key factors implicated in the high rate of AAGA in obstetrics (Pandit et al., 2014). The reasons for this are multifactorial, and a full evaluation regarding the most appropriate choice of induction drug for caesarean section is beyond the remit of this review. Briefly, the following issues have been identified.

- The majority of these cases are undertaken by trainees, who have less exposure to thiopentone than would have been the case previously, with 87% of anaesthetists using the drug less than monthly in one large activity survey (Murdoch et al., 2013).
- Inappropriately low doses of thiopentone were used in many cases of AAGA, with NAP 5 recommending a dosage of at least 5 mg/kg in non-compromised patients.
- Conversely, a recent maternal mortality report from MBRRACE commented on inappropriately large doses of thiopentone being administered to parturients compromised by shock (Knight et al., 2014).
- NAP 5 reported two cases of syringe swaps with antibiotics at induction due to the similarity of thiopentone and co-amoxiclav when reconstituted.
- The supply of thiopentone may not be robust, and it is currently more expensive than propofol (Rucklidge, 2013).

The obvious alternative to thiopentone is propofol, which is used extensively internationally in obstetric practice (it is the first-line agent in the USA; Murdoch et al., 2013). While concerns have been raised about potential effects on the neonate, these fears are not supported by the literature, which overall shows no adverse neonatal outcomes in comparison with thiopentone (Rucklidge, 2013; Valtonen et al., 1989; Devroe et al., 2015).

Propofol has definite advantages in terms of familiarity among practitioners, who are more likely to use it regularly for rapid sequence induction (RSI) outside obstetric practice. Its haemodynamic profile may be better suited to obstetrics, as it obtunds the cardiovascular response to laryngoscopy and intubation. The effect of propofol on airway reflexes may facilitate laryngoscopy and the placement of a supraglottic airway devices (SAD) in case of difficult airway. Propofol is much less likely to be implicated in syringe-swap drug errors than thiopentone and, although it cannot be drawn up in advance as is common practice with thiopentone, this also reduces the risk of reconstitution errors.

Whichever agent is used, it is good practice to have a second syringe available in order to maintain anaesthesia in case of a difficult airway (Pandit et al., 2014). In cases of cardiovascular instability due to major haemorrhage, the use of 1–2 mg/kg of ketamine may be preferable.

Muscle Relaxants

Suxamethonium continues to be the most widely used muscle relaxant in obstetric RSI due to its rapid onset of action. Its short duration of action has often been cited as a benefit in obstetric practice, as, theoretically, the patient could be woken prior to desaturation in case of failed intubation. This is unlikely to be the case in practice. In fact, the fasciculations caused by suxamethonium may increase metabolic oxygen demand and actually decrease the time to desaturation following induction. Care should be taken with dosing. For a dose of 1.5 mg/kg, a single 100 mg ampule is only sufficient for women weighing up to ~70 kg.

The combination of 1–1.2 mg/kg of rocuronium and reversal with sugammadex 16 mg/kg in the case of failed intubation provides an attractive alternative, particularly if the anaesthetist is concerned about potential difficult airway, with much reduced mean time to recovery of neuromuscular function than suxamethonium (Lee et al., 2009).

The 2015 OAA DAS obstetric airway guidelines recommend that in the 'can't intubate, can't oxygenate' situation, paralysis should be ensured (Mushambi et al., 2015). Given this advice, the use of an effective, long-acting, readily reversible agent from the outset is attractive.

Opioids

The routine use of opioids at induction has traditionally been avoided due to concerns around neonatal depression, as these agents readily cross the placenta. However, opinion may be shifting in this regard (the NAP 5 activity survey indicating 23.4% of obstetric RSI included an opioid). NAP 5 recommended the appropriate use of opioids in obstetric general anaesthesia as a means of reducing the risk of AAGA (Pandit et al., 2014).

Additional benefits include modulation of the maternal stress response during laryngoscopy and analgesia for skin incision. The presence of opioid at induction is also likely to improve intubating conditions. The available evidence suggests the use of short-acting opioids produces only transient neonatal depression with rapid recovery (Patel and Fernando, 2016). While there are clear maternal benefits to the use of opioids at induction, the neonatologist should be informed at delivery if they have been used.

Maintenance of Anaesthesia

In obstetrics, there is little time between intubation and start of surgery; therefore, careful attention must be paid to rapidly achieving an adequate end-tidal volatile concentration. High fresh-gas flow rates in combination with a high volatile agent concentration should be used in order to rapidly attain effective end-tidal concentrations (a pragmatic approach would be to set an initial fresh-gas flow of 8 l/min, with a sevoflurane dialled concentration of 5% in a nitrous oxide/oxygen mixture until the end-tidal concentration reaches at least 1.3% (Chin and Yeo, 2004)). Nitrous oxide should be used routinely (Pandit et al., 2014).

Airway Management

The 2015 OAA DAS obstetric airway guidelines (see Figure 24.1) (Mushambi et al., 2015) have provided advice and clarity in terms of airway management. Much of this, in terms of positioning, pre-oxygenation, choice of induction agents and gentle ventilation following induction has been discussed above.

The use of supraglottic airway devices, particularly second-generation devices, is now established as an airway rescue technique in cases of failed intubation in obstetric general anaesthesia. These guidelines also include a matrix to aid decision-making in terms of continuing to caesarean section or waking following a failure to intubate (see Figure 24.2).

Most obstetric theatres now have a dedicated video-laryngoscope, which can improve the view at laryngoscopy compared with a conventional laryngoscope, and practitioners should become familiar with the use of these devices.

Conclusion

The provision of general anaesthesia for caesarean section provides specific challenges to the anaesthetist due to a combination of the physiological changes of pregnancy increasing the risk of airway difficulty, accidental awareness and aspiration as well as the situational and human factors involved.

A classical RSI using thiopentone and suxamethonium remains the default choice for many anaesthetists, although recent publications have called this technique into question. It is likely that propofol will increasingly be used in place of thiopentone, in line with practice in other areas of anaesthesia. Other shifts in practice are likely to see increasing use of rocuronium and opioid at induction. The publication of the joint DAS/OAA guidelines, as well as improvements in equipment such as SADs, videolaryngoscopes and positioning devices, should make obstetric general anaesthesia a less daunting undertaking in future.

Bibliography

Bogod, D. and Plaat, F. (2015). Be wary of awareness – lessons from NAP5 for obstetric anaesthetists. *International Journal of Obstetric Anaesthesia* 24, 1–4.

Chin, K. J. and Yeo, S. W. (2004). A BIS-guided study of sevoflurane requirements for adequate depth of anaesthesia in Caesarean section. *Anaesthesia*, 59, 1064–1068.

Cook, T., Woodall, N. and Frerk, C. (Eds.). (2011). *The 4th National Audit Project (NAP4) on Major Complications of Airway Management in the UK: Results of the Royal College of Anaesthetists and the Difficult Airway Society*. London: RCoA & DAS.

Devroe, S., Van de Velde, M. and Rex, S. (2015). General anesthesia for caesarean section. *Current Opinion in Anesthesiology*, 28, 240–246.

Kinsella, S. M., Winton, A. L., Mushambi, M. C., et al. (2015). Failed intubation during obstetric anaesthesia: a literature review. *International Journal of Obstetric Anaesthesia*, 24, 356–374.

Knight, M., Kenyon, S., Brocklehurst, P., Neilson, J., Shakespeare, J. and Kurinczuk, J. J. (2014). *Saving Lives, Improving Mothers' Care – Lessons Learned to Inform Future Maternity Care from the UK and Ireland Confidential Enquiries into Maternal Deaths and Morbidity 2009–12 on Behalf of MBRRACE-UK*. Oxford: NPEU.

Lee, C., Jahr, J. S., Candiotti, K. A., Warriner, B., Zornow, M. H. and Naguib, M. (2009). Reversal of profound neuromuscular block by sugammadex administered three minutes after rocuronium: a comparison with spontaneous recovery from succinylcholine. *Anesthesiology*, 110(5), 1020–1025.

Lucas, D. N. and Yentis, S. M. (2015). Unsettled weather and the end for thiopentone? Obstetric general anaesthesia after the NAP5 and MBRRACE-UK reports. *Anaesthesia*, 70, 375–392.

Murdoch, H., Scrutton, M. and Laxton, C. H. (2013). Choice of anaesthetic agents for caesarean section: a UK survey of current practice. *International Journal of Obstetric Anaesthesia*, 22, 31–35.

Mushambi, M. C., Kinsella, S. M., Popat, M., et al. (2015). Obstetric Anaesthetists' Association and Difficult Airway Society guidelines for the management of difficult and failed tracheal intubation in obstetrics. *Anaesthesia*, 70, 1286–1306.

Pandit, J. J., Andrade, J., Bogod, D. G., et al. (2014). The 5th National Audit Project (NAP5) on accidental awareness during general anaesthesia. *Anaesthesia*, 69, 1078–1088.

Patel, S. and Fernando, R. (2016). Opioids should be given before cord clamping for caesarean delivery under general anaesthesia. *International Journal of Obstetric Anaesthesia*, 28, 76–82.

Rucklidge, M. (2013). Up to date or out of date: does thiopental have a future in obstetric general anaesthesia? *International Journal of Obstetric Anaesthesia*, 22, 175–178.

Valtonen, M., Kanto, J. and Rosenberg, P. (1989). Comparison of propofol and thiopentone for induction of anaesthesia for elective caesarean section. *Anaesthesia*, 44, 758–762.

Chapter

25

Antepartum Haemorrhage and Perimortem Caesarean Section

Kenneth Ma

Scenario in a Nutshell

Concealed abruption with hypovolaemic cardiac arrest requiring perimortem section in A+E.

Stage 1: Initial assessment of parturient with severe abdominal pain and reduced fetal movements.

Stage 2: Handover to MDT obstetric team, identification of placental abruption and activation of major haemorrhage pathway.

Stage 3: Cardiovascular collapse despite resuscitation.

Stage 4: Management of hypovolaemic PEA arrest and perimortem section.

Target Learner Groups

Appropriate members of the receiving A+E team and multidisciplinary obstetric team.

Specific learning opportunities
Knowledge of differential diagnosis of acute onset abdominal pain in pregnancy
Recognition of concealed haemorrhage
Knowledge of massive haemorrhage protocol
Knowledge of obstetric emergency equipment in A+E
Demonstrate safe, effective CPR with timely perimortem section

Suggested learners (to represent their normal roles)	In the room from the start	Available when requested
A+E nurse	√	
A+E ST3+	√	
Obstetric ST3+/Consultant		√
Midwife		√
Anaesthetic CT2/ST3+		√
Other responding members of A+E team		√
Neonatal resuscitation team (if able to run a simultaneous neonatal resuscitation scenario*)		√
Suggested facilitators		
Faculty to play role of triage nurse in A+E	√	

This scenario is written with an absent fetal heart beat from the start. However, if you wanted to involve the neonatal team, faculty can alter the scenario to include a live fetus.

Details for Facilitators

Patient Demographics

Name: Olivia

Age: 35

Gestation: 28

Booking weight: 60 kg

Parity: P0

Scenario Summary for Facilitators

Patient attends A+E with severe abdominal pain and reduced fetal movements.

Haemodynamically unstable, unresponsive to fluids.

When examined found to have hard, woody uterus.

If available, ultrasound confirms fetal death *in utero*.

Sonicaid shows no fetal heart beat.

Massive haemorrhage recognised and massive haemorrhage protocol activated. Before able to transfer to theatre, patient becomes less responsive and then suffers a hypovolaemic PEA cardiac arrest. Resuscitation with blood/blood products and perimortem section required.

Set-up Overview for Facilitators

Clinical setting	A+E resus bay
Initial monitoring in place	None – just arrived in resuscitation bay
Other equipment	Nil but all usual equipment available Intubation Catheterisation
Useful manikin features	Realistic CPR compression depth and resistance Supports abdominal incision and caesarean delivery

Medical Equipment

For core equipment checklist see Chapter 9.

Additional equipment specific to scenario		
Arterial line	Resuscitation trolley with defibrillator	Pads for defibrillation
Rapid fluid infuser	O-negative blood	Other simulated blood products
Drugs: Syntocinon Syntocinon infusion Haemobate Misoprostol Syntometrine Tranexamic acid	Surgical scalpel (disposable or handle and blade) 12 × 12 gauze swabs Antiseptic prep Sterile gloves Cord clamps Doppler machine/Fast Scan TA probe	

Information Given to the Learners

Handover to the A+E team from triage nurse (played by faculty member) who has brought patient straight to resus bay

Time: Midday

Situation: Pregnant patient presenting feeling faint with severe abdominal pain and reduced fetal movements

Background: 35 years old, heavy smoker, 28 weeks pregnant. Admitted with a small PV bleed a week ago, which settled and was discharged home. Started with abdominal pain about 1 hour ago – it is getting worse and she hasn't felt baby move since pain started. No PV loss.

Assessment: I will perform some observations and contact the obstetric emergency team.

Recommendation: Can you assess the patient please?

Scenario Schedule

Stage 1: Initial assessment of parturient with severe abdominal pain and reduced fetal movements	
Information given	**Expected actions**
Patient screaming in pain and holding her abdomen. Saying "My stomach really hurts and I can't feel my baby move!"	Take history
Patient too distracted to give much more of a history but says no history of trauma	
Airway clear, chest and heart sounds normal. Abdomen hard and very tender. No blood loss PV	ABCDE assessment and examination of patient
	Apply full monitoring, pulse oximeter, NIBP and ECG
	Apply Oxygen via non-rebreathing mask at 15 l/min whilst stabilising the patient (then titrate to SpO$_2$ 94-98%)
	Avoid aortocaval compression with manual uterine displacement
	Call for emergency obstetric team (Obstetrician / midwife / anaesthetist / neonatal response team)
	Secure 2x16G IV access and take blood for FBC, U+E, LFT, Coagulation including fibrinogen and X-match for 4u RBC

Observations	
A	Clear
B	RR 26/min SpO$_2$ 95% on air (99% on O$_2$)
C	HR 130bpm BP 90/60 CRT 4s
D	**A**VPU
E	Temp 36.5°C

Information given	Expected actions
ABG results if requested pH 7.25 pCO_2 4kPa pO_2 18kPa BE −10mmol/L HCO_3^- 17mmol/L Lactate 6 mmol/L Hb 70 g/L	Arterial/venous gas to include Hb
	Commence 250ml IV Hartmann's fluid bolus
	Locate A+E obstetric emergency trolley (if department has one)
	Consider potential causes for clinical condition including: Labour Abruption Amniotic fluid embolus Other intra-abdominal pathology

Progress to stage 2 once ABCDE assessment completed and initial resuscitation commenced

Stage 2: Handover to MDT obstetric team, identification of placental abruption and activation of major haemorrhage pathway

Information given	Expected actions
Obstetric team arrive – Obstetric registrar, anaesthetist and midwife	SBAR handover from A+E responders to the arriving obstetric team
Patient continues to complain of worsening abdominal pain. Abdominal examination reveals a tender, woody hard uterus. Vaginal examination reveals a closed cervix with no bleeding	Obstetric assessment and examination of patient
Sonicaid shows no fetal heart beat. U/S confirms fetal death in utero. No other abnormalities seen, difficult to perform with patient in pain	Assessment of fetal heart
	Repeat all observations
	Continue with oxygen and IV fluid boluses
	Discussion of differential diagnosis. Recognise and communicate to team that the most likely diagnosis is massive placental abruption and concealed haemorrhage. Aim to resuscitate and determine how to deliver
	If request venous or arterial blood gas see results in stage 1

Observations	
A	Clear
B	RR 29/min SpO_2 98% on O_2
C	HR 134 bpm BP 80/40 CRT 4s
D	AVPU
E	Temp 36.4°C

195

Information given	Expected actions
	Activate massive haemorrhage pathway
Blood arrive quickly from local fridge	Transfuse 2 units O-Negative blood
	Administer 1g Tranexamic acid IV
See stage 3 for TEG result	Request point of care testing for coagulation (TEG/ROTEM). Order cryoprecipitate (or fibrinogen concentrate) early once massive haemorrhage secondary to placental abruption is suspected
	Inform obstetric and anaesthetic consultants
Theatres are ready to receive the patient if needed	Contact theatre as may need caesarean section

Progress to stage 3 once diagnosis of placental abruption and massive haemorrhage protocol has been activated

Observations	
A	Clear
B	RR 35/min Sp0$_2$ 96% on 0$_2$
C	HR 140 bpm BP 78/40 CRT 5 s
D	A**V**PU
E	Temp 36.2°C

Stage 3: Cardiovascular collapse despite resuscitation

Information given	Expected actions
Patient now responds only to voice	Recognise that patient continues to deteriorate
	Repeat all observations
Massive haemorrhage pack arrives with 4 RBC 4 FFP	Resuscitate and treat coagulopathy with RBC/FFP/platelets/cryoprecipitate/fibrinogen concentrate/tranexamic acid / fluid (guided by results of TEG/ROTEM)
	Warm fluids and patient
Uterus remains woody and hard. Patient moans in pain during examination	Repeat examination

ABG
pH 7.19
pCO$_2$ 4 kPa
pO$_2$ 15 kPa
BE −18mmol/L
HCO$_3$− 15mmol/L
Lactate 8mmol/L
Hb 5g/L
K 4.0mmol/L

Repeat ABG

TEG result
Reaction time 12mins
Maximum amplitude 50mm

Progress to stage 4 once blood transfusion commenced, POCT testing back and plans for subsequent blood components made

Stage 4: Management of hypovolaemic PEA arrest and perimortem section

Information given	Expected actions
Patient now unresponsive	
No breath sounds no palpable pulse	Assess for signs of life
	Call for help-if more team needed
	Commence CPR as per ALS guidelines
	Maintain manual uterine displacement
PEA – narrow complex rate 130bpm with no output	Chest compressions 30:2 breathes Attach pads and connect to defibrillator Assess rhythm and confirm pulseless electrical activity (PEA) Adrenaline 1mg at time of diagnosis of PEA and every 3-5 minutes thereafter Reassess rhythm every 2 minutes
	Intubate and ventilate
4H's and 4 T's: Hypovolaemia- most likely, secondary to large placental abruption Hypoxia- ventilating well Hypothermia-temp 36⁰C Hyper/po kalaemia K+4mmol/L Thromboembolic - possible as patient pregnant so at risk Tension pneumothorax or cardiac tamponade or toxicity – no history or signs to support these diagnoses	Consideration of 4H's and 4T's
	Decision for perimortem caesarean section as soon as cardiac arrest recognised. Aim to start procedure at 4 minutes of maternal collapse with delivery of baby within 5 minutes or as soon as practicably possible
	Continue CPR until fetus delivered and blood products transfused
	Return of spontaneous circulation (ROSC) post perimortem caesarean section and further resuscitaion

Scenario ends with return of spontaneous circulation and decision to transfer to theatre for completion of wound closure and then transfer to ICU

Observations	
A	Intubated
B	RR as per ventilator setting SpO$_2$ 97% on FiO$_2$ 0.5
C	HR 120bpm BP 90/52 CRT 3s
D	AVP**U**
E	Temp 36⁰C (if actively warmed)

Suggested Topics for Debrief Discussion

- How well prepared do you think your A+E department is to receive obstetric emergencies?
- If you were transferring to theatre, how quickly could you get the patient there?
- Interpretation of point of care coagulation tests.

Discussion

Introduction

Cardiac arrest in pregnancy fortunately remains a rare event in the UK occurring in approximately 1 in 36,000 pregnancies (Beckett et al., 2017; Datner and Promes, 2006). It is one of the most dreaded and stressful events for all staff involved and optimal management requires clear leadership and effective communication between multiple specialities above the demands of a standard cardiac arrest. Thromboembolism and haemorrhage remain the leading causes of direct maternal deaths (Knight et al., 2016) and haemorrhage is the most common cause of maternal collapse (Royal College of Obstetricians and Gynaecologists, 2014). The majority of cardiac arrests in pregnancies occur in hospitals, where outcomes are better than those occurring at home or during ambulance transfer (Beckett et al., 2017).

Antepartum Haemorrhage

Antepartum haemorrhage (APH) is defined as bleeding from or in to the genital tract, occurring from 24+0 weeks of pregnancy and prior to the birth of the baby (Royal College of Obstetricians and Gynaecologists, 2011). APH complicates 3–5% of pregnancies and can be associated with significant maternal and fetal mortality and morbidity (Calleja-Agius et al., 2006). The causes of APH are shown in Box 25.1 (Luesley and Kilby, 2016). Pregnancies complicated by APH are at increased risk of adverse outcomes and increased risk of preterm delivery, stillbirth, fetal anomalies and decreased birthweight (Magann et al., 2005; McCormack et al., 2008).

Placental Abruption

Placental abruption is defined as premature separation of the placenta leading to bleeding. Although the aetiology for placental abruption is unclear, there

Box 25.1 Causes of Antepartum Haemorrhage

- Placenta praevia
- Placental abruption
- Others
  - Marginal placental bleeding
  - Show (blood-stained mucus plug)
  - Friable cervical ectropion
  - Genital infection
  - Varicosities
  - Genital tract tumours
  - Vasa praevia

are known risk factors for placental abruption. These include previous abruption (recurrence risk of 4.4% after one pregnancy complicated by placental abruption and 19–25% after two pregnancies complicated by placental abruption; Rasmussen and Irgen, 2009; Tikkanen, 2010), pre-eclampsia, fetal growth restriction, malpresentation, polyhydramnios, advanced maternal age, low maternal BMI, premature rupture of membranes, abdominal trauma, smoking and recreational drug use during pregnancy (Royal College of Obstetricians and Gynaecologists, 2011).

The diagnosis of placental abruption is clinical. The most important feature is massive haemorrhage, which may be concealed. The clinical features depend on the extent of placental separation and haemorrhage. This ranges from no symptoms associated with a retroplacental clot noted after delivery, mild pain associated with vaginal bleeding, to severe pain with a hard and tender uterus with/without hypovolaemic collapse secondary to massive haemorrhage. Ultrasonography has only limited sensitivity in identifying retroplacental haemorrhage and is therefore of limited use in the acute setting. However, it may be helpful in confirming fetal viability, assessing fetal growth and excluding placenta praevia.

Rapid recognition of concealed haemorrhage and subsequent resuscitation with fluids and blood products, as well as early decision for delivery is essential in minimising blood loss and maternal and fetal morbidity. Coagulopathy is likely and may be delayed.

Perimortem Caesarean Section

Perimortem caesarean section (PMCS) is defined as a caesarean delivery after cardiopulmonary resuscitation has been started. When performed in a timely fashion this can be a life-saving procedure for both the woman and her baby (Tikkanen, 2010). However, the focus remains on assisting maternal resuscitation. PMCS should be considered in cases of maternal cardiac arrest after 20 weeks gestation (Deakin et al., 2015) or in all women with an obviously gravid uterus, regardless of fetal condition if return of spontaneous circulation is not achieved within 4 minutes (American Heart Association, 2005).

From 20 weeks the gravid uterus causes aorto-caval compression and impedes venous return and cardiac output (Kerr, 1965). Cardiac compressions in non-pregnant women achieve 30% of normal cardiac output and this drops to 10% in pregnant women with aorto-caval compression (Katz et al., 1986). Uterine displacement is therefore critical to alleviate aorto-caval compression during resuscitation. The primary aim of PMCS is to deliver the fetus and placenta to improve venous return, cardiac output, to reduce metabolic demands and to facilitate chest compression and ventilation. In addition, there may be a chance of neonatal survival.

Irreversible anoxic brain injury occurs more quickly in pregnant women than non-pregnant women due to increased metabolic demands (Paterson-Brown and Howell, 2014); this occurs from 4 to 6 minutes into a cardiac arrest. The rationale for performing PMCS within 5 minutes of maternal arrest is to minimise anoxic brain injury. The current guidance from the Royal College of Obstetricians and Gynaecologists (UK) recommends that if return of spontaneous circulation is not achieved within 4 minutes of resuscitative efforts, caesarean delivery should be ideally achieved within 5 minutes of arrest. However, recent evidence suggests that decision for delivery should be made as quickly as possible and PMCS should not be delayed (Benson et al., 2016). Positive maternal and neonatal outcomes are possible outside of this window.

Setting and Equipment for PMCS

Once a peri-arrest is recognised, preparation should be made for PMCS at the scene of cardiac arrest, as transfer to other settings (e.g. operating theatre) would result in unnecessary delay. See Box 25.2 for a suggested checklist for personnel and equipment required for PMCS. Receiving units for unscheduled care should have robust pathways to call for appropriate help and physical equipment to facilitate PMCS, as well as subsequent neonatal resuscitation.

Box 25.2 Recommended Personnel and Equipment for PMCS

Recommended personnel for PMCS:

- Adult resuscitation team for the mother
- Obstetric consultant/registrar or A&E consultant/registrar to perform PMCS
- Neonatal resuscitation team
- Anaesthetic consultant/registrar as part of resuscitation team and to organise aftercare
- Midwife
- Others – scribe/porter/staff to coordinate care between blood bank/theatres/ICU

Recommended equipment list for PMCS:

(1) Protective equipment
   a. Sterile gloves
   b. Face mask
   c. Apron/gown

(2) Caesarean section equipment
   a. Scalpel (preferably disposable pre-loaded scalpel)
   b. Antiseptic skin preparation
   c. Scissors
   d. Clamps/haemostats/cord clamp
   e. Gauze/swabs
   f. Sutures/needle holder

(3) Neonatal resuscitation equipment
   a. Resuscitaire
   b. Neonatal bag valve mask
   c. Dry linen/neonatal airway supplies/suction/resuscitation drugs

---

Suggested Procedure for PMCS (Box 25.3)

Outcomes for PMCS

Both maternal and fetal outcomes following maternal cardiac arrest are scarce and are reported in case series only. The most recent data from the 2017 CAPS study, part of the UK Obstetric Surveillance System (UKOSS), showed in a three-year period there were 66 cases of maternal collapse requiring cardiac compressions. Within this group, 28 women died resulting in a mortality rate of 42% (Beckett et al., 2017). Cardiac output was restored in 48 of 66 women with 38 (58%) ultimately surviving their cardiac arrest. Forty-nine women underwent PMCS, with 11 cases performed in the emergency department. This is consistent with past data with approximately 50% of women surviving to

Box 25.3 Recommended Guide to Perform a PMCS

(1) Position: supine with manual uterine displacement until skill incision with ongoing CPR
(2) Apply antiseptic rapidly if available (do not delay PMCS if not available)
(3) Skin incision with scalpel
   a. Incision can be made via a midline vertical incision or a transverse horizontal approach
   b. Choose approach that will facilitate quickest delivery depending on operator
   c. For inexperienced operators, a midline vertical incision from umbilicus to symphysis pubis is recommended
(4) Continue incision through subcutaneous layer and rectus sheath (shiny white layer) until peritoneum is exposed
(5) Blunt dissection into the peritoneal cavity and use hands to pull peritoneum open laterally
(6) Identify uterus and make incision into uterine cavity
   a. Uterine incision can be performed vertically or horizontally. The quickest approach should be chosen and in inexperienced hands a vertical incision will give the most rapid access to achieve delivery
(7) Deliver baby, clamp + cut cord and pass baby to neonatal resuscitation team
(8) Deliver placenta and evacuate any clots
(9) Continue maternal resuscitation
(10) If maternal cardiac output is restored, the uterus and abdomen should be closed in the usual way to achieve haemostasis
   a. If no obstetric help available, temporary packing with large gauze may be appropriate

21 having no neurological complications (Katz et al., 1986). In the recent UKOSS case series 46 of 58 babies were born alive (Beckett et al., 2017). In this series, 96% of babies survived when PMCS was performed within 5 minutes compared with 70% of babies when PMCS was performed beyond 5 minutes. The longest reported interval between maternal cardiac arrest and a PMCS that resulted in the delivery of a child without neurological complications is 30 minutes (Capobianco et al., 2008). Although the timings in this case may not be accurate, PMCS should always be considered even if maternal cardiac arrest has occurred beyond the 5-minute time frame.

Bibliography

American Heart Association. (2005). American Heart Association Guidelines for Cardiopulmonary Resuscitation and Emergency Cardiovascular Care. Part 10.8: cardiac arrest associated with pregnancy. *Circulation*, 112, 150–153.

Beckett, V. A., Knight, M. and Sharpe, P. (2017). The CAPS Study: incidence, management and outcomes of cardiac arrest in pregnancy in the UK: a prospective, descriptive study. *British Journal of Obstetrics and Gynaecology*, 124, 1374–1381.

Benson, M. D., Padovano, A., Bourjeily, G. and Zhou, Y. (2016). Maternal collapse: challenging the four-minute rule. *EBioMedicine*, 6, 253–257. doi:10.1016/j.ebiom.2016.02.042

Calleja-Agius, J., Custo, R., Brincat, M. P. and Calleja, N. (2006). Placental abruption and placenta praevia. *European Clinics in Obstetrics and Gynaecology*, 2, 121–127.

Capobianco, G., Balata, A., Mannazzu, M. C., et al. (2008). Perimortem cesarean delivery 30 minutes after a laboring patient jumped from a fourth-floor window: baby survives and is normal at age 4 years *American Journal of Obstetrics & Gynecology*, 198(1), e15–e16.

Datner, E. and Promes, S. (2006). Resuscitation in pregnancy. In *Tintinalli's Emergency Medicine*, p. 254. New York, NY: The McGraw-Hill Co..

Deakin, C., Brown, S., Jewkes, F., et al. (2015). *Prehospital Resuscitation. Resuscitation Council (UK) Guidelines*. London: Resuscitation Council.

Einav, S., Kaufman, N., and Sala, H. Y. (2012). Maternal cardiac arrest and perimortem caesarean delivery: evidence or expert-based? *Resuscitation*, 83, 1191–1200.

Katz, V. L., Dotters, D. J. and Droegemueller, W. (1986). Perimortem caesarean delivery. *Obstetrics and Gynaecology*, 68, 571–576.

hospital discharge (Einav et al., 2012). Of note is the ongoing morbidity following survival, with 42% suffering complications such as postpartum haemorrhage, coagulopathy, renal and neurological complications. This highlights the importance for aftercare and anticipation of complications.

Fetal outcomes following PMCS appear to be related to the time from onset of maternal arrest to delivery and gestational age. The '4 minute rule' was first recommended by Katz et al. (1986), who found that babies born within 5 minutes were much less likely to develop neurological complications. Further literature review between 1985 and 2004 showed that of 38 PMCS deliveries there were 35 surviving infants, with

Katz, V., Balderston, K. and DeFreest, M. (2005). Perimortem cesarean delivery: were our assumptions correct? *American Journal of Obstetrics & Gynecology*, 192(6), 1916–1920.

Kerr, M. G. (1965). The mechanical effects of gravid uterus in late pregnancy. *Journal of Obstetrics and Gynaecology of the British Commonwealth*, 2, 513–519.

Knight, M., Kenyon, S., Brocklehurst, P., Neilson, J., Shakespeare, J. and Kurinczuk, J. J. (Eds.) on behalf of MBRRACE-UK. (2016). *Saving Lives, Improving Mothers' Care – Lessons Learned to Inform Future Maternity Care from the UK and Ireland Confidential Enquiries into Maternal Deaths and Morbidity 2009–14*. Oxford: National Perinatal Epidemiology Unit, University of Oxford.

Luesley, D. M. and Kilby, M. D. (2016). *Obstetrics & Gynaecology: An Evidence-based Text for MRCOG*, third edition. Boca Raton, FL: CRC Press.

Magann, E. F., Cummings, J. E., Niederhauser, A., Rodriguez Thompson, D., McCormack, R. and Chauhan, S. P. (2005). Antepartum bleeding of unknown origin in the second half of pregnancy: a review. *Obstetrical and Gynecological Survey*, 60, 741–745.

McCormack, R. A., Doherty, D. A., Magann, E. F., Hutchinson, M. and Newnham, J. P. (2008). Antepartum bleeding of unknown origin in the second half of pregnancy and pregnancy outcomes. *British Journal of Obstetrics and Gynaecology*, 115, 1451–1457.

Paterson-Brown, S. and Howell, C. (Eds.). (2014). *The MOET Course Manual. Managing Obstetric Emergencies and Trauma*. Cambridge: Cambridge University Press.

Rasmussen, S. and Irgens, L. M. (2009). Occurrence of placental abruption in relatives. *British Journal of Obstetrics and Gynaecology*, 116, 693–699.

Royal College of Obstetricians and Gynaecologists (RCOG). (2011). *Antepartum Haemorrhage. Green-top Guideline No. 63*. London: Royal College of Obstetricians and Gynaecologists (RCOG).

Royal College of Obstetricians and Gynaecologists (RCOG). (2014). *Maternal Collapse in Pregnancy and the Puerperium. Green-top Guideline No. 56*. London: Royal College of Obstetricians and Gynaecologists (RCOG).

Tikkanen, M. (2010). Etiology, clinical manifestations, and prediction of placental abruption. *Acta Obstetrica et Gynecologica Scandinavica*, 89, 732–740.

Chapter

Vasa Praevia

26

Shimma Rehman

Scenario in a Nutshell

Undiagnosed vasa praevia presenting with antepartum haemorrhage and fetal bradycardia in labour.
   Stage 1: PV blood loss and fetal bradycardia at the time of membrane rupture.
   Stage 2: Sustained fetal bradycardia, coordinate transfer to theatre.
   Stage 3: Category 1 caesarean section under general anaesthesia, vasa praevia diagnosed and neonatal resuscitation required.

Target Learner Groups

All members of the multidisciplinary obstetric team: anaesthetists, midwives, obstetricians, operating department practitioners/anaesthetic nurses and neonatal emergency response teams.

Specific learning opportunities
Knowledge of causes of APH
Recognition of vasa praevia as cause for APH
Team coordination to facilitate rapid delivery

Suggested learners (to represent their normal roles)	In the room from the start	Available when requested
Anaesthetic CT2/ST3+	√	
Obstetric ST3+	√	
Midwife Coordinator	√	
Midwife in room	√	
Full theatre team, Operating Department Practitioner (ODP)/anaesthetic nurse and scrub team		√
*Neonatal emergency team		√

Suggested learners (to represent their normal roles)	In the room from the start	Available when requested
Suggested facilitators		
Faculty to play role of student midwife giving handover at time of emergency buzzer	√	

This is a useful scenario to combine with neonatal team, resuscitation training (grossly anaemic, flat neonate for resuscitation).

Details for Facilitators

Patient Demographics

Name: Sarah	
Age: 28	
Gestation: 39+5	
Booking weight: 75 kg	
Parity: P1 (Prev NVD)	

Scenario Summary for Facilitators

Patient admitted to delivery suite for remifentanil PCA analgesia in labour 2 hours ago. Contracting 4 in 10. Fit and well. Mild asthma, previous normal vaginal delivery. Student midwife covering for a break.
Patient commences with PV bleed in labour and sudden-onset fetal bradycardia.
Emergency buzzer activated. Team arrive.
When examined, patient found to be 6 cm dilated, 150 ml blood loss on inco sheet, fetal heart rate 80 bpm.
Uneventful antenatal history. Her 21-week anomaly scan reported no fetal abnormalities with a posterior placenta, clear of the os.
Patient continues to bleed PV, sustained fetal bradycardia for 5 minutes.
Transferred to theatre for emergency category 1 caesarean section.
Uneventful intubation and delivery of fetus. Found to have velamentous insertion of umbilical cord and white flat fetus at delivery.

Set-up Overview for Facilitators

Clinical setting	On delivery suite in a delivery bed
Patient position	Semi-recumbent
Initial monitoring in place	Saturation monitoring
Other equipment	Remifentanil PCA (set as per local protocol) via 20G cannula
	16G cannula in other hand, IV Hartmann's attached and running at 80 ml/h
	Blood stained inco sheets
Useful manikin features	PV bleed
	Intubation

Medical Equipment

For core equipment checklist see Chapter 9.

Additional equipment specific to scenario
Drugs
Drugs for intubation
Syntocinon
Syntocinon infusion
Tranexamic acid

Information Given to the Learners

Emergency buzzer goes off, SBAR handover from student midwife to responding obstetrician, anaesthetist and midwife.

Time: 16:00
Situation: This is an emergency! The patient has started bleeding PV and there is a fetal bradycardia.
Background: 28-year para 1. Admitted in early labour. Midwifery-led care but on CDU for remifentanil which she started at 14:00. She has just ruptured her membranes and I noticed some PV bleeding and the fetal heart rate has been at 80 bpm for the last minute. She is contracting 4 in 10. Last examination was 2 hours ago, cervix was 4 cm dilated, membranes present and −2 above the spines.
Assessment: I have called for help and checked the CTG is not recording maternal pulse.
Recommendation: Please can you take over her care now?

Scenario Schedule

Observations	
A	Clear
B	RR 20/min SpO2 98% on air
C	HR 98bpm BP 110/74 CRT 2s
D	**A**VPU
E	Temp 36.8°C Inco sheet with 150ml blood
CTG	FHR 80bpm

Stage 1: PV blood loss and fetal bradycardia at the time of membrane rupture

Information given	Expected actions
Patient extremely anxious asking 'is my baby going to be alright?'	ABC approach, establish team leader and delegate tasks
	Apply oxygen to maintain saturations 94-98%
	Turn patient in left lateral position (or manual uterine displacement)
	Apply monitoring. Pulse oximeter (already on)/ NIBP
20G and 16G cannula already in situ. Bloods taken at time of cannulation earlier, FBC, group and save (including second sample)	Candidate may consider further IV access and repeat bloods
	Increase rate of IV Hartmann's
	Stop remifentanil

Information given	Expected actions
Abdomen is soft and non-tender. Blood loss is estimated to be 150mls. Vaginal examination: cervix 6 cm dilated, vertex presentation -1 above spines, membranes absent, persistent active bleeding.	Examination of patient, including vaginal examination
21-week anomaly scan reported no fetal abnormalities with a posterior placenta, clear of the os	Review of maternal notes and antenatal ultrasound scan for potential causes of APH

Progress to stage 2 once established APH (150ml) with prolonged fetal bradycardia

Observations	
A	Clear
B	RR 20/min SpO$_2$ 98% on air
C	HR 110bpm BP 100/68 CRT 2s
D	**A**VPU
E	Temp 36.8°C Inco sheet now 200ml blood
CTG	FHR 70bpm

Stage 2: Sustained fetal bradycardia, coordinate transfer to theatre

Information given	Expected actions
CTG now 70bpm. Sustained bradycardia since 1 minute prior to buzzer	By 5 minutes sustained fetal bradycardia, plan to transfer to theatre for category 1 caesarean section
	Verbal patient consent
Theatre are ready to receive patient	Communicate with theatre team
Neonatal team will attend	Fast bleep neonatal team
	Alert midwifery coordinator, senior obstetrician and anaesthetist if not already aware
A – No allergies M – No medications P - No past medical or surgical history L – Last ate 8 hrs ago, drinking isotonic drinks in labour E – Airway assessment looks straightforward	Anaesthetic history
	Transfer to theatre
	Consideration of causes of APH including vasa praevia, abruption, amniotic fluid embolism, DIC

Progress to stage 3 once decision made to transfer to theatre

Observations	
A	Clear
B	RR 20/min SpO$_2$ 98% on air
C	HR 110bpm BP 98/68 CRT 2s
D	**A**VPU
E	Temp 36.8°C Inco sheet now 200ml blood
CTG	FHR 70bpm

Stage 3: Category 1 caesarean section under general anaesthesia, vasa praevia diagnosed and neonatal resuscitation required

Information given	Expected actions
Arrival in theatre	
	Team brief for category 1 caesarean section
	Agree need for GA (see chapter 24)

Information given	Expected actions
Grade 1 intubation	RSI and intubation of patient whilst continued IV resuscitation with fluids
Baby very pale at delivery and flat No abruption seen	Rapid delivery of fetus
	Continues to bleed once placenta out
Bleeding settles quickly with uterotonics EBL in room 200ml in theatre 600ml	Syntocinon bolus and infusion. Administer tranexamic acid 1g IV
On inspection of placenta, noted to have velamentous insertion of cord	
Point of care coagulation tests normal if performed	
ABG result (if ABG requested) pH 7.34 CO_2 4.3 kPa O_2 19 kPa (on FiO_2 0.3) BE −4 mmol/L HCO_3− 22mmol/L Lactate 3mmol/L Hb 105g/L	
	Neonatal resuscitation ongoing (neonatal scenario)
	Wake and extubate patient

Observations	
A	Intubated
B	As per ventilator setting SpO_2 98%
C	HR 110bpm BP 90/68 CRT 2s
D	Anaesthetised
E	Temp 36.2°C

Scenario ends when uterotonics are administered, bleeding stops and anaesthetist decides to wake patient.

Suggested Topics for Debrief Discussion

- How was the communication between teams in the scenario?
- Would a communication prompt have helped with handover to the neonatal team? (See GAMES neonatal handover tool, Chapter 8.)
- Would you have administered tranexamic acid?

Discussion

Introduction

Vasa praevia is a rare condition with a reported incidence of about 1 in 500 to 1 in 6000, where the fetal blood vessels run freely through the membranes covering the internal cervical os beneath the presenting part. Vasa praevia can be divided into two subtypes. In type 1, there is a single-lobed placenta with a velamentous cord insertion; type II is a multilobed placenta with connecting vessels running over the internal cervical os. Unlike placenta praevia, vasa praevia is not associated with significant maternal risk. However, when the fetal blood vessels rupture during labour, spontaneous rupture of membranes or amniotomy, fetal bleeding can lead to fatal fetal consequences, the perinatal mortality rate in such circumstances being around 60%. As the fetal blood volume at term is around 80–100 ml/kg, even a small amount of bleeding can rapidly result in hypotension, fetal heart rate abnormalities and, within minutes, fetal death. Babies who are born alive have poor Apgar scores, need blood transfusions and more than likely have serious long-term sequel.

Predictive Risk Factors

A systematic review of predictive indicators of vasa praevia found at least 83% of cases had one or more risk indicators. The most-common risk factors identified were placenta praevia, bilobed and succenturiate-lobed placentas, velamentous insertion of the umbilical cord

205

and IVF pregnancy. Multiple pregnancy is reported in many case reports as a risk indicator, but data to support this were not found.

A strong association was found particularly between velamentous cord insertion and vasa praevia. Velamentous insertion of the umbilical cord is where the cord inserts onto the chorioamniotic membranes rather than the placental mass. The vessels are surrounded only by fetal membranes, unprotected by Wharton's jelly, before they come together into the umbilical cord. Incidence of velamentous cord in singleton pregnancies is 1.1%, whereas in twins it is 8.7%.

In this meta-analysis, some studies suggested that a second-trimester low-lying placenta, regardless of whether it has resolved at term, is a risk factor for vasa praevia. A potential explanation is that the placenta grows over the more vascular upper segment; the placental tissue in the lower segment atrophies, leaving the fetal blood vessels embedded in the cervical area unprotected, resulting in vasa praevia.

Can Antenatal Diagnosis Be Made?

Antenatal diagnosis (prior to rupture of membranes) has a significant impact in reducing neonatal morbidity and fetal demise. Transvaginal ultrasound with colour Doppler is the most accurate tool for diagnosis of vasa praevia with a sensitivity of 100% and specificity of 99–99.8%, and can be detected as early as 16 weeks gestation. In cases identified in the second trimester, imaging should be repeated in the third trimester because up to 15% resolve by term.

Prenatal detection of vasa praevia can be improved by routine evaluation of the umbilical cord insertion site, but there is insufficient evidence to support universal screening. The current recommendation is targeted transvaginal scanning in high-risk women including documentation of site of cord insertion, presence of velamentous vessels, and presence of extra-placental lobes.

MRI would diagnose vasa praevia antenatally, but is expensive and not readily available.

Rarely, diagnosis can be made by palpation of pulsating vessels in the membranes overlying the cervical os during vaginal examination or by direct visualisation using a speculum. More commonly, diagnosis is suspected when labour or rupture of membranes is associated with antepartum haemorrhage, followed by pathological CTG, severe fetal anaemia or fetal death. Very rarely, fetal heart rate abnormalities and compromise occur in the absence

of rupture of membranes due to the compression of the unprotected fetal vessels by the presenting part.

Histopathological examination of the placenta does not confirm vasa praevia; it may reveal velamentous cord insertion, but it is not possible to determine what position the placenta and cord were in while intrauterine.

Differential Diagnoses of Vasa Praevia

Differential diagnosis includes a normal loop of umbilical cord lying over the cervical os that can be mistaken for vasa praevia. This can be easily distinguished by changing the patient's position, shaking the uterus or reassessing after a short interval, as a normal loop of cord will float away. Other diagnoses include maternal cervico uterine vessels (which would have a rate consistent with maternal blood flow), marginal placental vascular sinus and amniotic band, which can be distinguished due to the lack of blood flow when colour Doppler is applied.

What are the Other Main Causes of APH?

Causes of antepartum haemorrhage can be largely divided into local causes and placental causes. The common cervical causes include cervical ectropion, cervicitis and benign cervical polyps. Cervical carcinoma presenting in pregnancy is uncommon and would require urgent referral to colposcopy. Placental causes include placental abruption, which can be associated with pain and bleeding or be concealed, and abnormal placentation (praevia, accrete, increta or percreta). Other causes to consider are uterine rupture, domestic violence resulting in abdominal trauma and hereditary coagulation defects.

How is Vasa Praevia Best Managed?

There is currently no agreed management pathway for vasa praevia due to the paucity of data available.

Current recommendations at most centres are to consider admitting women with prenatally diagnosed vasa praevia to a hospital with appropriate neonatal facilities from 28 to 32 weeks gestation until delivery and the administration of corticosteroids for lung maturity. Delivery by elective caesarean section should be considered from 35 to 37 weeks gestation. Where there is APH from suspected vasa praevia, delivery by urgent caesarean section is indicated. Appropriate discussion with the neonatal team should occur to ensure support is available for neonatal resuscitation and early arrangements for aggressive blood transfusion are made. Where APH is associated with acute fetal compromise, it is not appropriate to carry out ultrasonic assessments to establish diagnosis, as any delay can have fatal fetal consequences. At caesarean section, it is recommended that the umbilical cord is clamped as soon as possible after delivery, leaving the longer part attached to the neonate to facilitate umbilical artery catheterisation if required.

Bibliography

Amokrane, N., Waterfield, A., Datta, S. and Allen, E. R. F. (2016). Antepartum haemorrhage. *Obstetrics, Gynaecology and Reproductive Medicine*, 26(2), 33–37.

Oyelese, Y. and Smulian, J. C. (2006). Placenta previa, placenta accreta, and vasa previa. *Obstetrics and Gynecology*, 107, 927–941.

Royal College of Obstetricians and Gynaecologists. (2011, updated 2014). *Placenta Praevia, Placenta Accreta, Vasa Praevia: Diagnosis and Management; Green-top Guideline No. 27*. London: RCOG.

Ruiter, L., Kok, N., Limpens, J., Dereks, J. B., de Graaf, I. M. and Mol, B. W. J. (2015). Systematic review of accuracy of ultrasound in the diagnosis of vasa previa. *Ultrasound in Obstetrics and Gynecology*, 45, 516–522.

Ruiter, L., Kok, N., Limpens, J., et al. (2016). Incidence of and risk indicators for vasa praevia: a systematic review. *British Journal of Obstetrics and Gynaecology*, 123, 1278–1287.

Sinha, P., Kaushik, S., Kuruba, N. and Beweley, S. (2008). Vasa praevia: a missed diagnosis. *Journal of Obstetrics and Gynaecology*, 28(6), 600–603.

Swank, M. L., Garite, T. J., Maurel, K., et al. (2016). Vasa previa: diagnosis and management. *American Journal of Obstetrics and Gynecology*, 215, 223.e1–6.

27

Postpartum Haemorrhage

Pavan Kochhar and Stuart Knowles

Scenario in a Nutshell

Massive postpartum haemorrhage (PPH) following caesarean section, unresponsive to uterotonics, requiring hysterectomy.
Stage 1: Initial assessment of patient suffering with postpartum haemorrhage 6 hours after caesarean section.
Stage 2: MDT management of haemorrhage, commence algorithm for uterine atony and activate massive haemorrhage pathway.
Stage 3: Anaesthesia, surgical management of atony and correction of coagulopathy.

Target Learner Groups

All members of the multidisciplinary obstetric team: anaesthetists, midwives, obstetricians, operating department practitioners/anaesthetic nurses, theatre team.

Specific learning opportunities
Knowledge of risk factors for PPH
Knowledge of treatment algorithm for massive haemorrhage
Knowledge of interpretation of point of care testing

Suggested learners (to represent their normal roles)	In the room from the start	Available when requested
Anaesthetic CT2/ST3+		✓
Obstetric ST3+		✓
Postnatal ward midwife – responds first to the buzzer	✓	
Postnatal midwife shift lead/ other responding midwives		✓
Operating Department Practitioner (ODP)/ anaesthetic nurse/theatre team – scrub nurse/runner		✓

Suggested learners (to represent their normal roles)	In the room from the start	Available when requested
Suggested facilitators		
Faculty to play role of anxious husband (if enough faculty to allow for this)	✓	

Details for Facilitators

Patient Demographics

Name: Adenola

Age: 35

Gestation: 6 hours post elective LSCS

Booking weight: 92 kg

Parity: P2

Scenario Summary for Facilitators

35-year-old West African patient had an elective caesarean section performed 6 h ago. Indication for caesarean section – previous myomectomy for uterine fibroids 4 years ago and one previous emergency caesarean section for fetal distress.

The elective caesarean section had been uneventfully performed under spinal anaesthesia. Blood loss was 400 ml and postoperative uterine tone had been good. She was transferred to the postnatal ward.

The scenario starts 6 h post elective caesarean section. Patient has been trickling blood PV for 45 min and the bleeding has now become heavy. She appears to have lost 1.5 litres of blood and is feeling faint.

Following resuscitation, activation of massive haemorrhage pathway and commencement of uterotonics, she remains unstable and has ongoing uterine atony. She is transferred to theatre for GA, EUA but requires hysterectomy. Point of care testing shows marked coagulopathy.

Set-up Overview for Facilitators

Clinical setting	Postnatal ward, on a postnatal bed
Patient position	Sitting up in bed at 45°
Initial monitoring in place	None
Other equipment	16G cannula DRH but no fluids attached Urinary catheter (if hospital policy is to keep catheter in after surgery) Blood stained inco sheets under patient (1.5 l blood loss) All usual equipment available in postnatal ward
Useful manikin features	Bleeding Intubation Palpable uterine atony

Medical Equipment

For core equipment checklist see Chapter 9.

Additional equipment specific to scenario		
Arterial line	Rapid fluid infuser	Bakri balloon
Haemacue	O-negative blood	Other simulated blood products

Scenario Schedule

Additional equipment specific to scenario		
Drugs: Syntocinon Syntocinon infusion Haemobate	Syntometrine Ergometrine Misoprostol Tranexamic acid	Metaraminol Phenylephrine

Information Given to the Learners

Patient rings her buzzer to call for help. Facilitators inform postnatal midwife of information that she would have received from handover.

Time: 17:30

Facilitator explains to the first responding midwife:

The buzzer is going off in this bed space. From handover you know that this patient is 6 h post elective LSCS. Indication (if they ask) is previous myomectomy and previous emergency caesarean section. Her caesarean section today was uneventfully performed under a spinal anaesthetic. EBL 400 ml.

Her attending midwife is on her break and you are responding to the buzzer as you pass by the bed space.

Stage 1: Initial assessment of patient suffering with postpartum haemorrhage 6 hours after caesarean section	
Information given	**Expected actions**
Patient answers.......“I feel like blood is pooling between my legs and I am feeling faint and sick”	Attend the patient and ask if everything is ok?
	Commence ABCDE approach to patient
Patient talking	Perform airway assessment
	Apply Oxygen via non-rebreathing mask at 15 l/min
	Lie patient flat
	Pull buzzer and ask to fast bleep the MDT obstetric team
Once call for obstetricians and anaesthetists is made, more midwifery help arrives	

Observations	
A	Clear
B	RR 25/min SpO$_2$ 96% on air SpO$_2$ 99% on O$_2$
C	HR 110 bpm BP 110/50 CRT 3s
D	**A**VPU
E	Temp 36.5^{0}C

Information given	Expected actions
	Apply full monitoring
1x 16G IV access already in situ	Secure second IV access. Take bloods for FBC, U+E, coagulation including fibrinogen assay, cross match 4U RBC, check CBG (capillary blood glucose)
	Commence 500mls Hartmann's stat
If abdomen palpated, uterus well above the umbilicus and feels atonic. Over 1.5 litres of per vaginal (PV) blood loss already on the inco sheets	Exposes patient and examine abdomen
	Commences rubbing the uterus to encourage contraction
	Request emergency PPH drugs

Progress to stage 2 once ABCDE approach completed

Stage 2: MDT management of haemorrhage, commence algorithm for uterine atony and activate massive haemorrhage pathway

Observations	
A	Clear
B	RR 28/min SpO$_2$ 98% on O$_2$
C	HR 120bpm BP 90/60 CRT 3s
D	**A**VPU
E	Temp 36.0^{0}C

Information given	Expected actions
Midwifery shift leader, anaesthetist, obstetrician and available post-natal midwives arrive	Handover from midwifery team to emergency obstetric team (including indication for section, current findings and actions so far)
Patient complains of feeling faint, sick and passing blood PV	Repeat all observations
Over 2 litres blood loss PV now on inco sheet	Recognise that patient has significant ongoing blood loss
	Continue with Oxygen
	Continue with crystalloid resuscitation
	Activate Massive Obstetric Haemorrhage protocol
Blood arrives quickly	Request 2U O-ve blood from nearest blood fridge. Administer when arrives
	Discuss with team and examine to ascertain cause of haemorrhage: 4 T's Tone, Tissue, Thrombin, Trauma
Uterus remains atonic	Examination of patient
No evidence of vaginal / cervical trauma. Clots evacuated PV	
Operation note says placenta/membranes removed. Membranes not raggded	Review of operation note
	Uterine atony most likely cause for haemorrhage

Information given	Expected actions
	Commence uterotonics: 5u Syntocinon IV 1ml Syntometrine IM Syntocinon infusion (40u Syntocinon in 500mls Normal Saline at 125 mls/hr) 250 mcg Haemabate IM
No previous history of coagulopathy	Tranexamic Acid 1g bolus IV over 10 mins
Uterus remains atonic Clots removed from vagina Now 2.5L blood loss in total	Continue manual manoeuvres Uterine massage Evacuate clots PV Bimanual compression
	Ensure urinary catheter inserted (if not still in from theatre)
ABG result if requested pH 7.30 pCO_2 3.2kPa pO_2 18kPa BE -15mmol/L Lactate 3.4mmol/L Hb 68g/L	Estimate of Haemoglobin level (Haemacue or ABG)
	Blood sample for Point-of-Care testing (TEG or ROTEM)
	Ensure Consultant Obstetrician and Anaesthetist are aware
	Decision to transfer to theatre for EUA under GA
Theatres able to receive patient	Communication with theatres, massive obstetric haemorrhage requiring a GA and EUA
	Request theatre to prepare cell salvage, rapid fluid infusor, arterial line
Transfer to theatre (if scenario progressing this far or consider starting scenario at this point depending on team members' learning requirements)	Transfer to theatre with portable oxygen, transfer monitoring and ongoing bimanual compression

Progress to stage 3 once uterotonics have been administered and team transfer to theatre for EUA and proceed

Stage 3 – Anaesthesia, surgical management of atony and correction of coagulopathy

Information given	Expected actions
Arrival in theatre	Team brief for EUA / proceed for massive post-partum haemorrhage
EBL now > 3500 mls	

Observations	
A	Clear
B	RR 28/min SpO$_2$ 98% on O$_2$
C	HR 145bpm BP 80/50 CRT 4s
D	A**V**PU
E	Temp 35.8°C

Information given	Expected actions
Patient only responsive to voice	Apply all monitoring
	Rapid sequence induction (RSI) of anaesthesia. Consideration of most appropriate induction agent. (See chapter 24 for GA)
Grade 1 intubation	Intubation
	EUA commences once airway secure
	Consideration of surgical management of atony: uterine compression sutures (eg. B-Lynch) or balloon tamponade (eg. Bakri balloon)
	Repeat uterotonics Haemabate 250 mcg IM (every 15 mins) if required. Ensure Syntocinon infusion is ongoing. Consider misoprostol 1000mcg PR
	Recognition of extreme coagulopathy. Follow local TEG guidelines for management of PPH or massive obstetric haemorrhage if available
Lab results: Hb 61g/L WCC 15.3 x 10^9/L Platelets 65 x 10^9/L PT 37.5 secs APTT 64 secs Fib <0.6 g/l Results of TEG (Figure 27.1): No evidence of haemostasis.	Discussion with the on-call haematologist regarding the coagulopathy
Massive haemorrhage Pack 1 arrives (4 units RBC, 4 Units FFP) or as per local policy	Continue blood transfusion (packed red cells)
	Commence correction with FFP, Cryoprecipitate / Fibrinogen Concentrate, Platelets (as per local policy and discussion)
	Commence Tranexamic Acid infusion 1G over 8 hours (if 1g bolus not given in stage 2, give bolus first)
	Insert arterial line / consider central line once coagulation improved
	Liaise with critical care
Manual interventions to stop bleeding fail	Proceed to hysterectomy
EBL 5L	
	Commence antibiotics
	Actively warm patient

Information given	Expected actions
ABG (post-hysterectomy) FiO2 0.5 pH 7.31 pCO_2 4.2kPa pO_2 22 kPa BE -12mmol/L Lactate 3.5mmol/L Hb 89g/L Ca^{2+} 0.9mmol/L	
	Replace calcium with 10ml 10% calcium chloride
BP responds to vasopressors	Unstable cardiovascular parameters. Use of vasopressors (eg. Metaraminol or phenylephrine).
	Continual monitoring ongoing

Observations	
A	Intubated
B	RR as per ventilator setting SpO_2 98% on O_2
C	HR 120bpm BP 95/50 CRT 3s
D	Anaesthetisted
E	Temp 36.5⁰C if active warming

End of scenario with hysterectomy, final bloods and handover to critical care

Final blood loss 5 litres. Blood components replaced: 8u packed red cells, 6u FFP, 2 adult doses platelets, 3 adult doses (10 units) cryoprecipitate. If fibrinogen concentrate used then 3-5g needed depending on local policies, TEG/ROTEM testing or laboratory tests

Final blood results

Repeat TEG (Figure 27.2): MA 8.4, α-angle 55.5, MA 56.3

WCC 19.1 x10⁹/L

Hb 91g/L

Platelets 86 x 10⁹/L

PT 19.3sec

APTT 36sec

Fibrinogen 1.8 g/l

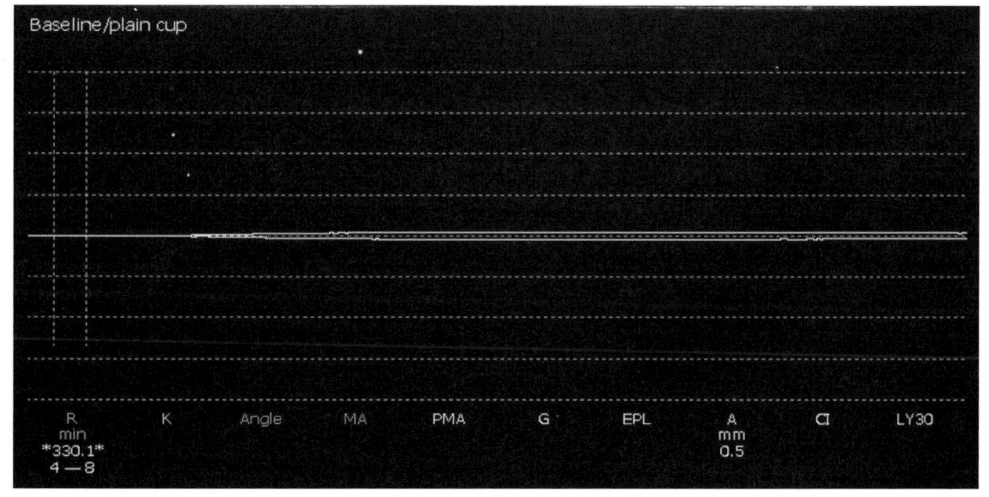

Figure 27.1 TEG.

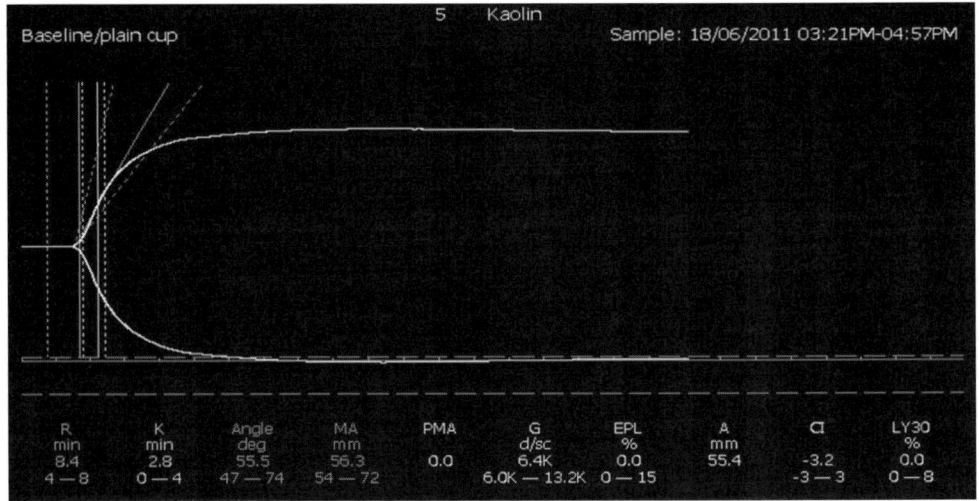

Figure 27.2 TEG.

Suggested Topics for Debrief Discussion

- How easy do you think it would be managing a postpartum haemorrhage on your postnatal wards?
- Would you have access to all the equipment that you would need?
- Would a checklist make this emergency easier to manage?

Discussion

Background

Postpartum haemorrhage (PPH) remains the leading cause of maternal mortality worldwide, causing approximately 127,000 deaths each year (Department of Making Pregnancy Safer, 2007).

There is no single accepted definition for PPH, but most literature agrees anything over 500 ml estimated blood loss (EBL) in the 24 hours following delivery (Mousa et al., 2014). Blood loss of 500 ml is unlikely to cause concern for maternal welfare in most scenarios, so major PPH may be a more useful term and this is defined as over 1000 ml EBL (Mavrides et al., 2017).

Risk factors for PPH include:

- abnormal placental implantation – estimated incidence of PPH in placenta praevia is 22% (Fan et al., 2017);
- multiple pregnancies;
- previous PPH;
- fetal macrosomia;
- failure to progress in second stage;
- prolonged third stage of labour;
- retained placenta;
- genital trauma;
- previous uterine surgery (e.g. myomectomy);
- general anaesthesia (Mavrides et al., 2017).

The most common method of recalling the causes of PPH are the four T's: **T**one (uterine atony), **T**rauma to the birth canal, **T**issue (retained) and **T**hrombin (coagulopathy). In clinical practice, atony accounts for approximately 70–80% of cases (Zelop, 2006). Coagulopathy may be pre-existing from haematological disorders or acquired from anticoagulant medication or other physiological processes (placental abruption, amniotic fluid embolus, pre-eclampsia or HELLP syndrome). In these cases, the clotting abnormality is likely to occur before a significant amount of blood is clinically revealed. Coagulopathy may occur due to haemodilution or inadequate resuscitation with appropriate blood products (Plaat and Shonfield, 2015).

The latest MBRRACE report and other studies (Knight et al., 2009, 2014) show a small increase in the incidence of maternal mortality from haemorrhage, including 13 direct deaths in the UK from PPH in the 2012–2014 triennium (Knight et al., 2014). While not statistically significant, it is concerning and is thought to be linked to an increased incidence of abnormally invasive placental implantation (Knight et al., 2014). The association between prior caesarean birth and placenta praevia, accreta, increta and percreta is well known (Fitzpatrick et al., 2012). Against a background of increasing rates of caesarean section, the increasing rate of abnormal placental implantation is inevitable.

Management

Early recognition of excessive blood loss is fundamental, with early initiation of more invasive therapies as appropriate. Visual estimation of blood volume is notoriously inaccurate (Mavrides et al., 2017), particularly when there is a large volume of liquor and hidden losses. Swab weighing can help but, in all cases, the maternal condition must be taken in context with estimated blood loss. Whenever signs of hypovolaemia such as tachycardia and tachypnoea or the late signs of agitation and hypotension occur then haemorrhage must be considered, even in the context of minimal visual blood loss (Knight et al., 2014).

It should be remembered that uterine blood flow can reach 700 ml/min at term so despite an expanded blood volume, increased heart rate, stroke volume and cardiac output, a major haemorrhage can occur extremely rapidly. With the effects of regional anaesthesia, the usual non-pregnant physiological values cannot be relied upon for estimating blood loss or reassuring stability (Plaat and Shonfeld, 2015) and the deteriorating clinical signs often indicate a more significant blood loss than in the non-pregnant population (Mavrides et al., 2017).

Uterotonics

Uterotonic agents are the mainstay of treatment for postpartum haemorrhage when atony is the cause. Various surgical interventions should be ongoing simultaneously in order to arrest bleeding, such as intrauterine balloon tamponade, compression suturing techniques, interventional radiology (if available) or ultimately hysterectomy. Tranexamic acid, an antifibrinolytic, should be considered alongside these therapies. The WOMAN trial has shown a survival benefit with the early administration of tranexamic acid, especially when given within three hours of giving birth (M.G. Foundation, 2017).

Syntocinon (synthetic oxytocin) is most commonly used as a prophylactic agent for the third stage of labour alone or combined with ergometrine. As well as uterine contraction, it causes vascular smooth muscle relaxation leading to a significant hypotension with reflex tachycardia. This response is directly related to the speed of injection so the initial 5 U bolus should be given slowly, often being followed by a 10 U/h infusion for 4 h. In cases where the cardiovascular effects would be particularly poorly tolerated, such as in significant cardiac disease, the initial bolus can be given slowly in a more dilute solution.

Ergometrine usually forms the second-line uterotonic agent and causes smooth muscle contraction in the uterus and vascular muscle. This can lead to prolonged hypertension; hence, it should be avoided in patients with pre-existing hypertension. Other side effects include nausea, vomiting and diarrhoea. It is usually administered intramuscularly, but can be given intravenously with a higher incidence of side effects (Saljoughian, 2011).

Carboprost (haemabate) is a synthetic prostaglandin which is also given by intramuscular injection at a dose of 250 μg. This can be repeated every 15 min to a maximum of eight doses, although in practice other methods of control should be sought before getting close to the maximum dose. The main concern is bronchospasm and pulmonary hypertension.

Misoprostol is a simple agent to administer as it can be administered by many routes and is relatively low-cost while being stable at room temperature (ideal in low-resource settings). The usual dose is 1000 μg rectally, so this can be given even without IV access. Side effects of note are diarrhoea, pyrexia and headaches (Saljoughian, 2011).

Fluids/Blood Products

Intravenous crystalloid is the initial resuscitation therapy of choice in haemorrhage, but once the scenario is recognised to be developing into a major PPH, blood products should be considered. Excessive crystalloid brings the risks of dilution of clotting factors, tissue oedema, poor oxygen delivery and metabolic acidosis (Plaat and Shonfeld, 2015). Activation of the obstetric major haemorrhage protocol is the quickest way to access appropriate blood products in the UK.

Clinical judgement must be used in the decision when to transfuse red blood cells. There are no specific accepted criteria for a transfusion threshold, but it should be given as soon as possible when clinical judgement indicates. If a full crossmatch is not available, then urgent type O rhesus negative red cells should be considered.

If a patient is known to have red cell antibodies, then blood should be crossmatched (at least 4 units) at the earliest opportunity. Cell salvage should also be considered in centres where it is available, especially in the elective setting.

Recent developments in the management of major obstetric haemorrhage have moved towards the earlier use of fresh frozen plasma (FFP) rather than just replacing red cells. If haemostatic tests are not immediately available then consider FFP at a dose of 12–15 ml/kg when coagulopathy is suspected, detection of PPH has been delayed or following transfusion of 4 units of red cells (Calkins, 2015; Mavrides et al., 2017).

It is recognised that fibrinogen is a vital component of the coagulation pathway and normal values in the obstetric population differ from the general population. Fibrinogen levels fall early in major haemorrhage and low levels have been shown to independently predict greater blood loss (Charbit et al., 2007). Although there is a small amount of fibrinogen in FFP, low levels should be replaced with pooled cryoprecipitate or fibrinogen concentrate where available (Plaat and Shonfeld, 2015). Fibrinogen should be maintained over 2 g/l when there is active bleeding (Mavrides et al., 2017).

Point-of-care (POC) haemostatic testing has the advantages of testing all aspects of clotting, often more quickly than lab-based testing. In a rapidly evolving haemorrhage situation, the delay in results from laboratory tests can make results meaningless. The most commonly used POC devices are thromboelastography (TEG) and rotational thromboelastometry (ROTEM) (Mallaiah et al., 2015).

The transfusion trigger for platelets should be 75×10^9/l to maintain a margin of safety over the target of 50 in the acutely bleeding patient (Calkins, 2015; Mavrides et al., 2017).

The following targets should be used for therapeutic goals in resuscitation (Mavrides et al., 2017).

Haemoglobin	> 80 g/l
Platelet count	> 50 × 10⁹/l
Prothrombin time (PT)	< 1.5× normal
Activated partial thromboplastin time (APTT)	< 1.5× normal
Fibrinogen	> 2 g/l

Hypothermia and acidosis can have independent negative effects on clotting and so must be actively managed. All intravenous fluids should be warmed, active body warming considered and invasive temperature monitoring instigated if possible. Anaesthetic technique is a multifactorial decision which can only be made by the managing clinician, but there are two distinct settings. In the elective setting where major blood loss is anticipated, such as with abnormal placental implantation, a regional technique is usually preferred with acknowledgement that there may need to be rapid conversion to general anaesthesia if blood loss is excessive. Usually invasive lines will be inserted before commencing surgery. In an emergency setting with cardiovascular instability or suspicion of a coagulopathy, a general anaesthetic will usually be preferable, although this decision should involve a senior member of the anaesthetic team.

When caring for a critically unwell patient such as this, all individuals must work together as a team and communicate effectively. This must be seen as equally important to the medical management. Protocol-based care has a role in improving outcomes, including in remote areas where recognition of limited facilities and appropriate transfer to expert centres is needed (Zelop, 2006).

Patient and relative communication is not the initial concern in a life-threatening situation, but the emotional toll must be appreciated and the patient and their relatives kept informed and reassured where possible.

Post PPH Management

When a massive obstetric haemorrhage has occurred there must be evidence of appropriate cardiovascular stability without ongoing bleeding before extubation is considered (Knight et al., 2014). If this is not the case, then ongoing management on a critical care unit is likely to be more appropriate.

Following a critical event, ensure that the appropriate documentation is completed. Time should be allowed for individual feedback, debrief of the team, patient and relatives, with identification of any learning opportunities identified. All PPH with an estimated blood loss of over 1500 ml should have a formal incident form completed (Mavrides et al., 2017).

Bibliography

Calkins, L. A. (2015). Blood transfusion in obstetrics and gynecology. *RCOG Greentop Guide*, 22(8) 704–707.

Charbit, B., Mandelbrot, L., Samain, E., et al. (2007). The decrease of fibrinogen is an early predictor of the severity of postpartum haemorrhage. *Journal of Thrombosis and Haemostasis*, 5(2), 266–273.

Department of Making Pregnancy Safer. World Health Organization. (2007). Reducing the global burden:

postpartum haemorrhage. *Making Pregnancy Safer. A Newsletter of Worldwide Activity World Health Organization*, pp. 1–8.

Dries, D. J. (2018). Tranexamic acid: is it about time? *The Lancet*, 391(10116), 97–98.

Fan, D., Xia, Q., Liu, L., et al. (2017). The incidence of postpartum hemorrhage in pregnant women with placenta previa: a systematic review and meta-analysis. *PLoS ONE*, 12(1), e0170194.

Fitzpatrick, K. E., Sellers, S., Spark, P., Kurinczuk, J. J., Brocklehurst, P. and Knight, M. (2012). Incidence and risk factors for placenta accreta/increta/percreta in the UK: a national case-control study. *PLoS ONE*, 7(12), e52893.

Knight, M., Callaghan, W. M., Berg, C., et al. (2009). Trends in postpartum hemorrhage in high resource countries: a review and recommendations from the International Postpartum Hemorrhage Collaborative Group. *BMC Pregnancy Childbirth*, 9(1), 55.

Knight, M., Kenyon, S., Brocklehurst, P., Neilson, J., Shakespeare, J. and Kurinczuk, J. J. (Eds.) on behalf of MBRRACE-UK. (2014). *Saving Lives, Improving Mothers' Care – Lessons Learned to Inform Future Maternity Care from the UK and Ireland Confidential Enquiries into Maternal Deaths and Morbidity 2009–12*. Oxford: National Perinatal Epidemiology Unit, University of Oxford.

M. G. Foundation. (2017). Effect of early tranexamic acid administration on mortality, hysterectomy, and other morbidities in women with post-partum haemorrhage (WOMAN). *Obstetrical and Gynecological Survey*, 72(9), 525–526.

Mallaiah, S., Barclay, P., Harrod, I., Chevannes, C. and Bhalla, A. (2015). Introduction of an algorithm for ROTEM-guided fibrinogen concentrate administration in major obstetric haemorrhage. *Anaesthesia* 70, 166–15.

Mavrides, E. T. A., Allard, S., Chandraharan, E., et al. (2017). Prevention and management of postpartum haemorrhage: Green-top Guideline No. 52. *British Journal of Obstetrics and Gynaecology*, 124(5), e106–e149.

Mousa, H. A., Blum, J., Abou El Senoun, G., Shakur, H. and Alfirevic, Z. (2014). Treatment for primary postpartum haemorrhage. *Cochrane Database of Systematic Reviews*, 2014(2), CD003249.

Plaat, F. and Shonfeld, A. (2015). Major obstetric haemorrhage. *BJA Education*, 15(4), 190–193.

Saljoughian, M. (2011). Uterotonic agents: an update. *US Pharmacist*, 36(5), 36–40.

Vogel, J. P., Oladapo, O. T., Dowswell, T. and Gülmezoglu, A. M. (2018). Updated WHO recommendation on intravenous tranexamic acid for the treatment of post-partum haemorrhage. *The Lancet Global Health*, 6(1), e18–e19.

Zelop, C. M. (2006). ACOG Practice Bulletin: Clinical Management Guidelines for Obstetrician–Gynecologists Number 76, October 2006: postpartum haemorrhage. *Obstetrics and Gynecology*, 108(4), 1039–1047.

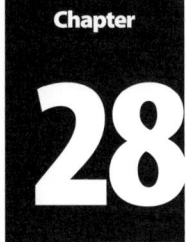

28

Group A Streptococcal Puerperal Sepsis

Laura Coleman and Melissa Whitworth

Scenario in a Nutshell

Postpartum woman develops Group A streptococcal septic shock.

Stage 1: Initial assessment with initiation of management for sepsis.

Stage 2: Deteriorating hypotensive patient not responding to fluid boluses – septic shock.

Stage 3: Commence vasopressors and plan for invasive monitoring and transfer to critical care.

Target Learner Groups

All members of the multidisciplinary obstetric team: anaesthetists, midwives, obstetricians, operating department practitioners/anaesthetic nurses.

Specific learning opportunities
Early recognition of a deteriorating septic patient
Knowledge of the management of sepsis with appropriate escalation of treatment
Effective team management of an acutely unwell obstetric patient with appropriate senior and multidisciplinary involvement

Suggested learners (to represent their normal roles)	In the room from the start	Available when requested
Anaesthetic ST3+		√
Obstetric ST3+	√	
Midwife coordinator		√
Midwife in room	√	
Operating Department Practitioner (ODP)/ anaesthetic nurse		√

Suggested learners (to represent their normal roles)	In the room from the start	Available when requested
Suggested facilitators		
Faculty to play role of ward midwife giving SBAR handover to midwife and obstetric ST3+ at start of scenario	√	

Details for Facilitators

Patient Demographics

Name: Eva
Age: 32
Gestation: 1 day post partum
Booking weight: 80 kg
Parity: P1

Scenario Summary for Facilitators

32-year-old, now P1 woman, had a normal vaginal delivery at 40+5 weeks, then had repair of a third-degree tear in theatre.

She is now 18 hours post-delivery with swinging temperatures, lower abdominal pain and foul smelling lochia.

She develops a tachycardia then hypotension.

Unresponsive to intravenous crystalloid infusion.

Diagnosis of septic shock.

Resuscitation with antibiotics, intravenous crystalloid and vasopressors.

Safe planning of transfer to critical care.

Set-up Overview for Facilitators

Clinical setting	On a postnatal ward bed
Patient position	Semi-recumbent
Initial monitoring in place	None
Other equipment	None

Medical Equipment

For core equipment checklist, see Chapter 9.

Additional equipment specific to scenario		
Antibiotics: (or as per local guidelines) Co-amoxiclav Benzypenicillin Clindamycin Tazocin	Local microbiology antibiotic guidelines	Arterial line
Cardiovascular drugs: Metaraminol Phenylephrine Noradrenaline	CVP line	

Information Given to the Learners

Information given to obstetric trainee and midwife who are taking over care of patient from the current ward midwife (facilitator)

Time: 15:00

The SBAR handover is as follows:

Situation: This is Eva, she has just called me because she is not feeling well.

Background: 32-year-old, previously fit and well primip who had a normal delivery yesterday at 40+5 weeks and then went to theatre for repair of a third-degree tear. She has no allergies.

She has started to feel generally unwell and has had some lower abdominal pain on and off today.

Action: I was just about to do some observations.

Recommendation: Are you OK to take over Eva's care?

Scenario Schedule

Observations	
A	Clear
B	RR 28/min SpO$_2$ 96% on air
C	HR 132bpm BP 110/61 CRT 1s
D	**A**VPU
E	Temp 38.4°C

Stage 1: Initial assessment with initiation of management for sepsis	
Information given	**Expected actions**
Patient is in the post-natal ward, complaining of feeling unwell with continuous lower abdominal pain	Commence ABCDE approach to patient: Apply full monitoring Consider sepsis early as part of differential diagnosis
If asked: Not unwell prior to delivery, toddler and husband have been under the weather with sore throat and cold Feels slightly short of breath today, no cough, no sputum, no sore throat, no earache, no facial pain No urinary symptoms No diarrhoea/vomiting Mild headache, no neck stiffness, no photophobia No breast pain Offensive-smelling lochia today – not previously. Low abdominal pain-was intermittent, now continuous.	Take history including looking for potential sources of sepsis (resp/abdo/urine/genital tract/central nervous system/breast/ sinuses/ears)
Chest clear, air entry bilateral, no added sounds Flushed, warm peripheries, bounding pulse, normal heart sounds Breast examination normal Abdomen soft, some tenderness lower abdomen, Normal bowel sounds present	Examine patient

Information given	Expected actions
Perineal wound looks swollen and inflamed	
	Secure IV access and take blood for FBC, U+E, LFT, Coagulation screen, CRP
	Genital tract sepsis most likely from history and examination
	Note 'red flags for sepsis' (see discussion, chapter 29)
	State emergency to the team: 'red flag sepsis - likely source genital tract'
	Call anaesthetic ST and inform obstetric and anaesthetic consultants, again stating 'red flag sepsis'
	Commence 'sepsis 6': • O_2 as required to maintain SpO_2 94-98% • Take blood cultures • Start IV antibiotics for genital tract sepsis as per local guidance • Check lactate • Administer IV crystalloid fluids – 500mls rapidly and assess response • Catheterise and monitor hourly urine output
ABG result on air: pH 7.3 pO2 12.9 kPa pCO2 3.5 kPa HCO3 14 mmols/L Lactate 4.6 mmols/L BE -10 mmol/L	
See Figure 28.1 for ECG if requested	
Pus evident when taking LVS	Commence septic screen: CXR, MSU, low vaginal swab (LVS), swab perineal wound
	Team recognise need to transfer to monitored bed – eg: obstetric HDU

Proceed to stage 2 once history and examination complete and sepsis 6 started

Stage 2: Deteriorating hypotensive patient not responding to fluid boluses – septic shock

Information given	Expected actions
Now on delivery unit, in obstetric HDU with midwife and obstetric ST3+ in the room	
Patient has become drowsy but is still responding to voice: GCS 14: E=3, V=5, M=6 No change from stage 1 if cardiorespiratory examination repeated	Reasses ABCDE
Anaesthetic ST3+ immediately available and attends	Urgently call for anaesthetic assistance if not arrived Restate the emergency and SBAR from ST3+ obstetrics to ST3+ anaesthetics
No response to fluid resuscitation	Further fluid boluses up to 30mls/kgSite 2nd large bore cannula
	Identify septic shock and state to team
Critical care Registrar agrees from history that patient needs transfer to critical care. They are busy with another emergency and can't attend immediately. They will try and arrange a bed but know that they are going to have to rearrange some patients – it may be several hours until a bed is available.	Recognise need for critical care – inform critical care team
	Request urgent assistance from ODP/anaesthetic nurse and anaesthetic consultant
Microbiologist suggests changing anitbiotics to broad-spectrum eg: IV tazocin (or as per local guidance) and addition of clindamycin to antibiotic regime to cover Group A streptococcus in view of rapid clinical deterioration	Ask team member to get urgent advice from Microbiology

Progress to stage 3 once adequate fluid bolus given and septic shock diagnosed

Observations	
A	Clear
B	RR 34/min SpO2 96% on O$_2$
C	HR 144bpm BP 80/32 CRT 2s
D	A**V**PU
E	Temp 38.7°C

Observations	
A	Clear
B	RR 32/min SpO$_2$ 96% on O$_2$
C	HR 140bpm BP 78/36 CRT 3s
D	A**V**PU
E	Temp 38.7°C

Stage 3: Commence vasopressors, plan for invasive monitoring and transfer to critical care

Information given	Expected actions
	Recognise urgent need for vasopressor administration: commence noradrenaline peripherally while preparing for central line insertion, (Alternatively, metaraminol or phenylephrine according to local practice)
ODP/anaesthetic nurse available if asked	This may require transfer to safe place to site CVP line and commence vasopressor treatment dependent on local guidelines – eg: obstetric theatres/recovery or in obstetric HDU room with anaesthetist and critical care nurse in continuous attendance. Appropriate treatment with vasopressors should **not** be delayed while waiting for a critical care bed to become available
	Arterial line insertion
ABG result: (on 15L/min O$_2$) pH 7.31 pO2 11.6 kPa pCO2 3.9 kPa bicarb 14 mmol/L BE -8 mmol/L lactate 4.1 mmol/L	Repeat arterial blood gas
More alert and feeling slightly better	Repeat observations
	Prepare for CVP line insertion
Initial blood results available: WCC 23 X10^9/L Hb 95g/L PLTs 98 X10^9/L CRP 298 mg/L	
Na+ 138 mmol/L K+ 4.1 mmol/L Urea 12.1 mmol/L Creat 144 µmol/L	
No coagulation result available as yet	
TEG/ROTEM normal	Send TEG/ROTEM while waiting for coagulation results
	Plan for transfer to critical care once bed available

Scenario ends once preparation for invasive monitoring and vasopressor commenced.
Inform team that next day Microbiology ring to say that perineal swab has grown Group A streptocoocus

Observations once vasopressor commenced	
A	Clear
B	RR 28/min SpO$_2$ 96% on O$_2$
C	HR 122bpm BP 108/ 56 CRT 2s
D	**A**VPU
E	Temp 38.6°C

Suggested Topics for Debrief Discussion

- Were the 'sepsis 6' completed in a timely manner?
- Was there early escalation of management to involve anaesthetics and intensive care and senior obstetricians and anaesthetists?
- Was there any problem locating any drugs/equipment needed: e.g. broad-spectrum IV antibiotics, clindamycin, noradrenaline?

Discussion

Sepsis

Sepsis is defined as a life-threatening organ dysfunction, which is due to a dysregulated host response to infection, organ dysfunction being identified by an increase of two points or more in the Sequential Organ Failure Assessment (SOFA) score (see Discussion and Table 29.1 in Chapter 29).

Sepsis in the presence of persistent hypotension requiring vasopressors to maintain MAP $\geq$ 65 mmHg or a lactate $\geq$ 2 mmol/l is known as septic shock, when the circulatory, cellular and metabolic abnormalities substantially increase mortality (Shankar-Hari et al., 2016).

Group A Streptococcal Puerperal Sepsis

Puerperal sepsis as defined by the World Health Organization is an infection of the genital tract occurring at any time between rupture of membranes or labour and the 42nd day postpartum (World Health Organization, 1992).

In the UK, approximately 50 women have life-threatening sepsis for each maternal sepsis death. While the largest proportion of severe sepsis cases are the result of *Escherichia coli* infection, outcomes are significantly worse for cases of group A streptococcal infection. There is an association between treatment with antibiotics in the perinatal period and severe sepsis. Therefore care must be taken to ensure that personnel recognise that treatment with antibiotics does not always prevent progression to severe sepsis and women need appropriate monitoring and follow-up to ensure improvement (Acosta et al., 2014).

Incidence

There is an increasing incidence of group A streptococcal puerperal sepsis leading to significant morbidity and mortality worldwide. In the UK, the incidence of severe group A *Streptococcus* is increasing and is currently 3.33 per 100,000 population, with 5% of all group A streptococcal infections in adults presenting as puerperal sepsis (Palaniappan et al., 2012). There is evidence of a re-emergence of virulent strains within

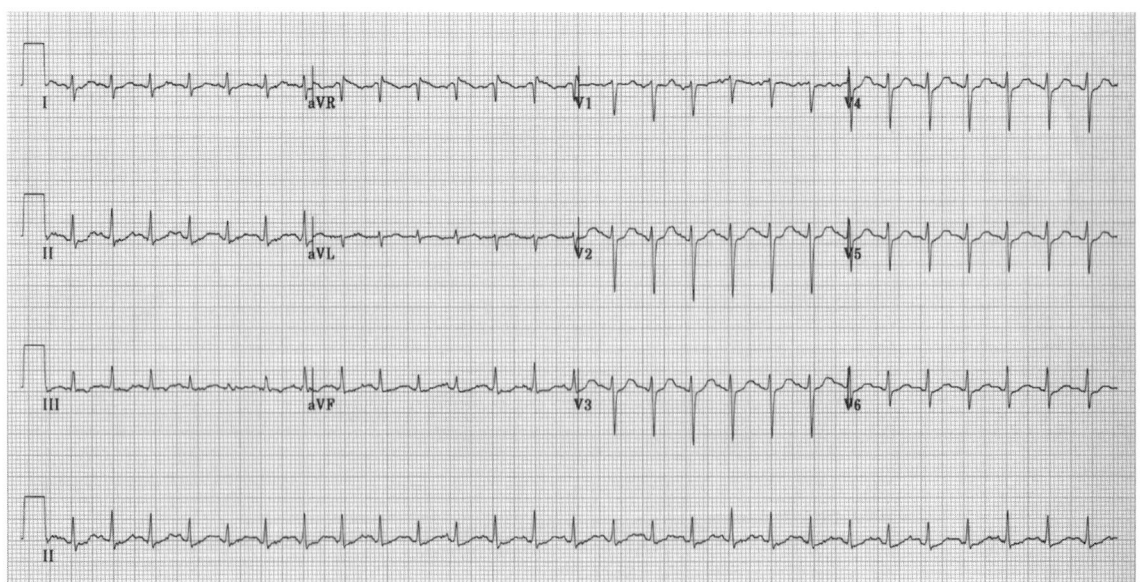

Figure 28.1 ECG.

developed countries, which can rapidly progress to toxin-mediated shock and multiorgan failure.

Unfortunately, although uncommon, puerperal sepsis remains a leading cause of maternal mortality, with group A streptococcal infection responsible for 75,000 maternal deaths per year globally (Shinar et al., 2016). Mortality rates for group A streptococcal-mediated septic shock are documented between 30% and 60% (Abouzeid et al., 2005; Byrne et al., 2009; Shinar et al., 2016) with a 7-day mortality of 20% (Palaniappan et al., 2012).

Transmission

Group A *Streptococcus*, also known as β haemolytic *Streptococcus pyogenes*, is a Gram-positive commensal of the throat and skin and can be present in the vagina. Transmission can be through inhalation or skin-to-skin contact.

If immunocompromised through a breach in the vaginal mucosa or perineal trauma during labour, bacterial invasion can occur and can reach the uterus and vasculature via the endocervix or tissue planes (Palaniappan et al., 2012).

Pathogenesis

Major virulence factors such as the M-protein type antigen (which provides resistance to phagocytosis) enable colonisation, multiplication and spread of infection (Byrne et al., 2009).

The pyrogenic exotoxin A influences the rapid onset of toxic shock (Abouzeid et al., 2005; Busowski et al., 2013) through inflammatory mediators such as tumour necrosis factor-alpha, interleukin-1-beta and interleukin 6, with these cytokines resulting in fever, tissue injury and shock (Byrne et al., 2009).

Clinical Presentation

Group A streptococcal infections range from mild respiratory, cutaneous and soft tissue infections to fatal invasive infections.

The clinical presentation of group A streptococcal sepsis is diverse, the most typical presentation is within the first 48 hours up to 7 days postpartum. There is often an insidious onset which can include a tachycardia, pyrexia, rigors, abdominal or limb or pelvic pain or foul-smelling lochia with the ability to progress rapidly to vasopressor-dependent shock and multiorgan failure (Abouzeid et al., 2005; Palaniappan et al., 2012; Busowski et al., 2013; Shinar et al., 2016).

A severe group A streptococcal infection is defined as isolation of group A *Streptococcus* from a sterile or non-sterile site with a clinical presentation of:

- toxic shock syndrome,
- necrotising fasciitis,
- pneumonia,
- puerperal sepsis,
- septic arthritis,
- meningitis (Palaniappan et al., 2012)

or those requiring:

- surgical exploration,
- an admission to the intensive care unit, or
- hospital length of stay of more than 14 days (Byrne et al., 2009).

Streptococcal toxic shock includes the presence of hypotension and two or more of:

- renal impairment,
- coagulopathy,
- liver involvement,
- adult respiratory distress syndrome (ARDS),
- erythematous rash, or
- necrotising fasciitis (Lamagni and Williams, 2009).

Pregnant women have a 20-fold increase compared to non-pregnant women for invasive group A streptococcal infections (where the bacteria are isolated from a normally sterile body site, such as blood), with risk factors including:

- upper respiratory tract infection with pharyngeal colonisation,
- contact with group A streptococcal carriers,
- prolonged rupture of membranes,
- mucosal damage,
- emergency caesarean section (Shinar et al., 2016).

A key characteristic of group A streptococcal sepsis is the rapid deterioration of a patient despite appropriate initial management (Palaniappan et al., 2012). Early recognition, diagnosis and prompt, aggressive treatment with the correct antibiotics are crucial.

Investigations

Investigations for suspected group A streptococcal sepsis include blood tests (full blood count, urea and electrolytes, C-reactive protein, coagulation, blood cultures, arterial blood gases), swabs (vaginal, placenta, wound) and further investigations to rule out any other potential sources (urine microscopy and culture, imaging of chest/abdomen/uterus) (Palaniappan et al., 2012; Busowski et al., 2013).

225

Management of Genital Tract Sepsis

Early recognition and prompt management of sepsis are key. Ongoing education for obstetric and midwifery staff on the symptoms and signs of sepsis and prompt initiation of the sepsis 6 can be aided by initiatives such as the UK Sepsis Trust Inpatient Maternal Sepsis Tool (UK Sepsis Trust, 2016) and raising staff awareness of maternal sepsis red flags (see Table 29.1).

Management remains largely supportive with intravenous fluids and intravenous antibiotics. High-dependency or intensive care may be required with multidisciplinary team involvement from midwives, obstetricians, physicians, anaesthetists and intensive care physicians in cases of multiorgan failure.

Treatment of severe peripartum sepsis requires antibiotics directed at likely causes:

* group A *Streptococcus*,
* *Staphylococcus aureus*,
* anaerobes,
* *E. coli.*

Penicillin is the antibiotic of choice in group A streptococcal infections, with clindamycin used in patients with a penicillin allergy, which can be added in streptococcal toxic shock to block toxin production (Abouzeid et al., 2005; Byrne et al., 2009; Busowski et al., 2013; Shinar et al., 2016). Microbiology advice should be sought as although group A *Streptococcus* remains sensitive to penicillin, a reduction in its efficacy has been observed in high colonisation rates (Byrne et al., 2009).

Surgery may be required for source control, for example: wound drainage and debridement, hysterectomy and adnexal tissue removal (Palaniappan et al., 2012) with early surgical intervention shown to improve morbidity (Byrne et al., 2009). The role of immunoglobulins still remains unclear (Anderson, 2014).

Bibliography

Abouzeid, H., Wu, P., Mohammed, N. and Al-Samarrai, M. (2005). Group A streptococcal puerperal sepsis: the return of a potentially fatal disease. *Journal of Obstetrics and Gynaecology*, 25, 806–808.

Acosta, C. D., Kurinczuk, J. J., Lucas, D. N., Tuffnell, D.J., Selters, S. and Knight, M., United Kingdom Obstetric Surveillance System (2014). Severe maternal sepsis in the UK, 2011–2012. A national case-control study. *PLoS Medicine*, 11(7), e100161672. doi: 10.1371/journal.pmed.1001672

Anderson, B. L. (2014). Puerperal group A streptococcal infection: beyond Semmelweis. *Obstetrics & Gynaecology*, 123(4), 874–882.

Busowski, M. T., Lee, M., Busowski, J. D., Akhter, K. and Wallace, M. R. (2013). Puerperal group a streptococcal infections: a case series and discussion. *Case Reports in Medicine*, 2003, 751329. Available from: http://dx.doi.org/10.1155/2013/751329.

Byrne, J. L. B., Aagaard-Tillery, K. M., Johnson, J. L., Wright, L. J. and Silver, R. M. (2009). Group A streptococcal puerperal sepsis: initial characterization of virulence factors in association with clinical parameters. *Journal of Reproductive Immunology*, 82, 74–83.

Lamagni, T. and Williams, C. on behalf of the national incident management team. (2009). *National Enhanced Surveillance of Severe Group A Streptococcal Disease: Protocol*. London: Health Protection Agency. Available from: www.hpa.org.uk/web/HPAwebFile/HPAweb_C/1234946226285

Palaniappan, N., Menezes, M. and Wilson, P. (2012). Group A streptococcal puerperal sepsis: management and prevention. *The Obstetrician & Gynaecologist*, 14, 9–16.

Shankar-Hari, M., Phillips, G. S., Levy, M. L., et al. (2016). Developing a new definition and assessing new clinical criteria for septic shock: for the third international consensus definitions for sepsis and septic shock (sepsis-3). *The Journal of the American Medical Association*, 315(8), 775–787.

Shinar, S., Fouks, Y., Amit, S., et al. (2016). Clinical characteristics of and preventative strategies for peripartum group a streptococcal infections. *Obstetrics & Gynecology*, 127(2), 227–232.

World Health Organization. (1992). The Prevention and Management of Puerperal Infections. Report of a Technical Working Group, Geneva, 20–22 May 1992. Available from: http://whqlibdoc.who.int/hq/1995/WHO_FHE_MSM_95.4.PDF

https://sepsistrust.org/wp-content/uploads/2017/08/Inpatient-maternal-NICE-Final-1107-2.pdf (accessed March 11, 2018).

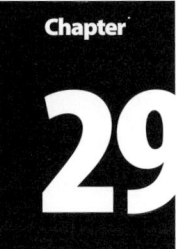

Chapter

29

Pneumonia and Respiratory Failure in a Pregnant Woman

James Hanison and Dougal Atkinson

Scenario in a Nutshell

> Antenatal viral pneumonia progressing to respiratory failure, requiring intubation. Then develops tension pneumothorax.
>   Stage 1: Initial assessment and commence sepsis 6.
>   Stage 2: Patient deteriorates with respiratory failure, requiring intubation.
>   Stage 3: Patient difficult to ventilate, develops tension pneumothorax.

Target Learner Groups

All members of the multidisciplinary obstetric team: anaesthetists, midwives, obstetricians and operating department practitioners/anaesthetic nurses.

Specific learning opportunities
Effective team management of two emergencies – respiratory failure and tension pneumothorax
Timely recognition of sepsis and consideration of viral pneumonia as a potential diagnosis
Efficient completion of the sepsis 6
Assess access on the delivery unit to: emergency intubation equipment, oseltamivir, chest drain insertion equipment

Suggested learners (to represent their normal roles)	In the room from the start	Available when requested
Anaesthetic ST3+		√
Obstetric ST3+		√
Midwife Coordinator		√
Triage midwife	√	
Operating Department Practitioner (ODP)/ anaesthetic nurse		√
Suggested facilitators		
Faculty to play role of patient's partner	√	

Details for Facilitators

Patient Demographics

Name: Rita	
Age: 35	
Gestation: 25+6	
Booking weight: 65 kg	
Parity: P2	

Scenario Summary for Facilitators

> 35-year-old 25-week pregnant multiparous woman. Telephoned antenatal ward and described a 4-day history of fever and shortness of breath. Advised to attend triage for assessment.
> Arrives in triage presenting with hypoxia, shortness of breath and pyrexia.
> Transferred to delivery unit high-dependency area.
> Rapidly deteriorates with worsening hypoxia and reduced level of consciousness.
> Intubation and ventilation is required, following which patient develops cardiovascular instability despite resuscitation.
> Tension pneumothorax. Requires decompression. Emergency chest drain.

Set-up Overview for Facilitators

Clinical setting	On triage trolley
Patient position	Semi-recumbent
Initial monitoring in place	None – just arrived
Other equipment	None
Useful manikin functions	Intubation Unilateral and bilateral chest movement Normal and abnormal breath sounds

227

Medical Equipment

For core equipment checklist, see Chapter 9, including advanced airway equipment.

Additional equipment specific to scenario

Anaesthetic drugs: Propofol Thiopentone Suxamethonium Rocuronium Opioid: fentanyl/ alfentanil Remifentanil/ propofol or other sedative infusions	Antibiotics/ antiviral drugs (or as per local guidelines): Co-amoxiclav Clarithromycin Oseltamivir/ zanamivir	Cardiovascular drugs: Metaraminol Ephedrine Phenylephrine Atropine Adrenaline 1:10,000

Doppler fetal monitor/pinard stethoscope

Aprons, gloves, surgical masks with eye protection, FFP3 face masks	Local microbiology antibiotic guidelines

Information Given to the Learners

Information given to the midwife starting in the room.

Time: 18:35

This handover is given by a facilitator playing the role of the midwife who has just brought the patient round from reception to a triage room because she looks unwell.

The SBAR handover is as follows:

Situation: This is Rita – I have brought her round as she was feeling unwell and looking short of breath in the waiting room.

Background: She is a 35-year-old, who is 25+6 weeks pregnant with her third child. Two previous normal vaginal deliveries. She doesn't have any allergies. She has mild asthma. She has been feeling generally unwell with a temperature for the last 4 days and has become short of breath over the last 24 hours.

Assessment: We've brought her straight round but haven't had a chance to do her observations yet.

Recommendation: The coordinator said you were free to take her – is that right?

Midwife handing over patient leaves.

Scenario Schedule

Stage 1: Initial assessment and commence sepsis 6

Information given	Expected actions
Patient is sat upright in bed, complaining of shortness of breath. She looks tired. Eyes closed but opening to voice.	Commence ABCDE approach to patient:
Patient can talk in short sentences. Cyanosed.	Perform airway assessment
	Apply oxygen via non-rebreathing mask at 15L/min
	Call for urgent help – co-ordinating midwife, obstetric ST and anaesthetic ST
	Apply full monitoring - activate emergency buzzer when severe cardiorespiratory compromise recognised
If asked: Generally unwell for last 4 days, hot and sweaty. Has also been feeling increasingly short of breath, particularly over last 24 hours. Has mild asthma, takes PRN salbutamol every few days. No hospital admissions for asthma.	Take brief history

Observations

A	Clear
B	RR 40/min SpO$_2$ 80% on air
C	HR 133bpm BP 90/60 CRT 4s
D	A**VP**U
E	Temp 38.5^{0}C

Information given	Expected actions
She also reports a dry cough. She reports that her other 2 children have been off school all week with "the flu". Not had flu vaccine. No chest pain, no haemoptysis, no leg swelling. No PV bleeding, no abdo pain	
	Secure IV access Take blood for FBC, U+E, LFT, CRP, G+S
CBG 6.1mmol/l	Check CBG (capillary blood glucose)
Obstetric and anaesthetic STs arrive	SBAR from midwife to obstetric and anaesthetic STs
Trachea central, chest expansion similar both sides, decreased air entry right base, normal breath sounds elsewhere, no wheeze Sweaty, heart sounds 1+2+0, mild oedema both feet Abomen soft, non-tender, bowel sounds present	Examine patient
	Request CXR
If candidate proceeds to treat for acute, severe asthma, no improvement seen	Identify sepsis and possible community acquired pneumonia or viral pneumonia
	Identify multiple red flags for maternal sepsis (see discussion)
	Initiate sepsis 6 management: Administer antibiotics as per local guidelines: for example, co-amoxiclav 1.2g IV and clarithromycin 500mg IV. Start oseltamivir(Tamiflu) 75mg bd. Take blood cultures (prior to antibiotics as long as this does not cause delay)
	Ask for microbiology advice once patient more stable
	Administer 500mls crystalloid bolus and assess response
ABG results on 15L/min O_2 (if requested): pH 7.25 CO2 6.0 kPa O2 9.2 kPa BE -6.0 mEq/L Lactate 4mmol/L	Perform arterial blood gas (ABG) and check lactate
	Catheterise and monitor hourly urine output

Information given	Expected actions
	Inform obstetric and anaesthetic consultants – communicate 'red flag sepsis'
CXR shows signs of right basal consolidation	Arrange transfer to monitored, high care bed such as obstetric HDU
	Note that isolation precautions are required: e.g. single room Staff to wear apron, gloves and surgical mask with eye protection or FFP3 mask if aerosol-generating procedure, eg: intubation, endotracheal suction
	Send throat swabs and sputum for C+S if any produced, urine for legionella and pneumococcal antigen.
Inform that first 500mls crystalloid is finished	Reassess observations once 500mls fluid bolus given. Commence further 500mls crstalloid.
See Figure 29.1 for ECG	Perform ECG
Fetal heart rate present	Listen to fetal heart

Proceed to stage 2 once initial assessment complete, sepsis 6 commenced and patient transferred to obstetric HDU

Observations	
A	Clear
B	RR 38/min SpO$_2$ 88% on O$_2$
C	HR 122bpm BP 115/62 CRT 4s
D	A**V**PU
E	Temp 38.5^{0}C

Stage 2: Patient deteriorates with respiratory failure, requiring intubation

Information given	Expected actions
Patient has arrived in obstetric HDU room and is monitored	
Anaesthetic ST3+ and obstetric ST3+ have come around to obstetric HDU with the patient	
Additional member of staff arrives – midwife co-ordinator	
Patient has stopped talking and is slumped over in bed	
Snoring	Reassess airway
	Perform airway-opening manoeuvres +/- insert oropharyngeal airway if tolerated. (Don't use nasopharyngeal airway as bleeding risk)
Airway now clear Trachea central, poor chest expansion but similar both sides, decreased air entry right base, normal breath sounds elsewhere, no wheeze audible	Reassess airway and breathing

Observations	
A	Obstructed
B	RR 45/min SpO$_2$ 80% on O$_2$
C	HR 100bpm BP 140/90 CRT 2s
D	AVP**U** then improves to A**V**PU once airway cleared
E	Temp 38.5^{0}C

Information given	Expected actions
	Identify hypoxia and need for endotracheal intubation.
	Consider optimising patient oxygenation with high-flow nasal oxygen (THRIVE) while preparing for intubation if equipment is located on/near delivery unit.
	Urgently call for assistance from ODP/anaesthetic nurse and senior anaesthetist
	Prepare drugs and equipment for rapid sequence induction
	Prepare emergency vasopressor dugs
	Inform obstetric and anaesthetic consultants of change in condition if not yet arrived
Additional member of staff arrives – ODP/anaesthetic nurse	Identify aspiration risk. Allocate team members roles for rapid sequence induction including; cricoid pressure, drugs, airway equipment and airway management
	Discuss airway plan A, B and C with team.
Grade 1 intubation ETCO$_2$ confirmed	Perform rapid sequence induction. Monitor with capnography
Critical care registrar agrees that patient requires critical care admission – no beds available at present, may take a couple of hours before bed becomes available	Inform critical care – contact ICU registrar on call. Arrange critical care transfer.
	Consider safest area to care for patient until ITU bed available – may need to move to obstetric theatre/recovery
	Establish sedative infusion or inhalational anaesthesia
Quite difficult to BVM ventilate from the outset, requires high inspiratory pressures but initially managing adequate tidal volumes.	Establish patient on a ventilator

Proceed to stage 3 once intubated and established on ventilator

Observations

A	Intubated
B	RR 18/min SpO$_2$ 94%, FiO$_2$ 0.8 ETCO$_2$ 8.2kPa
C	HR 118bpm BP 114/72 CRT 2s
D	Anaesthetised
E	Temp 38.3^{0}C

Stage 3: Patient difficult to ventilate, develops tension pneumothorax

Information given	Expected actions
Ventilator is alarming 'high airway pressure' and 'low tidal volumes' or patient becomes more difficult to ventilate if bag/valve/mask ventilation	Recognise that patient has deteriorated
	Recognise worsening hypoxia and cardiovascular collapse with hypotension and tachycardia
	Consider differential diagnosis including worsening sepsis, anaphylaxis, acute asthma and response to sedative medication.
	Reassess patient in ABCDE approach
ETT distance at lips unchanged Tracheal deviation to left, minimal chest expansion right side, resonant percussion note on right, absent breath sounds on right	Assess airway and respiratory system: Check ETT tube length Identify signs consistent with tension pneumothorax
	Recognise tension pneumothorax and proceed to emergency needle thoracocentesis.
	Do not wait for CXR to confirm diagnosis
	Prepare equipment including skin preparation and large bore intravenous cannula Identify location of needle insertion: 2nd intercostal space, mid-clavicular line
A soft hiss is audible when the cannula is inserted into the thorax	Needle thoracocentesis performed
The patient becomes easier to ventilate. Oxygen saturation improves. Heart rate reduces and blood pressure improves.	Identify need for definitive drainage of pneumothorax
	Prepare for insertion of intercostal drain

Scenario ends once need for intercostal drain is identified. Inform team that patient's throat swab was positive for Influenza A.

Observations (first)

A	Intubated
B	RR 18/min SpO$_2$ 80%, FiO$_2$ 1.0 ETCO$_2$ 4.2kPa
C	HR 140bpm BP 72/40 CRT 5s
D	Anaesthetised
E	Temp 37.8^{0}C

Observations (second)

A	Intubated
B	RR 18/min SpO$_2$ 96%, FiO$_2$ 1.0 ETCO$_2$ 7.1kPa
C	HR 112bpm BP 108/72 CRT 2s
D	Anaesthetised
E	Temp 37.5^{0}C

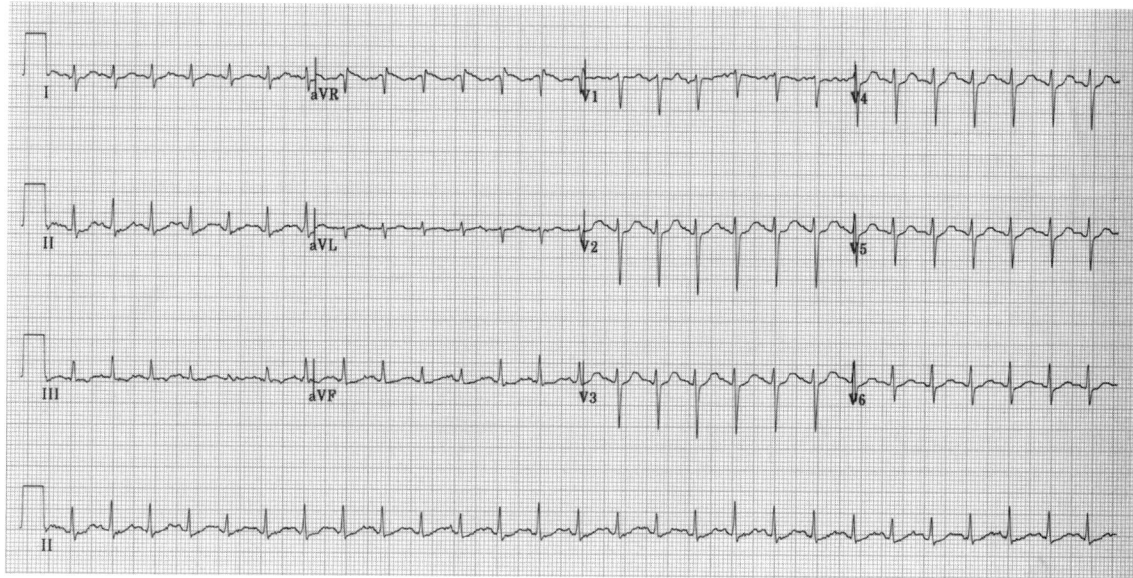

Figure 29.1 ECG.

Suggested Topics for Debrief Discussion

- Was viral pneumonia considered with appropriate investigations, patient isolation and antiviral therapy?
- Was the team confident with the recognition of tension pneumothorax and management?
- Were there any problems in locating drugs/equipment, e.g. high-flow nasal oxygen, chest drain, intubation equipment?

Discussion

Sepsis

In 2016, new consensus definitions for sepsis and septic shock were published (sepsis-3; Singer et al., 2016). The following provides a summary:

- Sepsis is defined as life-threatening organ dysfunction caused by a dysregulated host response to infection.
- Organ dysfunction can be identified as an acute change in total SOFA score ≥ 2 points consequent to the infection.
- The baseline SOFA score can be assumed to be zero in patients not known to have pre-existing organ dysfunction.

- A SOFA score ≥ 2 reflects an overall mortality risk of approximately 10% in a general hospital population with suspected infection. Even patients presenting with modest dysfunction can deteriorate further, emphasising the seriousness of this condition and the need for prompt and appropriate intervention, if not already being instituted.
- Patients with suspected infection who are likely to have a prolonged ICU stay or to die in the hospital can be promptly identified at the bedside with qSOFA – see Table 29.1.
- Septic shock is a subset of sepsis in which underlying circulatory and cellular/metabolic abnormalities are profound enough to substantially increase mortality.
- Patients with septic shock can be identified with a clinical construct of sepsis with persisting hypotension requiring vasopressors to maintain MAP ≥ 65 mmHg and having a serum lactate level > 2 mmol/l (18 mg/dl) despite adequate volume resuscitation. With these criteria, hospital mortality is in excess of 40%.

Table 29.1 qSOFA (quick SOFA) criteria.

Respiratory rate ≥ 22/min
Altered mentation
Systolic blood pressure ≤ 100 mmHg

Table 29.2 Maternal sepsis red flags (UK Sepsis Trust, 2016).

Any one of the following features represents a 'red flag' in a sick pregnant or postpartum woman with suspected infection:
Responds only to voice or pain/unresponsive
Systolic BP ≤ 90mmHg (or drop > 40 from normal)
Heart rate > 130 per minute
Respiratory rate ≥ 25 per minute
Needs oxygen to keep SpO_2 ≥ 92%
Non-blanching rash, mottled/ashen/cyanotic
Not passed urine in last 18 hours
Urine output less than 0.5 ml/kg/h
Lactate ≥ 2 mmol/l

Table 29.3 Risk factors for maternal sepsis.

Obesity
Impaired glucose tolerance
Impaired immunity
Anaemia
Vaginal discharge
History of pelvic infection
History of group B streptococcal infection
Amniocentesis and other invasive procedures
Cervical cerclage
Prolonged SRM
GAS infection in close contacts/family members
Black or other minority ethnic groups
Low socioeconomic status
Multiple pregnancy
Primiparity
Recent antibiotic treatment

(*Abbreviations*: MAP, mean arterial pressure; qSOFA, quick SOFA; SOFA, Sequential [sepsis-related] Organ Failure Assessment.)

Sepsis in Obstetrics

Sepsis remains an important cause of maternal death in the UK. Sepsis may result at any point during pregnancy and the puerperium with sources of infection including both obstetric and non-obstetric causes. Urinary tract infection and chorioamnionitis are common infections associated with septic shock in the pregnant patient. The most common organisms identified in pregnant women dying from sepsis are Lancefield group A beta-haemolytic *Streptococcus* and *Escherichia coli*.

The physiological changes of pregnancy may mask the clinical signs of sepsis and make the differential diagnosis of critical illness difficult. Early diagnosis and prompt management are essential with close liaison between senior clinical staff and critical care imperative. 'Red flags' for maternal sepsis have been defined (Table 29.2) and a maternity sepsis toolkit has been developed alongside new NICE guidance (National Institute for Health and Care Excellence, 2016). Risk factors for maternal sepsis are listed in Table 29.3.

The general principles of sepsis management apply to the obstetric patient, but must also take into account the physiological changes of pregnancy and associated conditions (e.g. pre-eclampsia).

The Sepsis-6 pathway should be administered to pregnant or postpartum women *within 1 hour* if there is suspected infection or they have clinical observations outside normal limits. This includes:

- administering oxygen to achieve saturation > 94%;
- checking blood lactate (venous ± arterial) – involve critical care if > 4 mmol/l;

Table 29.4 Differential diagnosis of respiratory failure in pregnancy.

Infection – bacterial, viral
Pulmonary oedema – cardiac, tocolytics, pre-eclampsia
Aspiration
Asthma
Venous air embolism
Amniotic fluid embolus
Thrombo-embolic disease
Neuromuscular conditions

- monitoring urine output – consider urinary catheter, fluid balance chart;
- administration of antibiotics according to local protocol;
- taking blood and other relevant cultures – peripheral blood, urine, sputum, vaginal swabs. Think source control and timing of delivery of baby – start CTG;
- administering IV fluids – 500 ml stat (up to 30 ml/kg if hypotensive or lactate raised > 2 mmol/l in first 3 h). Aim for MAP > 65 mmHg and normalisation of lactate with frequent reassessment.

Respiratory Failure in Pregnancy

Acute respiratory failure is a rare complication of pregnancy. Table 29.4 outlines the potential causes in pregnancy.

Community-acquired pneumonia is one of the more common causes of acute respiratory failure

Table 29.5 Risk factors for complicated influenza.

Pregnancy – especially second and third trimesters
Chronic cardiac, pulmonary, renal, hepatic or neurological disease
Morbid obesity (BMI $\geq$ 40)
Immunosuppression
- Severe primary immunodeficiency
- Current or recent (< 6 months) chemotherapy or radiotherapy for malignancy
- Solid-organ transplant recipients
- Bone marrow recipients
- High-dose systemic corticosteroids ($\geq$ 40 mg prednisolone per day for $\geq$1 week and within 3 months of stopping)
- Currently or recently (<6 months) receiving other immunosuppressive therapy
- HIV infection

Table 29.6 Presentation of influenza.

Uncomplicated influenza
Influenza presenting with fever, coryza, generalised symptoms (e.g. headache, malaise, myalgia) and sometimes gastrointestinal symptoms, but without any features of complicated influenza

Complicated influenza
Influenza requiring hospital admission and/or signs of low respiratory tract infection (e.g. hypoxaemia, dyspnoea, lung infiltrates), central nervous system involvement and/or significant exacerbation of an underlying medical condition

Table 29.7 Complications of influenza.

Septic shock and multiple organ failure
Disseminated intravascular coagulation
Myocarditis
Encephalitis and cognitive impairment
Venous thromboembolism
Bacterial superinfection
Physical and psychological complications of prolonged critical illness

in pregnant patients. The causative organisms are the same as those found in non-pregnant patients, e.g. *Streptococcus pneumoniae, Haemophilus influenzae, Mycoplasma pneumoniae* and *Influenza*. The reduction in cell-mediated immunity seen with pregnancy (especially during the third trimester) also places women at increased risk of atypical pathogens, e.g. herpes virus.

Influenza in Pregnancy

There is an increased risk of influenza in pregnancy. Although pregnant women have a similar incidence of influenza, hospitalisation rates are higher than for age-matched controls.

Infection is more common in second and especially third trimesters with risk further increased when other risk factors are present (Table 29.5). Pre-term delivery and the incidence of still birth or death in the first week of life are more likely in pregnant women admitted to hospital with influenza.

In the MBRRACE report published in 2016 (Knight et al., 2016) there was a decrease in deaths due to influenza. This was felt to be primarily due to a low level of influenza activity in 2012–2014 (compared with 2009 and 2010). The importance of increasing immunisation rates in pregnancy against seasonal influenza was also reinforced. Women at any stage of pregnancy can receive the vaccine.

Clinical Features

Influenza may be complicated or uncomplicated in presentation (Table 29.6). The complications of influenza are listed in Table 29.7.

Diagnosis

In uncomplicated cases this is often on clinical grounds. Diagnostic tests include viral culture, serology, rapid antigen testing, PCR and immunofluorescence assays dependent on local protocol. Samples include nasopharyngeal (NP) swab, nasal swab and nasal wash or aspirate. For rapid detection techniques, e.g. PCR, NP specimens are generally more effective.

Management
General Principles

1. There should be a low threshold for the hospital assessment/admission for pregnant women with suspected influenza and risk factors for and/or clinical symptoms of complicated infection.
2. Standard infection control measures should be instituted as set out in local guidelines (e.g. patient isolation, use of personal protective equipment: gloves/apron/surgical facemask with eye protection or FFP3 masks for aerosol-generating procedures such as intubation) in suspected cases.
3. Follow local guidelines for diagnostic testing for influenza virus and start treatment in suspected cases *before confirmation* if clinically indicated.
4. Exclude other pathologies (e.g. pneumonia, pulmonary oedema) and other causes of sepsis which may present with a similar clinical picture with appropriate investigations, e.g.

echocardiogram, sputum culture, blood cultures, MSU, urine for legionella and pneumococcal antigen.

5. Manage exacerbations of any pre-existing comorbid disease (e.g. asthma).

6. Early involvement of relevant medical specialities in complicated cases including obstetric, anaesthetic, medical and microbiology/virology teams.

7. Early involvement of critical care in complicated influenza. This should be based on clinical assessment and any local early warning score/escalation policy.

Antiviral Therapy for Treatment of Influenza in Suspected or Confirmed Influenza in Pregnancy

Current recommendations for treatment of influenza in the UK are for oseltamivir(Tamiflu) and zanamivir. These drugs are selective inhibitors of neuraminidase (NA) and prevent new virion release from infected cells. Oseltamivir PO 75 mg bd for 5 days, started within 48 h of symptoms where possible, is the first-line treatment for complicated and uncomplicated influenza. Zanamivir inhaled (Diskhaler) 10 mg bd is an alternative if resistance is present or when there is failure to respond.

Do not wait for laboratory confirmation before commencing treatment. Early administration of treatment within 48 h appears to confer a mortality benefit in the pregnant population and may reduce the risk of mortality even if started up to 5 days after onset.

In critically ill patients an increased dose is no longer recommended in patients with influenza. Early discussion about treatment with your local microbiologist or virologist is advised, especially in complicated cases.

Both oseltamivir and zanamivir may be administered to breastfeeding patients where clinically indicated.

Tension Pneumothorax

Tension pneumothorax results when there is progressive build up of air within the pleural space via a 'one-way valve' air leak from the lung or chest wall. This results in air escaping into the pleural space but does not allow return. The addition of positive pressure ventilation will exacerbate this one-way-valve effect.

As pressure within the pleural space builds, the lung on the side of the pneumothorax collapses, the mediastinum is pushed towards the opposite hemi-thorax

and venous return to the heart is obstructed, compromising cardiac output.

Causes include positive pressure ventilation in patients with a visceral pleural injury, complication of a simple pneumothorax or following blunt or penetrating chest trauma.

Clinical Signs

Classical signs include deviation of the trachea to the side opposite to the pneumothorax and an over-expanded chest with hyper-resonant percussion note which moves little with respiration and with a reduction/absence of breath sounds on the side of the pneumothorax. The central venous pressure may be raised but may also be low or absent. These classic signs may be absent or difficult to ascertain, especially when a patient is receiving positive pressure ventilation. The patient may suffer progressive cardiorespiratory compromise with tachycardia, hypotension, tachypnoea and respiratory distress and eventually cardiac arrest (PEA – pulseless electrical activity).

There is an association with recurrent spontaneous pneumothorax and pregnancy.

Cardiovascular collapse is likely to occur more rapidly in ventilated patients as compared to spontaneously breathing patients and they are more likely to proceed to cardiac arrest. Despite this it is often poorly recognised in critically ill patients. British Thoracic Society guidance suggests that tension pneumothorax is an emergency and treatment should not be delayed for a chest X-ray, but states that, when time is available, a chest X-ray is useful in confirming the diagnosis and lateralisation where uncertainty exists.

Management

Emergency needle thoracocentesis with a 14–16G needle in the second intercostal space in the mid-clavicular line of the affected hemi-thorax is the classic management when there is cardiorespiratory compromise with a tension pneumothorax suspected.

However, be aware this technique may be ineffective in larger patients, the needle may kink, block or dislodge and there is a risk of lung injury in addition. Up to one-third of patients have a chest wall thickness greater than 5 cm (standard cannula length) at the second intercostal space. In the absence of haemodynamic compromise it is sensible to obtain a chest X-ray first to confirm diagnosis.

Definitive management is with a formal chest drain. The cannula (if used) should remain *in situ* until a bubbling underwater seal is seen attached to the intercostal drain.

Bibliography

Knight, M., Nair, M., Tuffnell, D., et al. (2016). *Maternal, Newborn and Infant Clinical Outcome Review Programme 2016*. Oxford: National Perinatal Epidemiology Unit, University of Oxford.

MacDuff, A., Arnold, A., Harvey, J. and BTS Pleural Disease Guideline Group. (2010). Management of spontaneous pneumothorax: British Thoracic Society Pleural Disease Guideline 2010. *Thorax*, 65(Suppl 2), ii18–31.

National Institute of Health and Clinical Excellence. (2016). *Sepsis: Recognition, Diagnosis and Early Management*. NICE guideline. London: NICE.

Public Health England. (2016). PHE guidance on use of antiviral agents for the treatment and prophylaxis of seasonal influenza. Version 8.0, September 2017.

Rhodes, A., Evans, L. E., Alhazzani, W., et al. (2017). Surviving sepsis campaign: international guidelines for management of sepsis and septic shock: 2016. *Critical Care Medicine*, 45(3), 486–552.

Royal College of Obstetricians and Gynaecologists. (2012). *Bacterial Sepsis in Pregnancy. Green-top Guideline No. 64a*. London: Royal College of Obstetricians and Gynaecologists.

Singer, M., Deutschman, C. S., Seymour, C. W., et al. (2016). The third international consensus definitions for sepsis and septic shock (sepsis-3). *Journal of the American Medical Association*, 315(8), 801–810. doi: 10.1001/jama.2016.0287

The UK Sepsis Trust. (2016). Inpatient maternal sepsis tool. Available from: https://sepsistrust.org/wp-content/uploads/2016/07/Inpatient-maternal-NICE-Final-1107-2.pdf (accessed February 24, 2017).

Chapter

30

Chest Pain in a Pregnant Patient

Shahid Karim and Sarah Vause

Scenario in a Nutshell

Coronary artery dissection presenting to A+E.

Stage 1: Initial assessment of chest pain in 30-week primipara.

Stage 2: Severe chest pain with ST elevation on ECG, commence management for acute coronary syndrome (ACS).

Stage 3: Worsening acute myocardial infarction deteriorating to ventricular fibrillation (VF) arrest. Requiring advanced life support (ALS) and transferred to cardiac catheterisation lab for primary percutaneous coronary intervention (PCI).

Target Learner Groups

Appropriate members of the receiving A+E, cardiology and multidisciplinary obstetric teams.

Specific learning opportunities
Knowledge of differential diagnosis of chest pain in pregnancy
Recognition and management of acute myocardial infarction
Involve relevant specialities appropriately
Appropriate and timely management of VF arrest
Rapid decision-making and coordination to arrange transfer to cardiac catheter lab

Suggested learners (to represent their normal roles)	In the room from the start	Available when requested
A+E nurse	√	
A+E ST3+	√	
Cardiology ST6–7		√
Obstetric ST3+/ Consultant		√
Anaesthetic CT2/ST3+		√

Suggested learners (to represent their normal roles)	In the room from the start	Available when requested
Other responding members of A+E team		√
Suggested facilitators		
Faculty to play role of nurse in A+E performing handover on admission of patient to resus bay	√	

Details for Facilitators

Patient Demographics

Name: Helen Barker

Age: 37

Gestation: 30

Booking weight: 78 kg

Parity: P0

Scenario Summary for Facilitators

37-year-old primipara. (Stopped smoking at start of pregnancy. FH father had myocardial infarction (MI) in 40s. Intermittent cocaine use outside of pregnancy.)

Attends A+E with a 3-hour history of intermittent chest pain and shortness of breath.

Initial ECG unremarkable.

Further pain of greater severity and longer duration. ECG demonstrates ST elevation.

Given initial treatment for myocardial infarction after discussion with patient.

Constant severe pain with haemodynamic compromise and subsequent VF arrest.

Cardioverts with 1 DC shock, urgent referral and transfer for percutaneous coronary intervention.

Set-up Overview for Facilitators

Clinical setting	A+E resus bay
Patient position	Semi-recumbent on A+E trolley
Initial monitoring in place	None – just arrived in resuscitation bay
Other equipment	Nil but all equipment available
Useful manikin features	Defibrillation

Medical Equipment

For core equipment checklist see Chapter 9.

Additional equipment specific to scenario		
Arterial line	Resuscitation trolley with defibrillator	Pads for defibrillation
Drugs: GTN Aspirin Clopidogrel/ticagrelor Thrombolysis LMWH	Beta blocker ACE inhibitor Statin Eplerenone	

Information Given to the Learners

SBAR handover to the A+E team from the triage nurse who has brought patient straight to resus bay

Time: 14.00
Situation: Pregnant patient presenting with chest pain.
Background: 37-year-old primipara who is otherwise fit and well. 30 weeks pregnant. Intermittent chest pain for the last 3 hours with some shortness of breath.
Assessment: I was just about to perform some observations.
Recommendation: Can you please assess the patient?

Scenario Schedule

Stage 1: Initial assessment of chest pain in 30 week primipara	
Information given	**Expected actions**
History: Intermittent central chest discomfort, not related to posture/exertion. Feels like heavy weight on patient's chest, associated with shortness of breath. Patient not sure if due to advancing pregnancy or other reason. Stopped smoking after discovery of pregnancy. (If asked), reports some sporadic cocaine use before pregnancy and father had myocardial infarction in 40s.	Take full history
Examination: Chest: very mild crackles bibasally. CVS: short systolic murmur, loudest on inspiration in pulmonary area (common innocent murmur in pregnancy) and third heart sound present, otherwise unremarkable	Commence ABCDE approach and perform clinical examination
	Perform observations
	Apply Oxygen and titrate to SpO_2 94-98%

Observations	
A	Clear
B	RR 18/min SpO_2 96% on air
C	HR 110bpm BP 124/78 CRT 2s
D	<u>A</u>VPU
E	Temp 36.7°C

Information given	Expected actions
	Secure IV access. Take bloods for FBC, U+E, Troponin, Coagulation including fibrinogen and G+S
	Consideration of differential diagnosis for chest pain, including *MI, coronary artery dissection, aortic dissection, PE, musculoskeletal, reflux*
	Administer analgesia
ECG – Initially sinus tachycardia with no adverse features. See ECG 1, Figure 30.1.	Perform ECG
When candidate requests CXR, patient concerned re. radiation	Request portable CXR
	Respond to patient's concern regarding radiation exposure
	Call for appropriate help, senior cardiology and obstetric / anaesthetic team
Portable CXR – bibasal pulmonary congestion present	

Progress to stage 2 once initial assessment, ECG, bloods and CXR performed

Stage 2: Severe chest pain with ST elevation on ECG, commence management for acure coronary syndrome (ACS)

Information given	Expected actions
Cardiology, Obstetric and anaesthetic registrar arrive	Re-examine patient
Initial improvement in symptoms following analgesia to near pain free status	
If candidates assess fetal heart rate, sonicaid fetal heart rate 170bpm	
Then starts complaining of severe central chest pain	
ECG shows anterior ST elevation see ECG 2, Figure 30.2	Repeat observations Repeat ECG
	Explain situation and urgency to patient
	Attach to ECG monitoring (if not already on continuous monitoring)
	Attach defibrillator pads

Observations	
A	Clear
B	RR 24/min Sp0$_2$ 96% air (99% on 0$_2$)
C	HR 120bpm BP 110/86 CRT 2s
D	AVPU
E	Temp 36.7°C

Information given	Expected actions
Patient concerned re bleeding risk	Give initial therapy – Aspirin 300mg and Clopidogrel 300mg – answer concerns regarding bleeding risk
	Discuss need for coronary angiography
	Contact cardiac catheter lab
Patient concerned re risk of fetal exposure to contrast medium and radiation	Explain to the patient the life-threatening nature of this condition, the role of antiplatelet medications and Primary PCI. Explain that steps are taken to reduce fetal risk from ionising radiation where possible
Blood results: Hb 111g/L WCC 7.3 x 10^9/L Platelets 265 x 10^9/L Clotting / U+E normal Troponin level 50ng/ml	
	Give further analgesia
	Inform consultant cardiologist, obstetrician and anaesthetist

Progress to stage 3 once decision made to contact cardiac catheter lab (if in tertiary centre)

Stage 3: Worsening acute myocardial infarction (MI) deteriorating to ventricular fibrillation (VF) arrest. Requiring advanced life support (ALS) and transferred to cardiac catheter lab for primary percutaneous coronary intervention (PCI)

Observations	
A	Clear
B	RR 28/min SpO$_2$ 99% on O$_2$
C	HR 128bpm BP 90/55 CRT 2s
D	**A**VPU
E	Temp 36.7°C

Information given	Expected actions
Patient continues to complain of severe chest pain despite analgesia	Recognise patient deterioration Repeat observations Repeat ECG
ECG now shows marked rise in ST segments see ECG 3, Figure 30.3	
	Oxygen 15L via non-rebreathing mask if not already in place
Patient becomes unresponsive. No breath sounds, no pulse palpable	
	Recognise cardiac arrest

Information given	Expected actions
	Activate obstetric cardiac arrest call
	Follows ALS algorithm
	Lie patient flat and perform manual displacement of uterus
	Commence cardiopulmonary resuscitation (CPR)
	30 chest compressions to 2 breaths
	Attach defibrillator pads from defibrillator
Monitor / rhythm strip shows VF see ECG 4, Figure 30.4	Recognise VF rhythm on monitor
	Give immediate DC shock (as per defibrillator manufacturer's guidance)
	Consider 4H's 4T's
	Prepare for early intubation with cuffed endotracheal tube
	Team prepare for peri-mortem caesarean section. Plan to commence at 4 minutes post arrest, with delivery by 5 minutes.
	Reassess after 2 minutes of CPR
Reverts to sinus rhythm following 1st DC shock with return of spontaneous circulation (ROSC) and signs of life	
No ROSC until DC shock given	
Perimortem caesarean section not required if DC shock given within 5 minutes of onset of cardiac arrest. If delayed, perimortem section will be required	
Patient shows signs of life, opening eyes, moving arms and groaning	Reassess patient and perform observations
Team informed that cath lab are ready to receive patient	Decision to transfer to catheter lab as an emergency. Rapid, safe transfer organised

Observations	
A	Clear
B	RR 29/min SpO$_2$ 98% on O$_2$
C	HR 130bpm BP 89/58 CRT 3s
D	A**V**PU
E	Temp 36.3°C

Scenario ends with transfer to catheter lab. Proximal left anterior descending (LAD) artery dissection is discovered during angiography and treated with PCI.

This scenario assumes the patient has been assessed and treated at a cardiac tertiary centre with catheter lab on site. Depending on patient haemodynamic stability and distance from tertiary centre, if at a district general hospital, thrombolysis may need to be considered but is not the first choice of treatment. If in acute cardiogenic shock, striking a balance between achieving haemodynamic stability before transfer at the cost of potential further ischaemia is another point for discussion.

The patient has ROSC in the first cycle with 1 DC shock. If the team do not rapidly cardiovert the patient, then perimortem section should be commenced within 4 minutes of maternal collapse. This could prompt discussion regarding issues with anticoagulation immediately post surgery.

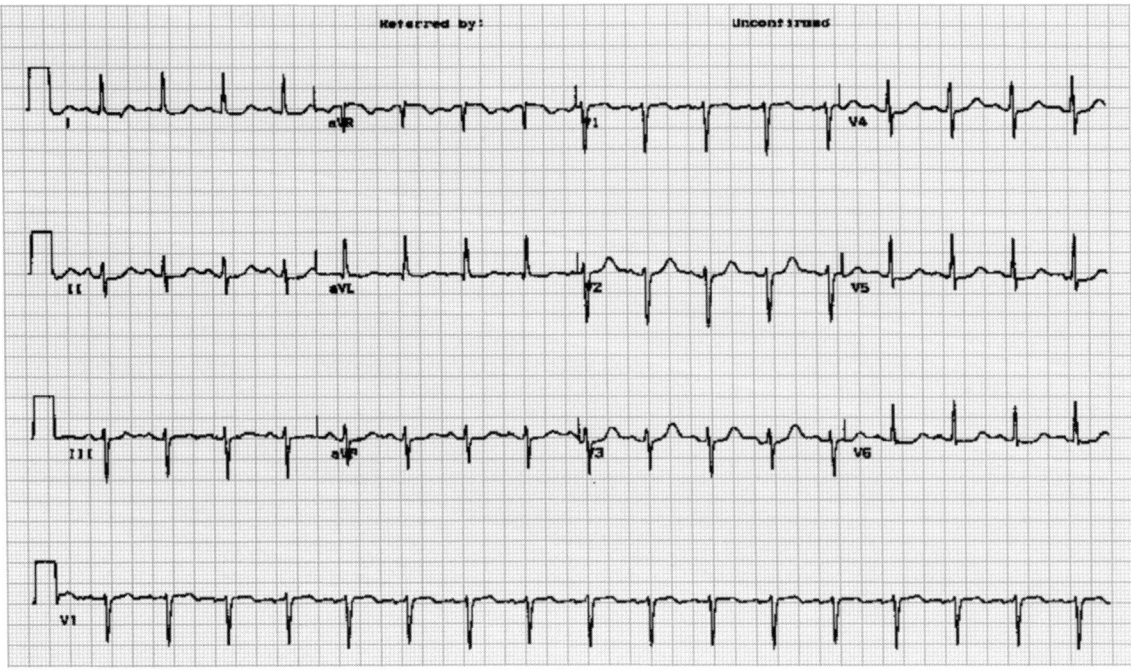

Figure 30.1 Sinus Tachycardia.

Suggested Topics for Debrief Discussion

- What were you thinking during the initial assessment?
- What do you think are her risk factors for myocardial infarction?
- Did you feel confident managing ACS in a pregnant patient?
- How easy was it to access the MDT help that you needed?

Discussion

Acute coronary syndrome covers a number of presentations of myocardial ischaemia from unstable angina to myocardial infarction. Typically, this results from rupture of an atherosclerotic plaque within a coronary artery followed by overlying thrombus formation occluding the coronary artery. Myocardial ischaemia can also occur from coronary artery dissection such as in this case. Atherosclerotic heart disease is associated with risk factors which may affect pregnant and non-pregnant patients alike. Using a multivariable regression model, the American National Inpatient Sample from 2000 to 2002 identified factors such as increasing maternal age at pregnancy (odds ratio (OR) 6.7 for women aged 30–34 and OR 15–16 for those over 35 years old), smoking (OR 8.4), obesity, dyslipidaemia, diabetes (OR 3.6), hypertension (OR 21.7), thrombophilia (OR 25.6), blood transfusion (OR 5.1) and postpartum infection (OR 3.2) as significant risk factors for pregnancy-related myocardial infarction (James et al., 2006).

The 2016 MBRRACE report found that 200 women from 2,341,745 maternities died from direct and indirect causes from 2012 to 2014. The overall maternal death rate was found to be 8.54 per 100,000 maternities. Fifty-one women died from cardiac causes – the largest cause of maternal deaths during this period (2.18 per 100,000). Deaths from cardiac disease have increased. The increase has been attributed to increasing maternal age and levels of obesity as well as more precise autopsy. Of women who died of cardiac causes from 2009 to 2014, 22% died from cardiac ischaemia. Most women who die of ischaemic heart disease have identifiable risk factors. Smoking and obesity are identified as two of the most preventable risk factors in pregnant women in the MBRRACE report and patient education regarding cardiovascular risk and symptoms to report is suggested (Knight et al., 2016).

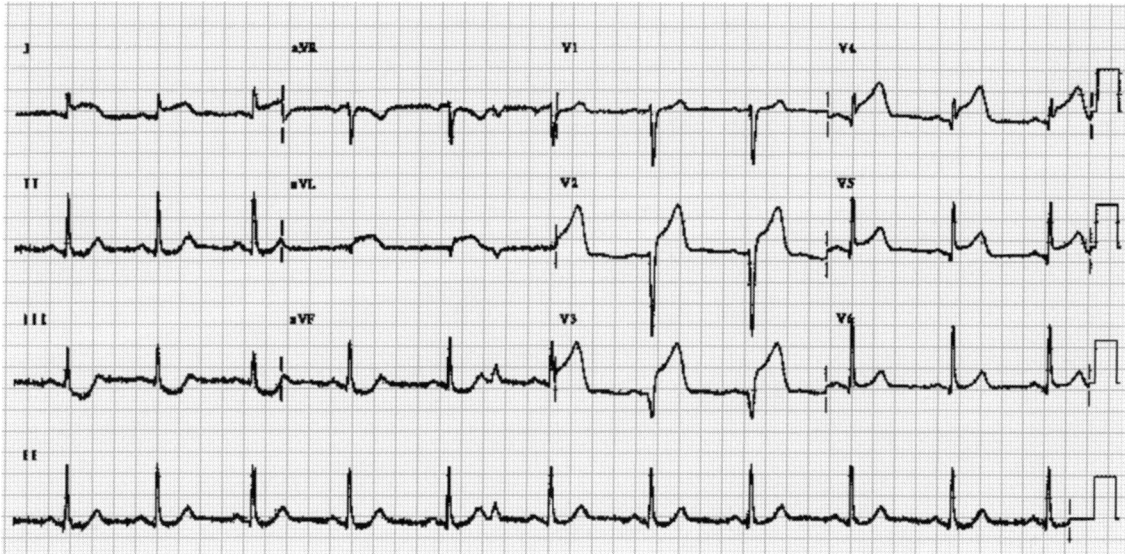

Figure 30.2 Anterior ST Elevation.

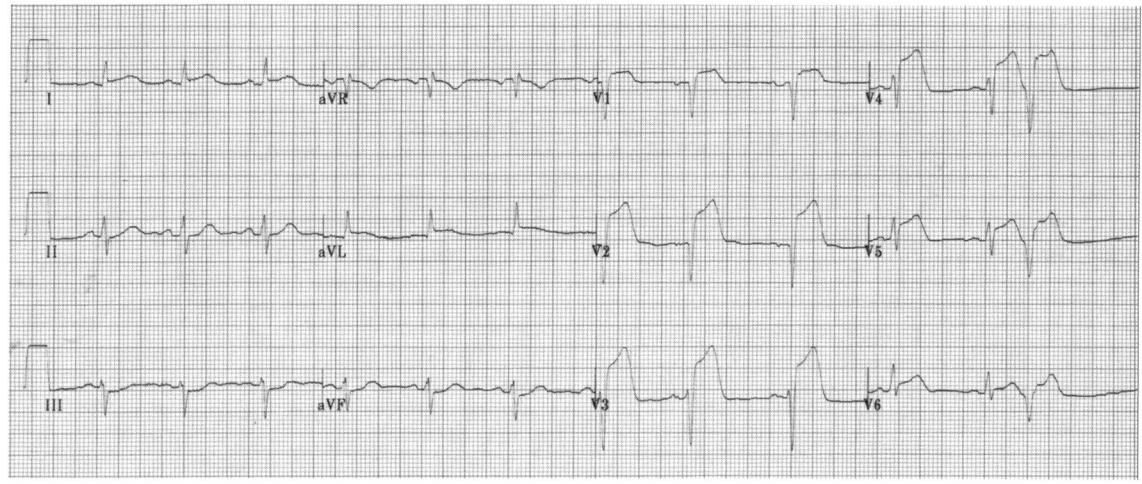

Figure 30.3 Extensive Anterior ST Elevation.

The MBRRACE report suggests early involvement of senior obstetric and cardiology clinicians when a pregnant or postpartum woman presents with suspected ischaemic heart disease, particularly if she presents to the A+E department. The NHS Services Seven Days a Week Forum Summary of Initial Findings (NHS England, 2013) suggests consultant-led maternity units should have 7-day access to ECG and echocardiographic facilities, with a focus on making a specific diagnosis rather than excluding others in women with chest pain and breathlessness. In the same way, women presenting with chest pain severe enough to require opiate analgesia ought to have a positive diagnosis rather than simply the exclusion of acute coronary syndrome or pulmonary embolism.

The differential diagnoses of myocardial infarction in pregnancy are similar to non-pregnant patients. Aortic dissection and pulmonary embolism should

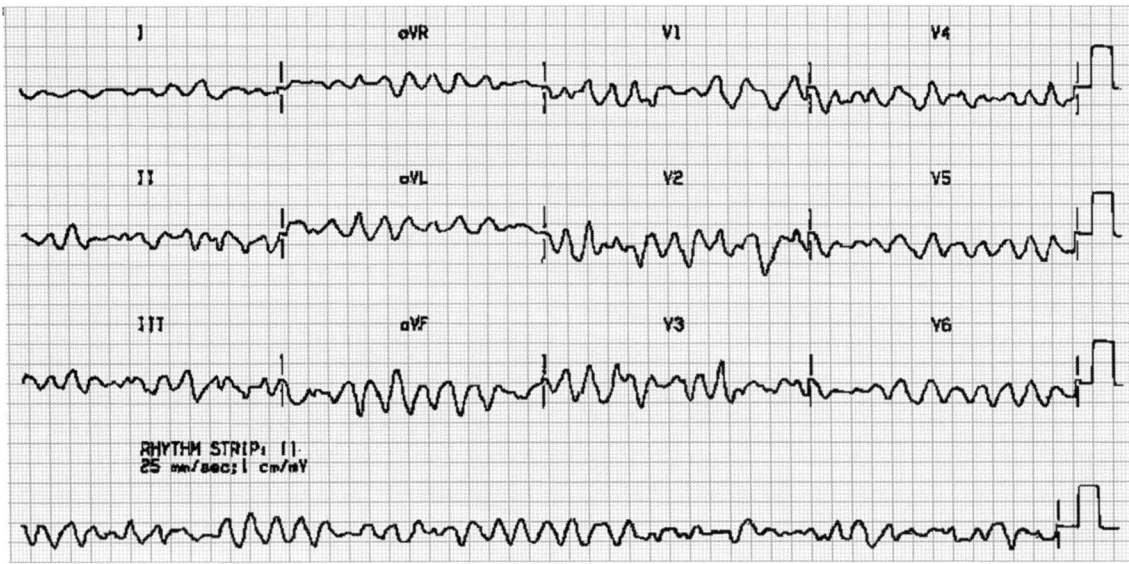

Figure 30.4 VF.

be considered as well as gastro-oesophageal reflux and musculoskeletal pain.

Ischaemic Heart Disease

Ischaemic heart disease can present with chest pain, ventricular arrhythmia as well as sudden cardiac death. While the patient in this case was successfully resuscitated within 2–3 minutes of cardiac arrest, perimortem caesarean section would need to be considered should resuscitation be more prolonged with caesarean section beginning 4 minutes from cardiac arrest with delivery accomplished by 5 minutes (see Chapter 25). Cardiac ischaemic pain is typically described as chest or epigastric discomfort which is often band-like or described as a pressure or weight on the chest. Radiation to the jaw, arms or shoulders may be experienced as well as breathlessness, nausea, sweating or even syncope.

The ECG may demonstrate a number of changes during the course of pregnancy. Left-axis deviation, q waves in leads II, III, aVF and flat or inverted T waves in leads III, V1–3 are more frequently observed in the pregnant versus non-pregnant population (Sunitha et al., 2014). ECG alterations can occur at the time of caesarean section for reasons including effects of anaesthesia administration, anxiety, hyperventilation, changes in autonomic tone during delivery and oxytocin administration (Moran et al., 2001). It is therefore important to interpret the ECG changes in the clinical context within which it is taken, as well as alongside

other clinical and biochemical features during assessment. ST segment elevation is not considered a normal finding during pregnancy and should prompt further urgent investigation.

A rise in troponin level is almost always associated with myocardial insult during pregnancy (Moran et al., 2001). Echocardiography may reveal regional wall motion abnormalities which are not expected during normal pregnancy and if found in conjunction with equivocal ECG changes should again prompt urgent investigation (Muscholl et al., 2002). The absence of regional wall motion abnormalities does not rule out acute coronary syndromes. Similarly, the lack of ECG changes and/or a rise in the troponin level does not exclude the diagnosis of an acute coronary syndrome.

Coronary Artery Dissection

Coronary artery dissection is recognised to have an association with pregnancy. The exact mechanism is unclear. It is suggested that increased physiological haemodynamic stresses or hormonal effects on coronary artery walls may be to blame (Petitti et al., 1997). There is an association with hypertension, but it should be noted that coronary artery dissection may occur in the absence of risk factors. There is also a recognised association with inherited vascular disorders such as Marfan or Ehlers Danlos syndromes.

The optimal treatment modality in coronary artery dissection is unclear. Diagnosis is made during angiography and usually with intravascular ultrasound (IVUS). In general, if the dissection flap is located distally within the coronary artery and the patient is pain-free at the time of angiography without haemodynamic compromise, a conservative approach may be taken with close monitoring of the patient and potentially with further cardiac artery analysis at later stages. Conservative management typically involves continuation of dual antiplatelet therapy alongside heparin, a beta blocker and, if postpartum, an ACE inhibitor. If the dissection is proximal, PCI with intracoronary stents may be preferred, typically with the use of bare metal stents (BMS) to limit the required duration of dual antiplatelet therapy (Regitz-Zagrosek et al., 2011). Where dissection involves the left main stem, coronary artery bypass grafting is usually preferred.

Aortic Dissection

Aortic dissection, another differential diagnosis of chest pain, has an extremely high rate of mortality in the acute phase. Patients often report sudden-onset severe chest pain which may be described as sharp and may radiate to the back or may be experienced in the back alone. Aortic dissection is typically classified by the involvement of the ascending aorta (Stanford Type A) or descending aorta (Stanford Type B), regardless of the site of primary intimal tear. A deficit between carotid, brachial or femoral pulses may indicate impaired peripheral blood flow by intimal flap or by compression from haematoma. Proximal aortic dissection may involve the aortic valve leading to a new diastolic murmur and may also lead to coronary artery involvement – typically the right coronary artery – leading to inferior territory ECG changes. Neurological changes in association with a history of acute chest pain should always alert the clinician to the possibility of aortic dissection. The lack of an abnormal ECG or chest X-ray is not sufficient to rule out aortic dissection, and other investigations such as echocardiography as well as CT scanning of the aorta should be considered if clinical suspicion is present. Treatment of aortic dissection is usually conservative in Type B dissections with careful monitoring and aggressive blood pressure control and surgical in Type A. It is important to rule out aortic dissection promptly if it is clinically suspected as mortality rises significantly with every hour that passes from the time of dissection and in cases where myocardial infarction is included in the list of differential diagnoses, as treatment with antiplatelet or anticoagulation medications may exacerbate the dissection and in turn increase the risk of mortality. If surgical treatment is required, depending on fetal gestation, MDT discussions will have to ensue regarding plans for delivery.

Treatment of Myocardial Infarction

Treatment of myocardial infarction in pregnancy is similar to the non-pregnant patient (Chaithiraphan et al., 2003). The mainstay of treatment is with antiplatelet medication before consideration of percutaneous coronary intervention (PCI), coronary artery bypass grafting (CABG) or 'conservative' management in select cases (Ismail et al., 2017). In acute myocardial infarction, dual antiplatelet medication is given before coronary angiography. Aspirin is considered safe in pregnancy and is accompanied by a $P2Y_{12}$ receptor blocker (clopidogrel, prasugrel, ticagrelor) in treatment of acute myocardial infarction. As data with prasugrel and ticagrelor during pregnancy are limited, clopidogrel is favoured. The addition of a $P2Y_{12}$ receptor blocker may lead to increased bleeding at the time of delivery. Management of the antiplatelet regimen will need to be individualised, taking into account the period of time since the myocardial infarction occurred and obstetric factors.

Heparin does not cross the placenta and so does not affect the fetus directly. It may, however, lead to increased risk of maternal bleeding, although regimens can be altered around the time of delivery or in cases of threatened excessive bleeding – placenta praevia, placental abruption, threatened miscarriage, for example. Beta blockers are considered safe during pregnancy and when breastfeeding. ACE inhibitors are not considered safe during pregnancy but may be used in the postpartum period including when breastfeeding. Statin therapy is generally contraindicated during pregnancy and breastfeeding, although in select cases, the benefits may be felt to outweigh potential risks, such as in cases of familial lipid disorders (Regitz-Zagrosek et al., 2011).

Coronary angiography with PCI is preferred to thrombolysis during acute myocardial infarction as it will also diagnose coronary artery dissection. Mean fetal radiation exposure during coronary angiography was found to be 3 mSv and much lower than doses reported to be associated with fetal malformations or an increased risk of malignancy (50–100 mSv) within the first trimester (Toppenberg et al., 1999). Measures should always be taken to minimise fetal radiation exposure such as abdominal shielding, using a radial artery approach (rather than femoral) and reducing fluoroscopy frame rates during image acquisition. Iodinated contrast agents are not known to be teratogenic and the risk of fetal congenital hypothyroidism is felt to be low and outweighed by the potential benefits to mother and baby.

Summary

Myocardial infarction should be considered in pregnancy as it would be in the non-pregnant patient. It is one of the leading causes of maternal death.

Care of the pregnant patient presenting with acute chest pain should be carefully coordinated between emergency, obstetric and cardiovascular teams.

Differential diagnoses should include, but not be limited to, PE, aortic dissection, reflux and musculoskeletal pain.

Bibliography

Chaithiraphan, V., Gowda, R. M., Khan, I. A. and Reimers, C. D. (2003). Peripartum acute myocardial infarction: management perspective. *American Journal of Therapeutics*, 10, 75.

Ismail, S., Wong, C., Rajan, P. and Vidovich, M. I. (2017). ST-elevation acute myocardial infarction in pregnancy: 2016 update. *Clinical Cardiology*, 40, 399–406.

James, A. H., Jamison, M. G., Biswas, M. S., et al. (2006). Acute myocardial infarction in pregnancy: a United States population-based study. *Circulation*, 113, 1564.

Knight, M., Nair, M., Tuffnell, D., et al. (Eds.) on behalf of MBRRACE-UK. (2016). *Saving Lives, Improving Mothers' Care – Surveillance of Maternal Deaths in the UK 2012–14 and Lessons Learned to Inform Maternity Care from the UK and Ireland Confidential Enquiries into Maternal Deaths and Morbidity 2009–14*. Oxford: National Perinatal Epidemiology Unit.

Moran, C., Ni Bhuinneain, M., Geary, M., Cunningham, S., McKenna, P. and Gardiner, J. (2001). Myocardial ischaemia in normal patients undergoing elective Caesarean section: a peripartum assessment. *Anaesthesia*, 56, 1051–1058.

Muscholl, M. W., Oswald, M., Mayer, C. and von Scheidt, W. (2002). Prognostic value of 2D echocardiography in patients presenting with acute chest pain and non-diagnostic ECG for ST-elevation myocardial infarction. *International Journal of Cardiology*, 84, 217–225.

NHS England. (2013). NHS Services, Seven Days a Week Forum Summary of Initial Findings. Available from: www.england.nhs.uk/wp-content/uploads/2013/12/forum-summary-report.pdf (accessed September 27, 2016).

Petitti, D. B., Sidney, S., Quesenberry, C. P. Jr and Bernstein, A. (1997). Incidence of stroke and myocardial infarction in women of reproductive age. *Stroke*, 28, 280.

Regitz-Zagrosek, V., Blomstrom, Lundqvist C., Borghi, C., et al. (2011). ESC Guidelines on the management of cardiovascular diseases during pregnancy: the task force on the management of cardiovascular diseases during pregnancy of the European Society of Cardiology (ESC). *European Heart Journal*, 32, 3147–3397.

Shivvers, S. A., Wians, F. H. Jr, Keffer, J. H. and Ramin, S. M. (1999). Maternal cardiac troponin I levels during normal labor and delivery. *American Journal of Obstetrics and Gynecology*, 180(1 pt 1), 122.

Sunitha, M., Chandrasekharappa, S. and Brid, S. V. (2014). Electrocardiographic Qrs axis, Q wave and T-wave changes in 2nd and 3rd trimester of normal pregnancy. *Journal of Clinical and Diagnostic Research*, 8(9), BC17–BC21.

Toppenberg, K. S., Hill, D. A. and Miller, D. P. (1999). Safety of radiographic imaging during pregnancy. *American Family Physician*, 59, 1813–1818, 1820.

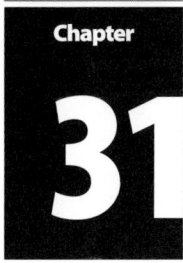

Chapter

31

Peripartum Cardiomyopathy

Omar Asghar and Sarah Vause

Scenario in a Nutshell

Peripartum cardiomyopathy complicated by cardiogenic shock.
 Stage 1: Initial assessment of new onset shortness of breath in the early postpartum period.
 Stage 2: Acute pulmonary oedema and impending cardiogenic shock.
 Stage 3: Management of cardiogenic shock.

Target Learner Groups

All members of the multidisciplinary obstetric team: postnatal ward midwifery staff, obstetricians, anaesthetists, cardiologists.

Specific learning opportunities
Knowledge of differential diagnosis of postpartum breathlessness
Knowledge of clinical presentation of peripartum cardiomyopathy
Demonstrate appropriate assessment and management of heart failure presenting in the early postpartum period

Suggested learners (to represent their normal roles)	In the room from the start	Available when requested
Anaesthetic ST3+	√	
Obstetric ST1/ ST3+	√	
Midwife Coordinator		√
Midwife	√	
Operating Department Practitioner (ODP)/anaesthetic nurse		√
Cardiology ST6+		√
Suggested facilitators		
Faculty to play the role of junior midwife on postnatal ward handing over	√	

Details for Facilitators
Patient Demographics

Name: Marian
Age: 35
Gestation: Postnatal
Booking weight: 95 kg
Parity: Now P1

Scenario Summary for Facilitators

A 35-year-old (now para 1) develops symptoms of breathlessness on the second day following an elective caesarean section delivery for breech. She suffers with mild asthma, using a salbutamol inhaler PRN. Initially she has signs of mild heart failure, but despite initial heart failure therapy, rapidly deteriorates to develop cardiogenic shock with severe pulmonary oedema requiring transfer to cardiac intensive care.
The patient has peripartum cardiomyopathy complicated by cardiogenic shock.

Set-up Overview for Facilitators

Clinical setting	On postnatal ward
Patient position	Semi-recumbent on postnatal bed
Initial monitoring in place	Nil monitoring
Other equipment	All usual equipment on postnatal ward is available
Useful manikin functions	Abnormal breath sounds (pulmonary oedema) Audible heart sounds (third heart sound) Intubation

Medical Equipment

For core equipment checklist, see Chapter 9.

Additional equipment specific to scenario		
Arterial line	Resuscitation trolley	Continuous positive airway pressure machine
Drugs: Furosemide GTN Hydralazine Levosimendan	Noradrenaline Dobutamine Adrenaline	Antibiotics Dalteparin

Information Given to the Learners

SBAR handover from faculty (playing the role of junior midwife on postnatal ward) to obstetric trainee and anaesthetic trainee

Time: Midday

Situation: I am a junior midwife on the postnatal ward. I am calling about Marian Khan who is getting increasingly short of breath.

Background: She is 35 years old. She is 2 days post elective caesarean section at 39 weeks gestation for breech, with an estimated blood loss of 500 ml. She is complaining of breathlessness which started earlier today.

Assessment: I have just performed her observations RR 24, SpO$_2$ 94% on air, BP 95/60 mmHg, HR 109.

Recommendations: Please can you come and assess her?

Scenario Schedule

Stage 1: Initial assessment of new onset shortness of breath in the early post-partum period

Information given	Expected actions
History from patient: Dyspnoea for a few hours - no relief from salbutamol inhaler. Worse when lying flat or walking around. 'Tickly' cough for about 1 week, not productive. No chest pain or palpitations. She has suffered with "fatigue and breathlessness" for the last few weeks, saw GP who said it was normal symptoms of pregnancy. Past medical history of mild asthma (no hospital admissions) not really changed in pregnancy. Uses reliever inhaler occasionally, no steroids. Asthma worse in cold weather. No other PMH. No other drugs apart from inhaler, no allergies.	Take history
Examination: Airway clear, mild SOB whilst talking. Bilateral fine inspiratory crackles at both lung bases, trachea central and no wheeze audible. Adequate pulse, JVP elevated, third heart sound audible. Mild ankle oedema. Abdomen soft, uterus small and non tender.	Perform examination
	ABCDE approach and perform observations
	Apply Oxygen via non-rebreathing mask at 15 l/min

Observations	
A	Clear
B	RR 24/min SpO$_2$ 94% on air (96% On O$_2$)
C	HR 109bpm BP 95/60 CRT 2s
D	**A**VPU
E	Temp 36.9°C

Information given	Expected actions
	Establish IV access with large bore cannula Take blood for FBC, U+E, CRP, coagulation and NT pro-BNP
	Check ABG
Investigations: ECG: sinus tachycardia, widespread T-wave inversion. (no old ECG to compare to)	Request ECG
	Request CXR
	Consideration of differential diagnosis Heart failure Pre-eclampsia Infective exacerbation of asthma (bacterial / viral) Pulmonary embolism Atelectasis Autoimmune disease
ABG (FiO$_2$ 0.21): pH 7.35 pO$_2$ 9kPa pCO$_2$ 4.2kPa HCO$_3^-$ 23mmol/L BE -4 mmol/L Lactate 0.9 mmol/l	
	Request consultant obstetrician and anaesthetist to attend
CXR: Radiographer declines to do CXR as "patient may need CTPA"	
Blood results awaited from lab	

Progress to stage 2 once differential diagnosis explored and examination and investigations performed

Observations	
A	Clear
B	RR 36/min SpO$_2$ 90% on 0$_2$
C	HR 120bpm BP 90/60 CRT 2s
D	**A**VPU
E	Temp 36.9°C

Stage 2: Acute pulmonary oedema and impending cardiogenic shock

Information given	Expected actions
Patient now very distressed. Sitting on the edge of the bed, very short of breath with cough productive of pink frothy sputum. Examination: widespread coarse inspiratory crackles and persistent cough. Tachycardic, JVP elevated, third heart sound audible	Re-examine cardiovascular system Repeat observations
	Suspect pulmonary oedema

251

Information given	Expected actions
	Continue with 15 l/min oxygen via non re-breathe mask If available, deliver high flow oxygen with CPAP
	Give stat dose IV furosemide 40mg
	Catheterise
Bloods: Hb 98g/dL WCC 15×10^9/L Platelets 225×10^9/L Na 142mmol/L K 4.6mmol/L Urea 3.8mmol/L Creatinine 50μmol/L CRP 30mg/L NT pro-BNP 8235 pg/ml Clotting normal	
	Call on-call cardiology registrar / consultant
Urgent target echocardiogram shows dilated left ventricle (LVEDd 6.1 cm) with severe global impairment of systolic function (LVEF 25%)	Request urgent echocardiogram
	Consider transfer to safe location for stabilisation depending on proximity theatre / HDU / CCU

Progress to stage 3 following diagnosis of heart failure (HF) and initial treatment with furosemide.
NB if candidate fails to recognise and treat as HF, patient goes into cardiorespiratory arrest and simulation ends after unsuccessful resuscitation.

Observations	
A	Clear
B	RR 40/min SpO$_2$ 88% on 15L 0$_2$
C	HR 125bpm BP 75/50 CRT 4s
D	A**V**PU
E	Temp 36.1°C

Stage 3: Management of cardiogenic shock

Information given	Expected actions
Patient very distressed Struggling to breath Cyanosed, and becoming drowsy	Reassess patient Repeat all observations
On examination: Florid pulmonary oedema, marked fine inspiratory crackles throughout. JVP elevated, third heart sound	Examine patient
	Recognises cardiogenic shock and initiates appropriate therapy.

Information given	Expected actions
	Handover to cardiologist on-call
	Inotropic/vasopressor therapy Arterial line insertion for continuous BP monitoring Trial of CPAP if not already facilitated
	Intubation and ventilation if worsening respiratory status Advanced HF therapies Transfer to cardiac ICU
	NB if candidate fails to recognise and treat as HF, patient goes into cardiorespiratory arrest and simulation ends after unsuccessful resuscitation.
Scenario ends when the team have successfully diagnosed cardiogenic shock and heart failure therapies have been commenced.	

Suggested Topics for Debrief Discussion

- What differential diagnosis were you thinking about when you first assessed the patient?
- Would this be easy to manage on your unit?

Discussion

Peripartum cardiomyopathy (PPCM) typically presents during the first week postpartum with dyspnoea; however, subtle preceding symptoms such as fatigue, cough, oedema and abdominal discomfort may have been mistakenly attributed to normal symptoms of pregnancy leading to delayed diagnosis. PPCM is a diagnosis of exclusion, defined as 'an idiopathic cardiomyopathy presenting with heart failure (HF) secondary to left ventricular systolic dysfunction (LVEF < 45%) towards the end of pregnancy or in the months following delivery, where no other cause is found' (Sliwa et al., 2014). Symptom onset may be gradual or sudden and clinical presentation may overlap with several other important diagnoses, thus emphasising the need for prompt assessment and diagnosis (Table 31.1). Once a diagnosis of acute HF has been established, careful assessment of the blood pressure, heart rate, respiratory rate, oxygen saturation and tissue/organ perfusion should be performed to determine the patient's haemodynamic and respiratory status as this will determine management strategy (Figure 31.1).

In the 2016 MBRRACE-UK report, PPCM accounted for 6% of all maternal cardiovascular mortality and 50% of cardiovascular mortality in women aged 30–40 years (Freedman and Lucas, 2015). The clinical course of PPCM is highly variable, ranging from mild reversible cardiac dysfunction, with subtle symptoms, to rapidly progressive end-stage HF requiring inotropic and mechanical support, or death (Bauersachs et al., 2016). Hence, it is vital for clinicians involved with the management of pregnant women to have knowledge of the presentation and management of PPCM.

In addition to conventional cardiovascular risk factors, several other risk factors have been identified for the development of PPCM. There is a strong association between maternal age and risk of PPCM, with over 50% of cases occurring in women over 30 years of age (Kolte et al., 2014; Arany and Elkayam, 2016). Other risk factors include Afro-Caribbean race, hypertension, anaemia, multiparity, multiple gestation and autoimmune disease; risk rising exponentially according to the number of risk factors present (Kao et al., 2013; Afana, 2016). Genetic factors may also contribute to the risk of developing PPCM (Kamiya et al., 2016; Ware et al., 2016). A history of PPCM in a previous pregnancy is a significant risk factor for developing PPCM in subsequent pregnancies (Elkayam, 2014). The risk of deterioration in left ventricular (LV) function and HF in a subsequent pregnancy is as high as 44% in women with persistent

Table 31.1 Cardiac causes of breathlessness during pregnancy.

	Heart failure	Acute coronary syndrome	Pulmonary embolus	Myocarditis
Presentation	Insidious (can be acute) Dyspnoea	Acute Chest pain (retrosternal)	Acute Chest pain (pleuritic)	Subacute Recent infection
Signs	Hypotension, tachycardia, tachypnoea Elevated JVP Inspiratory crackles S3	Normal (uncomplicated cases)	Tachypnoea Hypoxia	Fever Tachycardia S3
ECG	Rarely normal Non-specific repolarisation abnormalities	ST elevation/depression T-wave inversion LBBB/RBBB	Sinus tachycardia S1 Q3 T3 RBBB T-wave changes V1–3	T-wave changes LBBB Conduction abnormalities
CXR	Pulmonary congestion Cardiomegaly Pleural effusion	Normal	Normal	Normal
Biomarkers	Elevated BNP	Elevated troponin	Elevated D-dimer (BNP and troponin may be raised)	Elevated troponin ± BNP
Echocardiography	Global LV systolic impairment LVEF < 45% LV may be dilated or normal size	Regional LV systolic impairment (can be normal)	RV impairment (can be normal)	Global LV systolic impairment
Other investigations	CMR	Coronary angiography/ CMR	CTPA/VQ scan	CMR

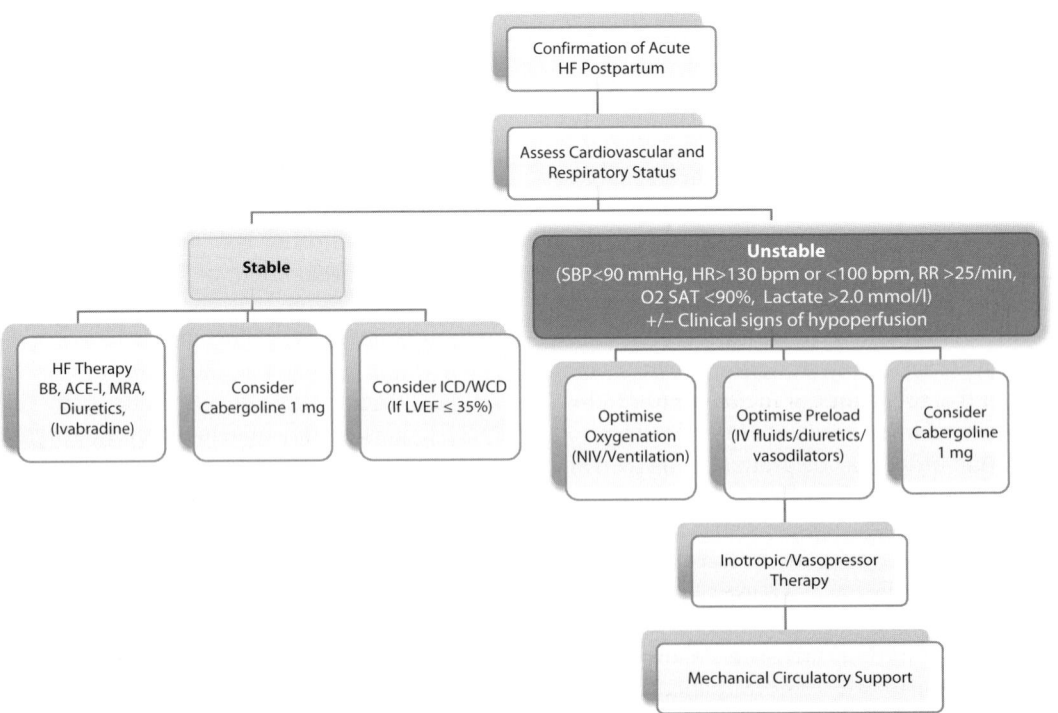

Figure 31.1 Treatment algorithm for acute heart failure in the postpartum patient.

LV dysfunction and 21% in those with complete recovery of LV function from their index pregnancy (Elkayam et al., 2001).

The initial treatment in acute PPCM with cardiopulmonary compromise is based on five key elements (Bauersachs et al., 2016) (Figure 31.1):

1. Optimisation of preload. Correction of volume status with intravenous fluids/blood in hypovolaemia or diuretics in fluid overload. Vasodilator therapy (nitrates, hydralazine) should be initiated where the systolic blood pressure is ≥ 110 mmHg.
2. Optimisation of oxygenation. Initially start oxygen at 15 l/min via a non-rebreather mask and then titrate administered oxygen to aim for target saturation of >95%. In respiratory distress secondary to pulmonary oedema, CPAP should be initiated. If despite CPAP respiratory status deteriorates or fails to improve, invasive ventilation is indicated.
3. Restoration of haemodynamics. In the setting of cardiogenic shock, inotropes or vasopressor therapy should be initiated. There is limited evidence suggesting that the use of catecholamines, such as dobutamine, is associated with adverse outcomes in PPCM (Stapel et al., 2017). However, levosimendan is a calcium-sensitising drug with positive inotropic and vasodilator properties, which causes rapid and profound haemodynamic improvement in patients with PPCM and should be considered where available (Labbene et al., 2017).
4. Urgent delivery. In cases of PPCM during pregnancy, there should be immediate assessment of fetal viability followed by multidisciplinary discussion to determine delivery and further management.
5. Adjunctive therapy. The peak incidence of PPCM occurs during the first week postpartum when plasma levels of prolactin and SFLT1 peak (Arany and Elkayam, 2016; MD et al., 2017). Prolactin is cleaved by the enzyme cathepsin D to produce a 16 kDa form, a potent antiangiogenic and proapoptotic molecule which plays an important role in the pathophysiology of PPCM (Hilfiker-Kleiner et al., 2007). Blockade of prolactin release by dopamine agonists, e.g. cabergoline, may improve outcomes in PPCM and should be considered in severe cases (Sliwa et al., 2010),

although cabergoline stops lactation and therefore the patient will not be able to breastfeed. In cases of PPCM refractory to medical treatment, mechanical circulatory support should be considered (Bauersachs et al., 2016). In addition, in the setting of severe LV dysfunction (LVEF ≤ 35%), anticoagulation therapy should be commenced and consideration given to determine whether a wearable cardiac defibrillator, an ICD or S-ICD is indicated to reduce the risk of sudden cardiac death (Duncker et al., 2014). When patients stabilise, standard HF therapy should be commenced. ACE inhibitors (enalapril and captopril) are considered safe in breastfeeding. In pregnancy, ACE inhibitors should only be used when it is judged that the benefits outweigh the risks to the fetus and safer alternatives have been considered.

Summary

- Various causes of breathlessness can occur in pregnancy; the team need to be alert to the possibility of PPCM.
- PPCM is a rare but potentially life-threatening obstetric emergency.
- Early recognition and prompt multidisciplinary management is essential to reduce maternal morbidity and mortality.
- A low threshold should be kept with a view to escalation to intensive care.

Bibliography

Afana, M., Brinjikji, W., Kao, D., et al. (2016). Characteristics and in-hospital outcomes of peripartum cardiomyopathy diagnosed during delivery in the United States from the Nationwide Inpatient Sample (NIS) database. *Journal of Cardiac Failure*, 22(7), 512–519.

Arany, Z. and Elkayam, U. (2016). Peripartum cardiomyopathy. *Circulation*, 133(14), 1397–1409.

Bauersachs, J., Arrigo, M., Hilfiker-Kleiner, D., et al. (2016). Current management of patients with severe acute peripartum cardiomyopathy: practical guidance from the Heart Failure Association of the European Society of Cardiology Study Group on peripartum cardiomyopathy. *European Journal of Heart Failure*, 18(9), 1096–1105.

Duncker, D., Haghikia, A., König, T., et al. (2014). Risk for ventricular fibrillation in peripartum cardiomyopathy with severely reduced left ventricular function-value of the wearable cardioverter/defibrillator. *European Journal of Heart Failure*, 16(12), 1331–1336.

Elkayam, U. (2014). Risk of subsequent pregnancy in women with a history of peripartum cardiomyopathy. *Journal of the American College of Cardiologists*, 64(15), 1629–1636.

Elkayam, U., Tummala, P. T., Rao, K., et al. (2001). Maternal and fetal outcomes of subsequent pregnancies in women with peripartum cardiomyopathy. *The New England Journal of Medicine*, 344(21), 1567–1571.

Freedman, R. L. and Lucas, D. N. (2015). MBRRACE-UK: saving lives, improving mothers' care – implications for anaesthetists. *International Journal of Obstetric Anaesthesia*, 24(2), 161–173.

Hilfiker-Kleiner, D., Kaminski, K., Podewski, E., et al. (2007). A cathepsin D-cleaved 16 kDa form of prolactin mediates postpartum cardiomyopathy. *Cell*, 128(3), 589–600.

Kamiya, C. A., Yoshimatsu, J. and Ikeda, T. (2016). Peripartum cardiomyopathy from a genetic perspective. *Circulation Journal*, 80(8), 1684–1688.

Kao, D. P., Hsich, E. and Lindenfeld, J. (2013). Characteristics, adverse events, and racial differences among delivering mothers with peripartum cardiomyopathy. *Journal of the American College of Cardiologists: Heart Failure*, 1(5), 409–416.

Kolte, D., Khera, S., Aronow, W. S., et al. (2014). Temporal trends in incidence and outcomes of peripartum cardiomyopathy in the United States: a nationwide population-based study. *Journal of the American Heart Association*, 3(3), e001056.

Labbene, I., Arrigo, M., Tavares, M., et al. (2017). Decongestive effects of levosimendan in cardiogenic shock induced by postpartum cardiomyopathy. *Anaesthesia Critical Care & Pain Medicine*, 36(1), 39–42.Sliwa, K., Blauwet, L., Tibazarwa, K., et al. (2010). Evaluation of bromocriptine in the treatment of acute severe peripartum cardiomyopathy: a proof-of-concept pilot study. *Circulation*, 121(13), 1465–1473.

Sliwa, K., Hilfiker-Kleiner, D., Petrie, M. C., et al. (2014). Current state of knowledge on aetiology, diagnosis, management, and therapy of peripartum cardiomyopathy: a position statement from the Heart Failure Association of the European Society of Cardiology Working Group on peripartum cardiomyopathy. *European Journal of Heart Failure*, 12(8), 767–778.

Stapel, B., Kohlhaus, M., Ricke-Hoch, M., et al. (2017). Low STAT3 expression sensitizes to toxic effects of β-adrenergic receptor stimulation in peripartum cardiomyopathy. *European Heart Journal*, 35(5), 349–361.

Ware, J. S., Li, J., Mazaika, E., et al. (2016). Shared genetic predisposition in peripartum and dilated cardiomyopathies. *The New England Journal of Medicine*, 374(3), 233–241.

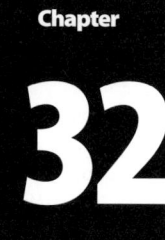

Chapter

32

Complete Heart Block in a Pregnant Patient

Anita Macnab and Kirsty MacLennan

Scenario in a Nutshell

Complete heart block in patient for TOP with known Mobitz type II requiring pacing.

Stage 1: Assessment of stable patient with known Mobitz type II heart block.

Stage 2: Bradycardia with adverse features necessitating medical management.

Stage 3: Bradycardia unresponsive to medical management, requires transcutaneous pacing.

Stage 4: Plan for temporary pacing wire insertion.

Target Learner Groups

All members of the multidisciplinary obstetric team: anaesthetists, midwives, obstetricians, HDU nurses (if part of the usual team), operating department practitioners and cardiologists.

Specific learning opportunities
Knowledge of appropriate medical management of bradyarrhythmia
Knowledge of risk factors for complete heart block
Recognition of need for pacing
Knowledge of transcutaneous pacing set-up

Suggested learners (to represent their normal roles)	In the room from the start	Available when requested
Anaesthetic CT2	√	
Anaesthetic ST3+		√
Obstetric ST3+		√
Midwife Coordinator		√
Midwife in room	√	
Operating Department Practitioner (ODP)/ anaesthetic nurse		√
Cardiology ST		√
Suggested facilitators		
Faculty to play role of antenatal midwife handing over	√	

Details for Facilitators

Patient Demographics

Name: Chloe

Age: 39

Gestation: 21

Booking weight: 80 kg

Parity: P0

Scenario Summary for Facilitators

Patient admitted to delivery suite for termination of pregnancy for severe fetal cardiac anomalies at 21 weeks pregnant.

She has a past history of Mobitz type II heart block.

She had mifepristone 24 hours ago and has received one dose of misoprostol PV on the delivery suite.

She complains of chest tightness, is bradycardic at 35 bpm and hypotensive.

She remains unresponsive to medical management (atropine/isoprenaline/adrenaline) and requires transcutaneous pacing and transfer for a temporary pacing wire.

Set-up Overview for Facilitators

Clinical setting	On delivery suite, on a delivery bed
Patient position	Semi-recumbent
Initial monitoring in place	None
Other equipment	No IV access All equipment available as per local unit set-up
Useful manikin features	Palpable pulses Pacing

Medical Equipment

For core equipment checklist, see Chapter 9.

Additional equipment specific to scenario		
Arterial line	Resuscitation trolley with defibrillator	Pads for pacing
Drugs: Atropine Ephedrine Adrenaline Isoprenaline	Drugs for sedation	

Information Given to the Learners

SBAR handover from faculty (playing the role of a midwife from the antenatal ward) to midwife and anaesthetic trainee on delivery suite

Time: 10:00

Situation: This patient, with a known heart problem, is having TOP for fetal cardiac anomalies at 21 weeks.

Background: 39-year-old, primipara who is 21+0 weeks pregnant. She has had one dose of mifepristone 24 hours ago and I have just given her misoprostol PV now. She has Mobitz type II heart block and has a letter in her notes from her last cardiology appointment 6 months ago. She is otherwise well with no allergies.

Assessment: I have brought her to the delivery suite for monitoring of her cardiac condition during her induction and delivery.

Recommendation: We need a plan for her care. Would you like to see the letter from cardiology? (See Figure 32.1.)

Cardiology Clinic
6 months earlier

Dear General Practitioner,

Regarding Chloe Brown

Diagnosis: Asymptomatic congenital heart block with intermittent Mobitz Type II noted on a 24 hr tape.

Chloe was diagnosed with intermittent 2:1 AV block approximately 3 years ago. This was picked up following screening, as a family member had also been diagnosed with congenital heart block requiring a pacemaker.

At the time of Chloe's diagnosis, she was found to have intermittent 2:1 AV block on 24 hr tape. HR 57 bpm and narrow QRS complexes. Structurally and functionally normal heart was confirmed on echo. Chloe was offered a permanent pacemaker but refused because her relative had suffered with infective complications requiring pacemaker explant.

Although Chloe declined a permanent pacemaker, she does understand that she runs the risk of developing complete AV block in the future.

We monitor her with annual 24 hr tapes and we have not seen any progression so far.

She is currently planning for a baby. If she becomes pregnant, we would need to have a further discussion regarding prophylactic intrapartum temporary pacing. An emergency pacemaker may be required if she has any haemodynamic compromise with heart block. The cardiology on-call team should be contacted for in-reach support during her admission.

She has a back-up appointment to see me in 8 months' time. She is aware of the need to contact me sooner if she becomes symptomatic with dizziness, syncope, breathlessness or chest pains.

Yours sincerely

Consultant Cardiologist

Figure 32.1 Letter from Cardiology Clinic.

Scenario Schedule

Stage 1 – Assessment of stable patient with known Mobitz type II heart block	
Information Given	**Expected Actions**
History from patient: Diagnosed with Mobitz type II heart block following family screening. Never been symptomatic. Refused pacemaker as sister had bad infection and needed hers removing. She has not told her cardiologist that she is pregnant as she has felt fine throughout and she has not seen any other cardiac team. No cardiac symptoms. Good exercise tolerance.	Take a full cardiac history and inform senior obstetrician and anaesthetist that patient is on the delivery suite

Observations	
A	Clear
B	RR 18/min SpO$_2$ 98% on air
C	HR 89bpm BP 121/70 CRT 2s
D	<u>A</u>VPU
E	T. 36.8°

Information Given	Expected Actions
	Apply monitoring. Pulse oximeter / ECG / NIBP
Letter from cardiologist available (Figure 32.1) ECG 1 – Mobitz type II rhythm strip (available if requested). Figure 32.2 ECG 2 – Mobitz type II chest lead ECG (available if requested). Figure 32.3	
	Establish IV access as precaution Take bloods for FBC, U+E, Magnesium, G+S
If cardiology are contacted, they are busy in cardiac catheter lab	Alert cardiology that patient is on the unit

Progress to stage 2 once history taken / ECG seen and cardiac letter has been reviewed

Stage 2: Bradycardia with adverse features necessitating medical management

Observations	
A	Clear
B	RR 25/min SpO$_2$ 93% on air, poor trace
C	HR 35bpm BP 75/40 CRT 3s
D	<u>A</u>VPU
E	T. 36.8°C

Information Given	Expected Actions
Patient complaining of chest pain – feeling heavy in the chest and dizzy	Reassess patient. Repeat observations. Recognise fall in HR and BP
ECG on monitor shows rate of 35bpm with p waves dissociated from QRS complex. Faculty can also show ECG 3 Figure 32.4 – Complete heart block rhythm strip, although HR has fallen since this has been recorded	Reassess cardiac rhythm
	Apply Oxygen via non-rebreathing mask at 15 l/min whilst stabilising the patient (then titrate oxygen to SpO$_2$ 94-98%)
	IV access if not already established Commence IV Hartmann's 250ml bolus
	Commence medical management for bradycardia Consult ALS bradycardia algorithm
No improvement in HR with atropine	Atropine 500mcg IV with flush, to a maximum of 3mg in total
Cardiology will call back when available – they are scrubbed in cardiac catheter lab	Call cardiology for urgent assistance

Information Given	Expected Actions
	Consider other medical management. Commence isoprenaline 4mcg/ml concentrations. Example drawing up regime...1mg in 250ml of 5% Dextrose, (ie 10 ampoules each containing 100mcg). Start at a rate of 15ml/hr (1mcg/min) and titrate up to 30/45/60/75 ml/hr (ie increase by 15ml/hr) every 3 mins until Hr>60bpm. Usual max required is 150ml/hr
No HR response to isoprenaline	
Adrenaline infusion may not be candidate's first choice as it is not tolerated well in the awake patient	Commence Adrenaline infusion at 2-10mcg/minute IV as per ALS algorithm (4mg in 50ml N saline or 5% Dextrose (80mcg/ml) run at 1.5-7.5ml/hr)

Progress to stage 3 once medical management has been attempted and no resolution of bradycardia

Stage 3: Bradycardia unresponsive to medical management, requires transcutaneous pacing

Information Given	Expected Actions
Patient still complaining of chest pain and feeling faint	Explain situation to patient. Medications have not improved the HR so will need transcutaneous pacing which can be painful
Patient has not eaten for over 10 hours and only had sips of water.	Discuss the need for sedation / anaesthesia
Patient responds well to small amount of sedation (If candidate chooses GA for patient, will need transfer to theatre)	
	Commence temporary pacing as per ALS guidelines
HR remains 35bpm with p waves dissociated from QRS complex	Attach ECG monitoring from defibrillator. Ensure skin is dry. Apply pads. May consider use of Anterior-Posterior (AP) postion of pads
	Turn pacer on. Demand mode. Pacing rate 60-90bpm. Gradually increase the current output until each pacing spike on ECG is followed by QRS complex and a T wave (typically 50-100mA). This is electrical capture

Observations pre pacing	
A	Clear
B	RR 28/min SpO$_2$ 95% on O$_2$ (poor trace)
C	HR 35bpm BP 70/42 CRT 4s
D	**A**VPU
E	T. 36.8°C

Information Given	Expected Actions
Tolerates transcutaneous pacing well	Confirm mechanical capture with palpation of pulse
	If electrical capture but no mechanical capture, increase current
	If remains hypotensive, increase the HR on pacer setting
Progress to Stage 4 once pacing established and BP improved	

Observations on pacing	
A	Clear
B	RR 20/min SpO$_2$ 98% on O$_2$
C	HR - as per pacing setting BP 100/70 CRT 2 s
D	A**VP**U (If sedated)
E	T. 36.8°C

Stage 4: Plan for temporary pacing wire insertion	
Information Given	**Expected Actions**
Cardiology available	Contact cardiology with SBAR handover
Cardiologist able to insert pacing wire in cardiac catheter lab now	Arrange urgent transfer to cardiology for temporary transvenous pacing wire insertion
	Full monitoring of patient including insertion of arterial line for continuous BP and HR monitoring
	Pause termination of pregnancy until temporary pacing wire in place and patient stable
Scenario ends when handover to cardiology performed and plans for transfer to cardiac catheter lab.	

Suggested Topics for Debrief Discussion

- Did you feel confident managing this scenario?
- Do you feel competent to initiate transcutaneous pacing?
- If a similar case presented on your unit, would it be useful to run this scenario on the day to help improve knowledge and team-working?

Discussion

Heart Block in Pregnancy

Bradycardia, defined as a heart rate less than 60 bpm, is uncommon during pregnancy in the absence of structural heart disease, even in athletic parturients.

The most prevalent arrhythmia in childbearing-age women is supraventricular tachycardia. Bradyarrhythmias, although uncommon in this age group, can occur with a prevalence of approximately 1 in 20,000 (Regitz-Zagrosek et al., 2011; Metz and Khanna, 2016).

Bradyarrhythmias are typically considered according to the location of the deficit: sinus node dysfunction, atrioventricular block or intraventricular conduction block.

- *Sinus node dysfunction* is said to occur when the SA node is unable to generate a heart rate commensurate with the patient's physiological requirements.

Atrioventricular blockade can be further described.

- *First-degree* atrioventricular heart block can occur as a normal variant, in athletes and in pregnancy, in the absence of underlying heart disease. Although there is prolongation of impulse transmission through the left atrial conduction system (PR interval > 220 ms), all impulses are transmitted, so every P-wave is followed by a normal QRS complex. No intervention is required for this type of heart block.

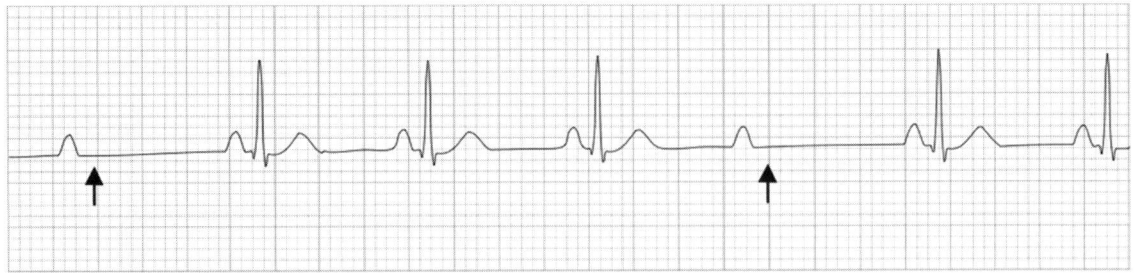

Figure 32.2 ECG 1

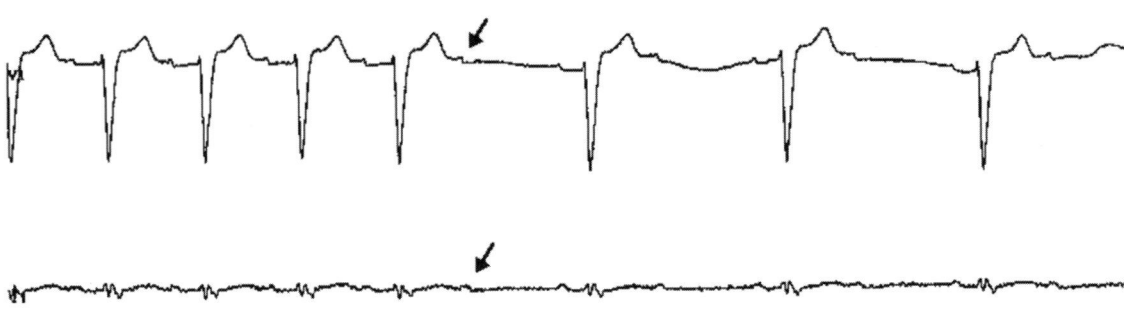

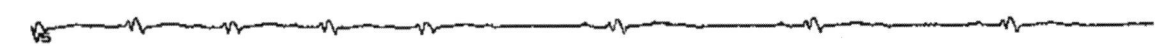

Figure 32.3 ECG 2

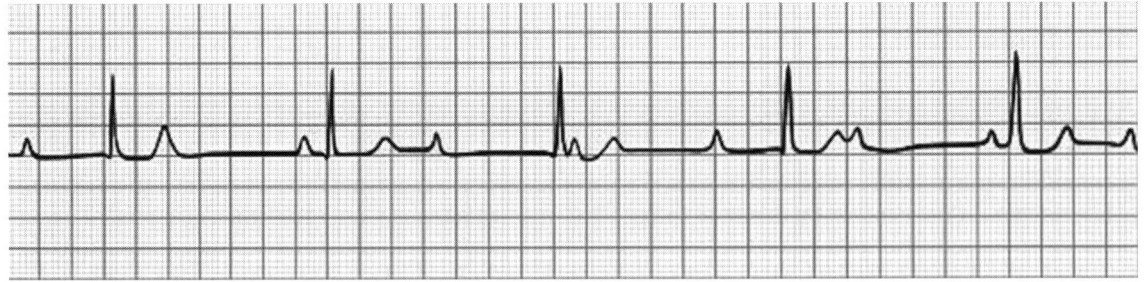

Figure 32.4 ECG 3

Second-degree heart block usually occurs in association with structural heart disease (e.g. repaired TOF or VSD) or drug therapy.

- *Second-degree AV block type 1* or Mobitz type 1 (Wenckebach) accounts for most cases of second-degree heart block in pregnancy and can be more common during sleep. It is characterised by progressive lengthening of the PR interval until there is failure of passage of an impulse through the AV node and thus no subsequent QRS complex until the PR interval shortens again and the cycle restarts. This is regarded as a benign block and does not require intervention. It is not usually associated with structural heart disease.

262

Table 32.1 Common causes of heart block.

Structural heart disease
Medications – beta blocker, calcium channel blockers
Congenital – autoimmune (e.g. maternal lupus with transplacental antibody transfer)
Acquired – degeneration of the conduction tissues, connective tissue disease, levo-transposition of the great arteries or following surgery (e.g. valve replacement or VSD repair)

- *Second-degree AV block type 2* or Mobitz type 2 occurs in cases where regular atrial electrical activity occurs with variable passage through the AV node. As is the case in this scenario, it can lead to symptoms and higher degrees of heart block.
- *Third-degree* or complete heart block occurs when there is complete failure to transmit atrial rhythms through the AV node. This is most often seen in pregnancy in association with corrected congenital heart disease.

Of note, 30% of congenital AV blocks are not diagnosed until adulthood; as such, the first presentation could be during pregnancy (Regitz-Zagrosek et al., 2011). For common causes of heart block, see Table 32.1.

Management Plan for Complete Heart Block

Complete heart block presenting with narrow QRS complexes is likely to have a block limited to the AV node level and a left ventricular escape rhythm originating close to it. Higher heart rates can be expected and therefore less haemodynamic instability. Patients are better able to increase their heart rate response to stress, exercise and atropine when compared with those who have the block extending past the AV node into the bundles of HIS.

For management of bradycardia algorithm see Figure 32.5.

Anaesthetic Assessment

A thorough anaesthetic assessment with multidisciplinary cardiology, obstetric and anaesthetic team planning of such cases is imperative.

Anaesthetic history should focus on preconception and current functional capacity. Symptoms of fatigue, dizziness, shortness of breath, syncope or any other signs of reduced end-organ perfusion.

A history covering risk factors for complete heart block should be explored (previous cardiac surgery, family history including connective tissue disease, concomitant medication, e.g. beta blockers or calcium channel blockers).

ECG and baseline echo (to rule out structural heart disease and to observe ejection fraction) should be performed (Sundaraman et al., 2016).

Delivery Plan

Parturients with complete heart block (CHB) are unable to increase their cardiac output with an increase in heart rate. Any increase is dependent on an increase in stroke volume. See Table 32.2 for changes in cardiac physiology during pregnancy.

Although CHB does not preclude a parturient from having a normal vaginal delivery, it is recommended that labour is augmented to shorten the active labour phase and instrumental delivery is performed to reduce the time spent straining. Parturients with CHB are at risk of syncopal attacks and convulsions as a result of bradycardias associated with Valsalva manoeuvres and forceful uterine contractions (Suri et al., 2009). Although asymptomatic CHB presenting in labour can be managed conservatively (Suri et al., 2009), temporary pacing and cardiology expertise needs to be on standby.

Epidural analgesia alone or combined with low-dose spinal analgesia is advocated for labour analgesia.

For caesarean section, the risks and benefits of both neuraxial and general anaesthesia must be considered.

Significant haemodynamic changes can occur with both general induction agents and inhalational anaesthetics. In those parturients without pacing, induction agents that are less likely to cause bradycardias should be considered, e.g. ketamine.

Although neuraxial anaesthesia is the usual anaesthetic technique of choice, caution must be exercised, as rapid-onset high-block sympathetic block can further exacerbate the bradycardia. A combined low-dose spinal with slow epidural top-up can reduce the risk of a sudden decrease in preload and strong vagal activity. Regarding vasoconstrictor of choice, ephedrine may be a preferred alternative to phenylephrine, thus avoiding the reflex bradycardia. Atropine, adrenaline and isoprenaline must also all be available.

Pacing

In asymptomatic patients with good functional capacity, a permanent pacemaker can be avoided. Likewise, temporary pacing may also be avoided, but this must be decided on an individual patient basis. If the decision has been made to manage the patient conservatively,

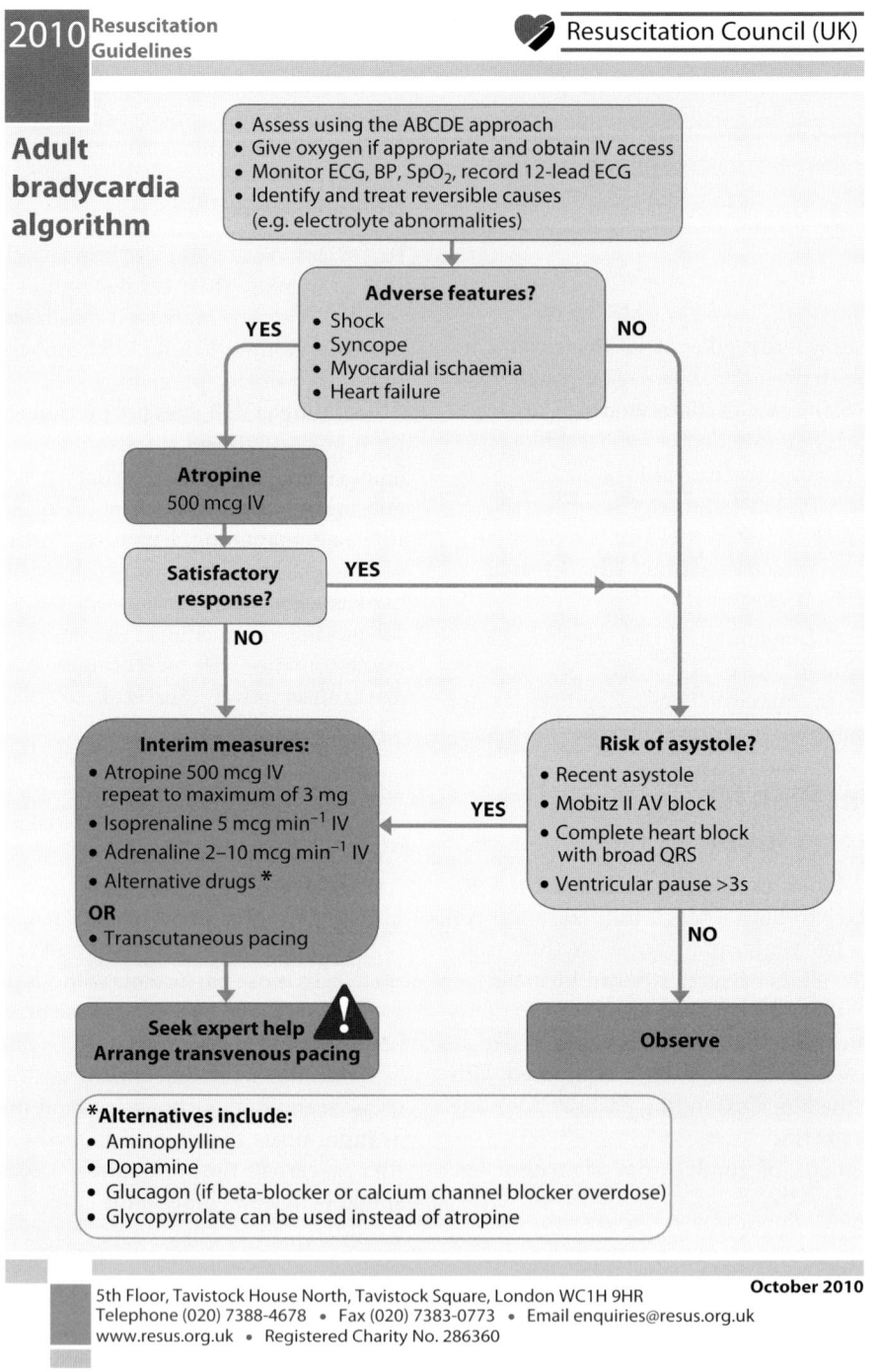

Figure 32.5 Adult bradycardiac algorithm, Resuscitation Council UK.

Table 32.2 Normal HR/SV changes during pregnancy.

Heart rate	Increases by 25%	Increases by 5 weeks reaching maximum at approx. 32 weeks
Stroke volume	Increases by 40–50%	Increases by 8 weeks reaching maximum at approx. 20 weeks

transcutaneous pacing pads can be applied if urgently required, until transvenous pacing can be sited and commenced. Cardiology support needs to be on standby and the team caring for the parturient need to be well-briefed, ideally having rehearsed the eventuality of malignant bradycardia. Temporary pacing during delivery is recommended for those patients who are symptomatic and at risk of severe bradycardia or syncope (Regitz-Zagrosek et al., 2011).

The period of time immediately post-delivery sees the highest cardiac output for the parturient, as the autotransfusion from the contracted uterus adds to the circulating blood volume. This time period is critical and observations must not be relaxed in the immediate postpartum period. Following discharge from hospital, close cardiology contact must be maintained as patients may become symptomatic in the early postpartum period (Sundaraman et al., 2016).

Risks of temporary pacemaker insertion must also be considered, including irradiation, bleeding, infection, pneumothorax and embolism (Hidaka et al., 2006).

To perform transcutaneous pacing, it is recommended that the pads be placed in an anterior–posterior position (Bektas and Soyuncu, 2016); first, establish electrical capture by increasing the current until a broad QRS complex is seen after each pacing spike. Then assess for mechanical capture by feeling for a pulse and recording a blood pressure. If blood pressure remains low, increase the heart rate. Analgesia and sedation may be required, but use with caution in the pregnant patient, remaining mindful of the inherent risks of airway compromise. Most non-obstetric patients requiring transcutaneous pacing need sedation (e.g. midazolam and fentanyl) as it is not a well-tolerated therapy, so it is only useful as a holding measure for a couple of hours.

How long can the temporary wire stay in for? There is evidence showing microscopic, subclinical infection on wires within 48 hours. Infection risk is worse from a groin puncture and this is often the preferred site in an emergency as it is quick, requires less training and

leaves the subclavian untouched for the permanent system. The wires also have a tendency to float and lose contact, so the outputs have to increase and the patients start to feel diaphragmatic twitches.

Typically, temporary wires are switched to a permanent system as soon as possible; however, there are two exceptions to this. Temporary wires are left in for a longer period following inferior MI (where the AV node recovers around day 3 with reperfusion) and following aortic valve replacement (where the AV node recovers around day 5).

Pacemaker Settings for Pregnancy

If a patient already has a pacemaker, there is no specific guidance on settings during pregnancy. If the parturient is atrially paced then the heart rate can be increased to 80 bpm in the second trimester and further increased to 100 bpm at the time of delivery (Metz and Khanna, 2016).

Rate-responsive pacemakers that react to minute ventilation should respond appropriately in labour.

Bibliography

Bektas, F. and Soyuncu, S. (2016). The efficacy of transcutaneous cardiac pacing in ED. *The American Journal of Emergency Medicine*, 34(11), 2090–2093.

Hidaka, N., Chiba, Y., Kurita, T., Satoh, S. and Nakano, H. (2006). Is intrapartum temporary pacing required for women with complete atrioventricular block? An analysis of seven cases. *British Journal of Obstetrics & Gynaecology*, 113(5), 605–607.

Metz, T. D. and Khanna, A. (2016). Evaluation and management of maternal cardiac arrhythmias. *Obstetrics and Gynecology Clinics*, 43(4), 729–745.

Regitz-Zagrosek, V., Blomstrom Lundqvist, C., Borghi, C., et al. (2011). ESC guidelines on the management of cardiovascular diseases during pregnancy: the Task Force on the Management of Cardiovascular Diseases during Pregnancy of the European Society of Cardiology (ESC). *European Heart Journal*, 32(24), 3147–3197.

Sundararaman, L., Cohn, J. H. and Ranasinghe, J. S. (2016). Complete heart block in pregnancy: case report, analysis, and review of anesthetic management. *Journal of Clinical Anesthesia*, 33, 58–61.

Suri, V., Keepanasseril, A., Aggarwal, N., Vijayvergiya, R., Chopra, S. and Rohilla, M. (2009). Maternal complete heart block in pregnancy: analysis of four cases and review of management. *Journal of Obstetrics and Gynaecology Research*, 35(3), 434–437.

Cardioversion in a Pregnant Patient with Corrected Tetralogy of Fallot

Kailash Bhatia

Scenario in a Nutshell

Patient with known repaired Tetralogy of Fallot (ToF) suffers new-onset, regular, narrow complex tachycardia which is unresponsive to medical management requiring DC cardioversion under general anaesthesia.

Stage 1: Initial assessment of narrow complex tachycardia in labouring parturient with adult congenital heart disease (ACHD).

Stage 2: Correction of electrolytes, perform vagal manoeuvres, administer adenosine for continued tachyarrhythmia.

Stage 3: Medical management for tachyarrhythmia unsuccessful, adverse features now present.

Stage 4: DC cardioversion and caesarean section.

Target Learner Groups

All members of the multidisciplinary obstetric team: anaesthetists, midwives, obstetricians, operating department practitioners and cardiologists.

Specific learning opportunities
Assessment of narrow complex tachycardia in adult congenital heart disease (ACHD) patients
Knowledge of algorithm for management of tachyarrhythmia
Consideration of anaesthetic plan for DC cardioversion in pregnancy
Importance of senior MDT obstetric and cardiology input in ACHD parturients

Suggested learners (to represent their normal roles)	In the room from the start	Available when requested
Anaesthetic ST3+	√	
Obstetric ST3+	√	
Midwife Coordinator		√
Midwife in room	√	

Suggested learners (to represent their normal roles)	In the room from the start	Available when requested
Operating Department Practitioner (ODP)/anaesthetic nurse		√
Cardiology ST		√
Suggested facilitators		
Faculty to play role of student midwife giving handover at time of emergency buzzer	√	

Details for Facilitators

Patient Demographics

Name: Michelle

Age: 29

Gestation: 36

Booking weight: 64 kg

Parity: P0

Scenario Summary for Facilitators

29-year-old 36-week primipara woman, with history of repaired Tetralogy of Fallot, attends delivery suite in spontaneous labour. She has been complaining of sudden onset of palpitations and feels her heart is racing. She has a confirmed narrow complex tachyarrhythmia on the monitor.

Her past surgical history is repaired TOF with Waterston shunt, followed by a repair of pulmonary valve and closure of VSD. Recent echo shows signs of moderate pulmonary regurgitation and mild RV dysfunction. She attended the joint obstetric, cardiac, anaesthetic clinic 6 weeks ago. (For the Anaesthetic letter see Figure 33.1. For the echocardiogram report see Figure 33.2.)

On arrival on the delivery suite, she is reviewed by the team. All investigations performed and bloods taken. Potassium and magnesium corrected.

Although initially stable with tachyarrhythmia, it does not respond to vagal manoeuvres, adenosine or beta blockers.

Patient then becomes hypotensive and complains of chest pain. Decision made for DC cardioversion in theatre.

The patient is intubated and cardioverted successfully. CTG remains suspicious, the obstetric team proceed to perform an emergency LSCS.

Set-up Overview for Facilitators

Clinical setting	In a delivery room, on a delivery bed
Patient position	Semi-recumbent
Initial monitoring in place	No monitoring – has just arrived on delivery suite
Other equipment	No IV access or maternal/fetal monitoring but all equipment available
Useful manikin features	Intubation Defibrillation and cardioversion

---

Anaesthetic clinic
6 weeks earlier

Dear Obstetrician

Thank you for referring Michelle to our obstetric anaesthetic clinic. She is a 29-year-old primipara, now 30 weeks pregnant.

She was diagnosed with Tetralogy of Fallot (TOF) after birth, having a Waterston shunt in infancy followed by repair of TOF. There is no family history of any cardiac problems.

During pregnancy she has been well. No history of palpitations, chest pain, ankle oedema or dizzy spells. She can climb a flight of stairs without any problem but reports mild dyspnoea on exertion, especially on walking uphill.

She has no allergies and takes no regular medication. On examination, she is Mallampati class 2, with good neck movements and Calder score A.

She has been seen in obstetric cardiac clinic and is aiming for a normal vaginal delivery with a planned induction at 37 weeks.

Her ECG today shows normal sinus rhythm with a heart rate of 78/min. Echocardiogram today suggests good LV function but mild RV dysfunction with mild–moderate pulmonary and tricuspid regurgitation.

We discussed various analgesic options for labour. I have recommended an epidural and have discussed the benefits and risks as per OAA leaflet. She will have SpO_2/ECG/NIBP monitoring throughout and may need invasive arterial BP monitoring. Regarding oxytocics, I recommend a slow syntocinon infusion and avoidance of syntometrine. Misoprostol and mechanical methods should be other preferred techniques in case of uterine atony.

If she requires operative intervention, a regional technique would be preferable. If she requires a GA, I suggest a propofol/rocuronium/alfentanil technique and avoidance of tachycardia/hypoxia/acidosis/hypothermia/hypotension. Phenylephrine should be used as a vasopressor and enoximone and beta blockers should be available. Strict attention to fluid balance and thrombo-prophylaxis are needed.

Please alert the on-call consultant anaesthetist when Michelle arrives on the delivery suite.

Yours sincerely
Consultant Anaesthetist

Figure 33.1 Anaesthetic Clinic Letter.

Echocardiogram Report
1) Left Ventricle (LV) – LV cavity is normal in size. LV is normal in thickness. Overall LV function is good
2) Right Ventricle (RV) – Dilated RV with TAPSE 1.6 cm suggesting reduced longitudinal function. Tricuspid Annular displacement is 1.75 cm suggestive of RV dysfunction
3) Left Atrium (LA) – Normal in size 3.9 cm
4) Right Atrium (RA) – Mildly dilated
5) Aortic Valve – Normal trileaflet in appearance, thin and mobile
6) Aortic Root – 3 cm
7) Mitral Valve – mobile no obvious abnormality noted
8) Pulmonary valve – mobile leaflets, mild–moderate pulmonary regurgitation noted
9) Tricuspid Valve – Mild–moderate tricuspid regurgitation noted
10) Both Atrial/Ventricular septae are intact and no pericardial effusion is noted

Summary
1) RV function reduced with RV dysfunction
2) Dilated RA with mild–moderate pulmonary and tricuspid regurgitation noted
3) Good LV function

Figure 33.2 Patient's echocardiogram report.

Medical Equipment

For core equipment checklist, see Chapter 9.

Additional equipment specific to scenario		
Arterial line	Resuscitation trolley with defibrillator	Pads for defibrillation
Drugs: Adenosine Beta blockers – Metoprolol Digoxin Diltiazem	Magnesium Potassium Drugs for intubation	

Information Given to the Learner

SBAR Handover by faculty (playing the role of midwife) to the obstetric and anaesthetic on-call team

Time: Midday

Situation: 29 years old. 36 weeks primipara in spontaneous labour. She has a past history of adult congenital heart disease and is now complaining of palpitations.

Background: She was diagnosed with Tetralogy of Fallot in childhood and has had surgical repair. She has been seen in obstetric anaesthetic clinic (see Figure 33.1). She has been symptom-free in pregnancy until yesterday, when she started suffering with palpitations. She has just arrived in hospital and is in spontaneous labour, which commenced about 3–4 hours ago.

Assessment: I was just about to perform some observations but thought it best to get you immediately.

Recommendations: Would you like me to get the clinic letter while you meet Michelle?

Scenario Schedule

Stage 1: Initial assessment of narrow complex tachycardia in labouring parturient with ACHD	
Information given	**Expected actions**
Patient complaining that heart is racing. Had one similar episode yesterday, which settled spontaneously. Nothing makes it better or worse. No chest pain or dizziness. Had mild SOB for last 2 weeks but assumed this was due to pregnancy. Apart from heart condition no other medical problems.	Commence ABCDE approach whilst taking a full history

Information given	Expected actions
Examination: Speaking in full sentences. Chest clear. Tachycardic, heart sounds normal. No oedema. No PV bleeding. Cervical Dilatation 2 cm, fully effaced. Intermittent contractions 3 in 10 started 4 hours ago. No analgesia requested yet. Has just eaten lunch	Examination of patient including obstetric examination to rule out bleeding
	Apply Oxygen via non-rebreathing mask at 15 l/min whilst stabilising the patient (then titrate oxygen to SpO$_2$ 94-98%)
ECG sinus rhythm on monitor	Apply ECG / pulse oximeter / NIBP monitoring
	Secure IV access and take blood for FBC, U+E, Magnesium, LFT, Coagulation including fibrinogen (TEG) and G+S. Check CBG and venous blood gas
	Give Hartmann's bolus 250 ml
U/S scans in pregnancy showed posterior placenta clear of os.	Review antenatal investigations
Give all information Figures 33.1, 33.2, 33.3	Review clinic letter (Figure 33.1). Review echocardiogram report (Figure 33.2). Request 12 lead ECG (Figure 33.2)
	Call for senior obstetric / anaesthetic / cardiology help

Observations

A	Clear
B	RR 22/min SpO$_2$ 96% on air SpO$_2$ 99% on O$_2$
C	HR 140-150bpm BP 110/60 CRT 2s
D	**A**VPU
E	Temp 36.6°C
CTG	Normal FHR 130bpm

VBG:

pH 7.34
pCO$_2$ 3.9 kPa
pO$_2$ 4 kPa
BE -3 mmol/L
HCO$_3$ 23mmol/L
Lactate 1.9 mmol/L
K 3.6 mmol/L
Na 136 mmol/L
CBG 5.3 mmol/L
Hb 122g/L

Progress to stage 2 once history taken, ABC approach completed

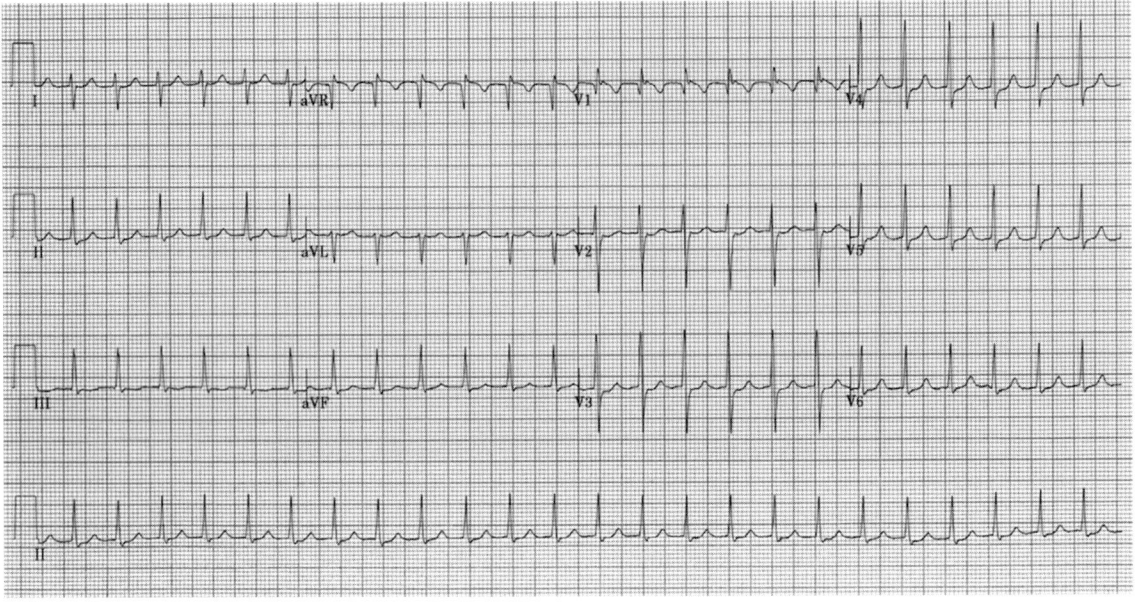

Figure 33.3 12-Lead ECG of patient.

Observations	
A	Clear
B	RR 24/min SpO$_2$ 98% on 0$_2$
C	HR 150bpm BP 110/50 CRT 2s
D	**A**VPU
E	Temp 36.6°C
CTG	Baseline 160-170bpm

Stage 2: Correction of electrolytes, perform vagal manoeuvres, administer adenosine for continued tachyarrhythmia

Information given	Expected actions
Cardiology registrar will attend as soon as he can and advises to follow the tachycardia algorithm	Continue with Oxygen. Consult ALS tachycardia algorithm (if available)
	10-20 mmol of potassium chloride in 1000ml of normal saline may be considered intravenously at 125ml/hr -200ml/hr
Patient still complaining of heart racing	2g Magnesium Sulphate over 30 minutes may also be considered
	Bring emergency trolley with cardiac defibrillator into delivery room
If monitoring applied, rhythm strip shows narrow complex tachycardia	Connect to monitor and record rhythm strip
	Commence ALS algorithm for management of narrow complex regular tachycardia
No effect with carotid sinus massage / Valsalva	Carotid sinus massage either side or Valsalva manoeuvre used initially (Vagal manoeuvres)
Michelle feels a bit odd following adenosine. Heart rate initially slows but reverts to 150–160/min after each of the 3 adenosine boluses	Administer Adenosine 6mg IV with flush, followed by 12mg and another 12mg IV when remains in SVT

Progress to stage 3 once vagal manoeuvres attempted and adenosine given.

Stage 3: Medical management for tachyarrhythmia unsuccessful, adverse features now present

Information given	Expected actions
Cardiology registrar arrives	
Patient still c/o palpitations. Rhythm strip shows narrow complex tachycardia 150-160bpm	Cardiology registrar reviews ECG / clinic letter / notes
	As BP stable, give metoprolol 0.1mg/kg
No change in HR from metoprolol.	Consider repeating 250ml bolus of Hartmann's
Patient now complaining of chest pain and feeling dizzy. Observations now as per the start of stage 4	Suggest proceed to DC cardioversion in view of symptoms
	Discussion re where to perform cardioversion between cardiologists/ anaesthetists/obstetrician
If examined again, cervical dilatation is 2-3 cm. CTG suspicious	
	Agree to proceed with cardioversion in theatre (full stomach, aspiration risk)
	Alert theatre team re plan for cardioversion +/- caesarean section depending on CTG
Theatres happy to receive patient	Transfer to theatre with portable oxygen and full monitoring

Progress to stage 4 once attempted rate control and now showing adverse signs

Observations pre beta-blocker

A	Clear
B	RR 24/min SpO$_2$ 98% on 0$_2$
C	HR 150bpm BP 98/45 CRT 3s
D	**A**VPU
E	Temp 36.6°C
CTG	Baseline 180bpm, reduced variability, variable decelerations

Stage 4: DC cardioversion and caesarean section

Information Given	Expected Actions
A – No allergies M – No medications P – Previous cardiac surgery no anaesthetic problems L – Last ate 30 min ago E – Airway assessment looks straightforward	Take anaesthetic history
	Administer Ranitidine 150mg IV + 30ml 0.3M Sodium citrate
	Apply monitoring and defibrillator pads.
	Attach CTG
Grade 1 intubation, easy to ventilate	Perform GA (see chapter 24)

Observations

A	Clear
B	RR 26/min SpO$_2$ 98% on 0$_2$
C	HR 150bpm BP 79/39 CRT 3s
D	**A**VPU
E	Temp 36.6°C

Observations	
A	Intubated
B	RR as per ventilator setting SpO$_2$ 98%
C	HR 100bpm BP 95/55 CRT 2s
D	Anaesthetised
E	Temp 36.1°C
CTG	Baseline 180bpm, reduced variability, variable decelerations

Information given	Expected actions
	Vasopressor support with phenylephrine if needed
	Commence DC cardioversion, 100J Energy
Patient reverts to Sinus rhythm with first DC shock	Sync button activated and cardioversion performed
	Obstetrician decides to perform an LSCS and deliver the baby

Scenario ends once DC cardioversion performed and decision to caesarean section confirmed.

Suggested Topics for Debrief Discussion

- How confident would you be handling this emergency?
- Consider what you would have used for induction of anaesthesia.
- Were all teams clear what the plan was at all times?

Discussion

Heart Disease in Pregnancy and Corrected Tetralogy of Fallot

Heart disease is the one of the leading causes of maternal mortality in the UK. As per the 2016 MBRRACE report, 2 women per 100,000 die from heart disease. This rate has not changed much since 2003 and is the leading cause of indirect deaths in pregnancy. Tetralogy of Fallot (ToF) is one of the most common forms of congenital cyanotic heart disease (1:3600 live births) and represents 5–6% of all cases of congenital heart disease (CHD). The four main characteristics of Tetralogy of Fallot are:

1. Pulmonary stenosis.
2. Ventricular septal defect (VSD) of the membranous portion.
3. Over-riding of aorta.
4. Right ventricular hypertrophy (RVH) due to the shunting of blood from left to right.

ToF results in a reduction in pulmonary blood flow (PBF) at birth. Temporary palliative surgery such as Waterston shunt (shunt between ascending aorta and right pulmonary artery) is initially used to increase the PBF. Full surgical repair usually follows which involves the removal of some thickened muscle below the pulmonary valve or opening or widening the pulmonary valve and enlarging the peripheral pulmonary arteries that go to both lungs and closure of the VSD.

During pregnancy, blood volume slowly increases by 40–50%. Cardiac output increases by about 50%, mostly with maximum values being attained at 20–24 weeks and maintained thereafter in the lateral position until term. The systemic vascular resistance (SVR) also slightly decreases due to smooth muscle relaxation caused by elevated progesterone.

Although pregnancy is well tolerated in ToF, the increase in blood volume/cardiac output could affect both ventricles, especially in the presence of diastolic dysfunction. One study demonstrated that the normal increase in ejection fraction (EF) was less in patients with corrected ToF. LV end diastolic dimension (LVEDD) was significantly smaller in this group compared to normal parturients, which can lead to increased maternal and neonatal peripartum complications. Corrected ToF falls under class II modified World Health Organization (WHO) risk (see Table 33.1).

Supraventricular arrhythmias, heart failure and endocarditis are the most common cardiovascular

Table 33.1 Modified WHO classification of maternal conditions.

Risk class of pregnancy by medical condition	
I	No detectable increased risk of maternal mortality and no/mild increase in morbidity
II	Small increased risk of maternal mortality or moderate increase in morbidity
III	Significantly increased risk of maternal mortality or severe morbidity. Expert counselling required. If pregnancy is decided upon, intensive specialist cardiac and obstetric monitoring needed throughout pregnancy, childbirth and the puerperium
IV	Extremely high risk of maternal mortality or severe morbidity; pregnancy contraindicated. If pregnancy occurs, termination should be discussed. If pregnancy continues, care as for class III

Table 33.2 Causes of palpitations in pregnancy and investigations.

Lifestyle	Excessive caffeine, smoking, alcohol, cocaine, cannabis
Emotional	Stress, anxiety
Cardiac	Heart disease – congenital, acquired, familial, ischaemic, valvular, hypertension, arrhythmias, heart failure, cardiomyopathy
Haematologic	Anaemia
Endocrine	Pregnancy, thyrotoxicosis, diabetes, hypoglycaemia, phaeochromocytoma
Obstetric	Pre-eclampsia, sepsis, haemorrhage, thrombo-embolism
Electrolyte imbalance	Hyper/hypokalaemia, hypomagnesemia, acidosis, renal failure
Medications	Beta 2 agonists, anti-depressants, nifedepine

complications in pregnancy affecting 4.5–18% of all corrected ToF patients. Pulmonary regurgitation, RV dysfunction and use of cardiac medications were some of the predictors of cardiovascular events in this population.

Maternal complications include:

- postpartum haemorrhage (~10%),
- preterm labour (<5%) and
- delivery by caesarean section (~20%).

Palliative surgery, use of cardiac medications and maternal cardiac events are significant predictors of fetal outcomes. Fetal complications include:

- miscarriage (~15–20%),
- preterm birth (~17%),
- small for gestational age (19%) and
- perinatal mortality (~6%).

Multidisciplinary team (MDT) input from the obstetrician, cardiologists and anaesthetists as per European Society of Cardiology (ESC) and Royal College of Obstetricians (RCOG) recommendations are essential. The main causes of palpitations in pregnancy are highlighted in Table 33.2.

Discussion

Management of Patients With Narrow Complex Tachycardia

When managing arrhythmias in this group of patients, cardiology input is required and the adult Advanced Life Support (ALS) tachyarrhythmia algorithm needs to be adhered to (see Figure 33.4).

Vagal Manoeuvres

- The *modified Valsalva manoeuvre* is most commonly used (exhale forcefully against a closed glottis after a normal inspiratory effort).
- *Supine repositioning* (15 seconds of passive leg raise at a 45-degree angle).
- *Carotid sinus massage* (pressure is applied to one carotid sinus for 5–10 seconds).

If vagal manoeuvres are unsuccessful and the parturient remains medically stable, proceed to pharmacological management.

The main drugs used to treat stable narrow complex tachycardia are highlighted in Table 33.3.

DC Cardioversion

DC cardioversion is recommended in unstable patients with adverse features (shock, syncope, myocardial infarction or heart failure). This will require sedation or general anaesthesia. Sedation in a labouring parturient has inherent risks, including further haemodynamic instability, aspiration and risk of LSCS. Although not without its risks, administration of general anaesthesia with securing of the airway with an endotracheal tube seems to be the safest choice.

Electrical cardioversion has been performed without complications in all stages of pregnancy to treat both atrial and ventricular arrhythmias. No significant effects are expected on the fetus, as they have a high fibrillation threshold, and the amount of current that reaches the uterus is usually very small. Electrical cardioversion does not result in compromise of blood

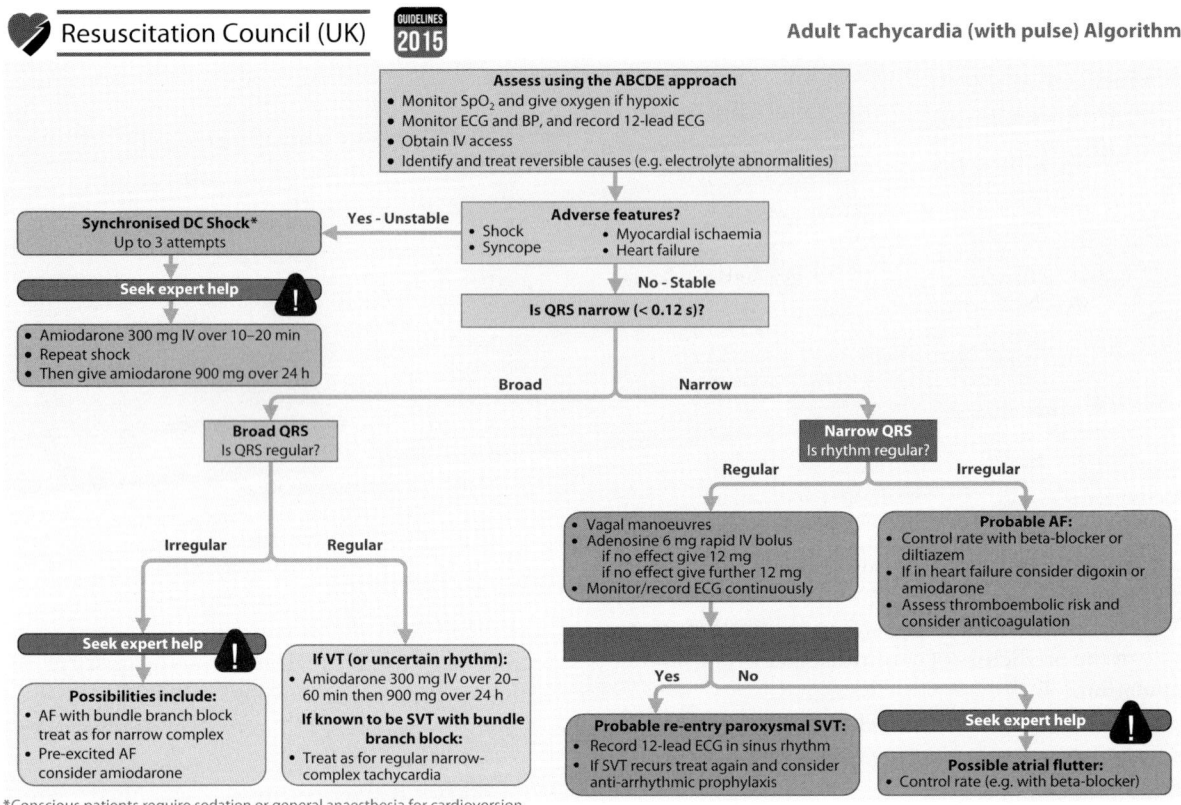

Figure 33.4 Adult Advanced Life Support narrow and broad complex tachycardia algorithm.

Table 33.3 Drugs available used to terminate narrow complex tachycardia in pregnancy.

Medication	Mechanism of action	Use	Breastfeeding safety	Fetal effects
Adenosine	Nucleoside, blocking AV node	SVT	Yes	None
Beta blockers (metoprolol, propranolol, atenolol, bisoprolol)	Decrease conduction across SA, AV node	SVT, AF	Yes (atenolol concentration higher in breast milk)	Mild hypotension (IUGR, prematurity noted when used during second and third trimesters). Monitor for hypoglycaemia
Calcium channel blockers (diltiazem, verapamil)	Decrease conduction across AV node	SVT	Yes	Verapamil used to treat fetal arrhythmias
Amiodaraone	Potassium channel blocker	SVT in WPW, VT	Best to avoid as long half-life Risks vs. benefits need to be taken into consideration	Fetal goitre, hypothyroidism IUGR, prematurity birth defects
Digoxin	Inhibits Na/K ATPase	SVT	Yes	Mild growth restriction but overall safe
Flecainide	Sodium channel blocker	SVT	Yes	Limited information available, used for treatment of fetal arrhythmias
Sotalol	Potassium channel blocker	SVT	Yes	Limited information, bradycardia (other beta blockers preferable)

Abbreviations: SVT, supraventricular tachycardia; SA, sino-atrial; AV, atrio-ventricular; IUGR, intrauterine growth retardation; WPW, Wolf Parkinson-White.

flow to the fetus. Fetal heart rate monitoring is recommended because of reported cases of emergency caesarean delivery due to fetal arrhythmias. A review of the literature suggests that when cardioversion is considered, the obstetrician must be prepared for a LSCS. Hence the parturient should be consented for LSCS, especially after 24 weeks of gestation, and the neonatal team be alerted.

Although anterior–posterior defibrillation pads placement may be favoured over anterior–lateral, there is no evidence that pad position is a critically important factor in DC cardioversion success (Kirkland et al., 2014).

The energy to be selected for the first DC shock is 100 J for biphasic shocks. A lower energy can be selected for atrial flutter starting between 70 and 120 J. The 'sync' button needs to be on during cardioversion to decrease the risk of ventricular fibrillation (R on T phenomenon). If the first shock does not lead to electrical cardioversion then subsequent shocks should be delivered at 150 J. Also check manufacturer guidelines for your local defibrillator.

MBRRACE reports remind us that when dealing with obstetric cardiac patients, you must continue to consider the whole picture. Non-cardiac causes for presentation of tachycardia must be considered, such as hypovolaemia. The decision on where to perform the cardioversion requires MDT discussion and balancing of risk and benefit.

Bibliography

Balci, A., Drenthem, W., Mulder, B. J. W., et al. (2011). Pregnancy in women with corrected tetralogy of Fallot: occurrence and predictors of adverse events. *American Heart Journal*, 161(2), 307–313.

Barnes, E. J., Eben, F. and Patterson, D. (2002). Direct current cardioversion during pregnancy should be performed with facilities available for fetal monitoring and emergency caesarean. *British Journal of Obstetrics and Gynaecology*, 109(12), 1406–1407.

De Silva, R. A., Graboys, T. B., Podrid, P. J. and Lown, B. (1980). Cardioversion and defibrillation. *American Heart Journal*, 100, 881–895.

European Society of Gynecology, et al. (2011). European Society of Cardiology Guidelines on the management of cardiovascular diseases during pregnancy. *European Heart Journal*, 32, 3147–3197.

Hidaka, Y., Akagi, T., Himeno, W., Ishii, M. and Matsuishi, T. (2003). Left ventricular performance during pregnancy in patients with repaired tetralogy of Fallot: prospective evaluation using the Tei index. *Circulation Journal*, 68(2), 682–686.

Kirkland, S., Stiell, I., AlShawabkeh, T., Campbell, S., Dickinson, G. and Rowe, B. H. (2014). The efficacy of pad placement for electrical cardioversion of atrial fibrillation/flutter: a systematic review. *Academic Emergency Medicine*, 21(7), 717–726.

Knight, M., Nair, M., Tuffnell, D., et al. (Eds.) on behalf of MBRRACE-UK. (2016). *Saving Lives, Improving Mothers' Care – Surveillance of Maternal Deaths in the UK 2012–14 and Lessons Learned to Inform Maternity Care from the UK and Ireland Confidential Enquiries into Maternal Deaths and Morbidity 2009–14.* Oxford: National Perinatal Epidemiology Unit, University of Oxford.

Royal College of Obstetricians and Gynaecologists. (2011). *Cardiac Disease and Pregnancy. Good Practice No. 13.* London: Royal College of Obstetricians and Gynaecologists.

Resuscitation Council (UK). (2015). Advanced Life Support Guidelines. Available from: www.resus.org.uk/resuscitation-guidelines/peri-arrest-arrhythmias/ (accessed April 2017).

Schroeder, J. S. and Harrison, D. C. (1971). Repeated cardioversion during pregnancy: treatment of refractory paroxysmal atrial tachycardia during three successive pregnancies. *American Journal of Cardiology*, 27, 445–446.

Toff, N. J. (2010). Human factors in anaesthesia: lessons from aviation. *British Journal of Anaesthesia* 105(1), 21–25.

Wang, Y. C., Chen, C. H., Su, H. Y. and Yu, M. H. (2006). The impact of maternal cardioversion on fetal haemodynamics. *European Journal of Obstetrics, Gynecology, and Reproductive Biology*, 126(2), 268.

Chapter

Diabetic Ketoacidosis in Pregnancy

Samantha Bonner and Jonathan Schofield

Scenario in a Nutshell

Diabetic ketoacidosis (DKA) in pregnancy.
Stage 1: Initial assessment of acutely unwell pregnant woman and diagnosis of DKA.
Stage 2: Emergency management of DKA and consideration of abnormal CTG.
Stage 3: Ongoing management and monitoring of DKA 1 hour after initiation of treatment.

Target Learner Groups

Obstetricians, anaesthetists and midwives.

Specific learning opportunities
Assessment and resuscitation of the acutely unwell pregnant patient
Recognition of diabetic ketoacidosis (DKA) in pregnancy
Demonstrate the emergency management of the acutely unwell pregnant woman with DKA
Demonstrate appropriate senior multidisciplinary involvement

Suggested learners (to represent their normal roles)	In the room from the start	Available when requested
Midwife in room	√	
Midwife Coordinator		√
Obstetric ST3+	√	
Anaesthetic ST3+		√
Suggested facilitators		
Faculty to play role of obstetric ST2	√	

Details for Facilitators

Patient Demographics

Name: Emma
Age: 25
Gestation: 34+4
Booking weight: 65 kg
Parity: P0

Scenario Summary for Facilitators

A 25-year-old primigravida presents at 34 weeks gestation to the obstetric triage department with a 3-day history of feeling generally unwell. This lady is a known type 1 diabetic. She has been compliant with antenatal care and has had negative screening for both microvascular and macrovascular complications.
Apart from diabetes, she is otherwise fit and well and has been well in the antenatal period.
She presents with suprapubic abdominal pain and vomiting. Although usually compliant with her insulin regime she does say that she has not been taking her insulin properly over the last 24 hours due to persistent vomiting and anorexia.
On examination: she appears pale and clammy and unwell. She is tachypnoeic and her breath has a ketotic odour.
Her urine shows significant ketonuria (4+), nitrites and protein and her initial capillary blood glucose is 17.0 mmol/l.
This woman has diabetic ketoacidosis, probably triggered by a urinary tract infection.
She is unwell on triage. Emergency treatment of DKA is initiated and she is moved to obstetric HDU.
CTG is abnormal. Mother stabilised prior to consideration of delivery.
Trigger for DKA sought. Investigations and treatment for sepsis.
After 1 hour of treatment with insulin and fluids, review biochemistry to check for adequate improvement.

Set-up Overview for Facilitators

Clinical setting	In a triage room on a trolley
Patient position	Semi-recumbent
Initial monitoring in place	ECG, NIBP, SpO$_2$
Other equipment	None

Medical Equipment

For core equipment checklist, see Chapter 9.

Additional equipment specific to scenario		
Vomit bowl	Urinalysis multistix	Blood ketone monitor and testing strips
Human soluble insulin (e.g. Actrapid) – syringe, giving set, drug labels	Normal saline (0.9% sodium chloride) and giving set	10% glucose
IV broad-spectrum antibiotics	Arterial line	IV paracetamol

Information Given to the Learners

Handover from ST2 Obstetrics (faculty) on for triage to ST3+ Obstetrics

The SBAR handover is as follows:

Situation: This is Emma, who has come into triage with a 3-day history of abdominal pain, vomiting and feeling generally unwell.

Background: She is a 25-year-old, primiparous woman who is 34+4 weeks pregnant. She is a known type 1 diabetic on insulin. She only took a small dose of her insulin yesterday as she hardly ate anything all day and hasn't had any insulin today as she has been vomiting and unable to keep any food or fluids down. She has no allergies.

Assessment: We are just doing a first set of observations now.

Recommendation: Could you help me?

Scenario Schedule

Observations	
A	Clear
B	RR 32/min SpO$_2$ 96%
C	HR 118bpm BP 91/42 CRT 4s
D	A**V**PU
E	Temp 37.8°C

Stage 1: Initial assessment of acutely unwell pregnant patient and diagnosis of DKA

Information given	Expected actions
Looks unwell – pale, cool and clammy Intermittently retching	Call for help (obstetric consultant/ anaesthetist/ midwife co-ordinator)
Eyes closed but opening them to voice	Perform observations and repeat regularly Commence ABCDE approach to patient:
	Position with left lateral tilt or semi-recumbent
Can speak, airway clear	Perform airway assessment
	Apply Oxygen via non-rebreathing mask at 15 L/min whilst stabilising the patient (then titrate oxygen to SpO$_2$ 94-98%)
As examines patient, notices sweet, pear drop smell Kussmaul breathing - deep, laboured Trachea central, symmetrical chest expansion, good air entry bilaterally, no added sounds	Examine respiratory system
Cool, shut down peripheries HS 1+2+0	Examine cardiovascular system
Uterus is appropriate size for gestation. Her abdomen is soft, although she does have some generalised abdominal pain, worse over the suprapubic area. There are no signs of an acute abdomen	Examines abdomen

Information given	Expected actions
	Secure IV access (ideally 2 large bore cannulae)
CBG 17.0 mmol/L	Check capillary blood glucose (CBG) with glucometer
	Take blood for FBC, U+E, LFT, serum glucose, bone profile, Magnesium and G&S.
Urinary ketones 4+, protein 2+, nitrites Capillary ketones – 5.0 mmol/L	Measure blood or urinary ketones
	Start fluid replacement immediately (0.9% sodium chloride) initially 1000 ml in 1st hour, then 500 mls / hr for next 4 hours with continuous review
ABG (or VBG) result: (on air) pH 7.26 (7.23 if venous gas) pO2 13 kPa (5.3kPa if venous gas) pCO2 2.2 kPa (3.0 kPa if venous gas) HCO3 7.2 mmol/LBE -18 mmol/L Na+ 135 mmol/L K+ 5.4 mmol/L Glu 17.8 mmol/L Lactate 2.3 mmol/L	Perform venous (VBG) or arterial blood gas (ABG) Doesn't give bicarbonate
	Diabetic ketoacidosis (DKA) recognised as likely diagnosis and stated to team
	Arrange immediate transfer to delivery suite and HDU care (All pregnant women with DKA should be cared for in a level 2 facility (National Institute for Health and Clinical Excellence, 2015))

Proceed to stage 2 once initial assessment and diagnosis of DKA made, rapid IV fluids commenced and decision made to transfer to obstetric HDU

Stage 2: Urgent management of DKA and consideration of abnormal CTG	
Information given	Expected Actions
Patient now in obstetric HDU room	Urgent commencement of insulin therapy (weight-based fixed rate intravenous insulin infusion (FRIII) according to local policies, eg: 0.1 UNITS insulin/kg/hr (Joint British Diabetes Societies recommend using current weight rather than booking weight)– initial rate not exceeding 14 units of insulin/hr)
	Doesn't give a 'priming' bolus of insulin prior to insulin infusion but ensures there is no delay in commencing FRIII

Observations	
A	Clear
B	RR 30/min SpO2 97%
C	HR 120bpm BP 101/60 CRT 4s
D	A**V**PU
E	Temp 38.4°C
CTG	Baseline 170 bpm baseline variability 5-10bpm decelerations

Information given	Expected Actions
Senior co-ordinating midwife and anaesthetic registrar arrive.	SBAR to anaesthetic registrar and senior midwife co-ordinator
	Repeat observations
	Catheterise and monitor hourly urine output
	Contact consultant anaesthetist, diabetic inpatient specialist team (medical registrar on-call if out of hours) and obstetric consultant if not called earlier
	Commence CTG and note abnormal
	Recognise that fetal heart rate abnormalities will usually correct with correction of maternal hyperglycaemia and ketosis. Recognise that the patient must be stabilised before giving consideration to delivering the fetus
3 day history of suprapubic abdominal pain and vomiting. She also has reduced fetal movements. No diarrhoea. Urinary frequency **++** and dysuria for 2 days. Feeling generally unwell and lethargic. No chest pain No headache or neck stiffness. Vision feels a bit blurry today. No PV discharge No respiratory symptoms except feels a bit short of breath today	Identify and treat any precipitating factors for DKA– full systemic enquiry
	Consider urinary tract infection as likely triggering factor for DKA
	Start IV broad spectrum antibiotics (according to local policies) or as per Microbiology advice
	Perform septic screen: • MSU (midstream specimen of urine) • Blood cultures • HVS (high vaginal swab) • Throat swabs • CXR if clinically indicated (not indicated here as chest clear and symptoms and urinalysis suggest urinary tract infection)

Information given	Expected Actions
	Ensure the 'Sepsis Six' have been completed: • Titrate oxygen to SpO2 ≥94% • Take blood cultures • Administer intravenous antibiotics • Measure serum lactate • Intravenous fluids • Catheterise and commence accurate urine output measurement
	IV paracetamol
	Reasonable if anaesthetist suggests arterial line as patient unwell with likely sepsis. Routinely, for DKA, venous blood gases are fine for monitoring progress of DKA (British Joint Diabetes Societies Inpatient Care Group, 2013, 2017)– arterial line recommended only if required for monitoring critically unwell patient, eg: concurrent sepsis
	Critical care team made aware of patient and potential for transfer if deteriorates
Is more alert and says she is feeling a little better after first litre of saline given	
Proceed to stage 3 once FRIII commenced, precipitating factors for DKA looked for and treatment for probable sepsis commenced	

Observations	
A	Clear
B	RR 28/min SpO2 96%
C	HR 112bpm BP 110/70 CRT 3s
D	**A**VPU
E	Temp 38.1°C
CTG	Baseline 165bpm baseline variability 5-10bpm still some decelerations

Observations	
A	Clear
B	RR 26/min SpO2 96%
C	HR 108bpm BP 102/72 CRT 3s
D	**A**VPU
E	Temp 38.1°C
CTG:	Baseline 155bpm baseline variability 5-10bpm still some decelerations

Stage 3: Ongoing management and monitoring of DKA 1 hour after initiation of treatment

Information given	Expected Actions
1 hour has now passed since initiation of treatment for DKA	
Examination results not changed from stage 1	Reviews ABCDE assessment and rechecks observations
CBG now 13.8mmol/L	Checks CBG
	Commences 10% glucose at 125mls/hr in addition to 0.9% sodium chloride now that CBG <14mmol/L
ST2 Obstetrics (facilitator) suggests decreasing the rate of insulin infusion rather than giving IV dextrose as well	Team recognise need for continued IV insulin therapy to clear ketonaemia – continue FRIII at same rate as improvements in CBG, blood ketones and bicarbonate are all occurring at a reasonable rate (see blood gas result)

281

Information given	Expected Actions
ABG (or VBG) result: pH 7.28 (7.25 if VBG) pO2 13.1kPa (5.4 kPa if VBG) pCO2 3.2 mmol/L (4.0mmol/L if VBG) HCO3- 11 mmol/L BE -14.2 mmol/L K+ 4.2mmol/L	Checks arterial/venous blood gas and compares to blood gas result from 1 hour ago
Blood ketones 4.3 mmol/L	Checks blood ketones
	Team happy that rate of biochemical improvement has been satisfactory over the first hour (see discussion)
FBC and U+Es results now available: Na+ 140mmol/L K+ 4.3mmol/L urea 9.9mmol/L creatinine 98 µmol/L WCC 14.3 X 10 9/L Hb 126 g/L PLTs 402 X10 9/L	If first 1000mls of 0.9% saline has been administered, then next 1000mls 0.9% saline should be commenced with 40mmol KCL over 2hrs
ST2 obstetrics (facilitator) notes that 0.9% saline has finished and asks what fluid should be given next and how fast? If asked: Urine output 55 mls in first hour	If first 1000mls of 0.9% saline has been administered, then next 1000mls 0.9% saline should be commenced with 40mmol KCL over 2hrs Ask for early expert senior help - management of fluid therapy can be difficult in the pregnant patient with DKA
Patient could prompt by saying 'I usually take my Lantus about now but I haven't had anything to eat and I suppose I am already getting insulin by the drip.'	Ensure usual dose of subcutaneous long-acting (basal) insulin analogues have been given as well as insulin infusion (see discussion)
	If suggest a dose of corticosteroid for fetal lung maturation – this should be a consultant decision between obstetrician and diabetes specialist and only considered once there is some clinical and biochemical improvement of the DKA
Woman could prompt CTG review by asking if baby OK	Recognise that CTG may take 4-6 hours to improve as mother's condition improves
	Decision to deliver and timing of delivery must be made on an individual basis by consultant multidisciplinary team: obstetrician, obstetric anaesthetist, physician, neonatal team +/- critical care
Patient is alert, less clammy and starting to feel better	

Scenario ends when medical registrar/diabetes team arrives to assess the patient

Suggested Topics for Debrief Discussion

- How did you diagnose DKA?
- How easy was it to find the guidelines for the appropriate IV insulin regime for a pregnant woman with DKA? Could this be improved on your unit?
- Is a blood ketone monitor available on your delivery unit? If not, where is the nearest available monitor and person trained in its use?

Discussion

Definition of DKA

Diabetic ketoacidosis (DKA), although preventable, remains a frequent and life-threatening complication of type 1 diabetes. DKA is a complex, disordered metabolic state characterised by the biochemical triad of:

1. Ketonaemia >3.0 mmol/l or ketonuria >2+ on urine dipstick
2. Hyperglycaemia > 11.0 mmol/l or known diabetes
3. Acidaemia (bicarbonate <15.0 mmol/l and/or pH <7.3).

DKA in Pregnancy

DKA in pregnancy poses specific challenges. It remains a significant clinical problem in spite of improvements in antenatal diabetes care. Mortality rates have fallen significantly in the last 20 years but DKA in pregnancy continues to result in significant morbidity and mortality for both the mother and fetus. Maternal mortality is now less than 1% and is usually related to severe hypokalaemia, adult respiratory distress syndrome and comorbid states such as sepsis. The fetal mortality associated with DKA ranges between 9% and 36%. The fetal effects are related to maternal dehydration and acidosis with reduced uteroplacental perfusion.

Aetiology

DKA usually develops as a consequence of absolute or relative insulin deficiency accompanied by increased counter-regulatory hormones. These changes enhance hepatic gluconeogenesis and glycogenolysis resulting in severe hyperglycaemia. Enhanced lipolysis increases serum-free fatty acids which are then metabolised as an alternative energy source in the process of ketogenesis. This results in the accumulation of large quantities of ketone bodies and subsequent metabolic acidosis.

DKA has traditionally been considered to be indicative, or even diagnostic, of type 1 diabetes, but cases in ketone-prone type 2 diabetes and gestational diabetes are increasingly being recognised. The initial treatment is the same. Pregnancy is associated with physiological changes including respiratory alkalosis and insulin resistance that can predispose a pregnant woman with any form of diabetes to DKA.

Clinical Presentation

DKA is more common in the second and third trimesters because of increased insulin resistance, but may be the first presentation of diabetes. DKA in pregnancy can also be precipitated by corticosteroid treatment, hyperemesis, infections, insulin non-compliance or pump failure, and starvation. β_2-agonists can also stimulate gluconeogenesis, glycogenolysis and lipolysis leading to hyperglycaemia and ketosis. Recognition of the condition that precipitates DKA is essential for its management. An elevated white cell count is commonly observed in DKA, but is often secondary to dehydration rather than infection.

Common presenting symptoms and signs of DKA in pregnancy include:

- nausea/vomiting,
- abdominal pain,
- dry mucous membranes,
- hyperventilation with ketotic breath,
- hypotension,
- polydipsia,
- polyuria,
- tachycardia,
- muscle weakness,
- blurred vision,
- altered consciousness,
- abnormal CTG.

Euglycaemic diabetic ketoacidosis is not uncommon in pregnancy and should not be forgotten when glucose levels are not particularly raised. Improved patient education with increased blood glucose and ketone monitoring has also led to partial treatment of DKA prior to admission, resulting in lower blood glucose levels at presentation.

Management

The most important initial therapeutic intervention in DKA is appropriate fluid replacement followed by insulin administration.

283

IV Fluids

The main aims for fluid replacement are:

- restoration of circulatory volume,
- clearance of ketones,
- correction of electrolyte imbalance.

Fluid depletion in DKA occurs secondary to several mechanisms:

- osmotic diuresis due to hyperglycaemia,
- vomiting,
- as DKA progresses – inability to take in fluid due to a diminished level of consciousness.

Fluid replacement with isotonic saline should be commenced immediately as most patients have a negative fluid balance of about 100 ml/kg of body weight. Assuming a systolic blood pressure greater than 90 mmHg, initial fluid resuscitation should be with normal saline 1000 ml over 1 h, then 500 ml/h for 4 h.

Particular attention needs to be paid to fluid replacement in:

- pregnancy,
- young adults aged 18–25 (higher risk of cerebral oedema in DKA),
- renal failure,
- cardiac failure.

Triggers for DKA

It is important that the precipitating factor for the DKA is sought and treated concurrently:

- protracted vomiting,
- hyperemesis gravidarum,
- starvation,
- infections,
- non-compliance with insulin therapy,
- Medications: e.g. sympathomimetics or corticosteroids,
- subcutaneous insulin pump failure,
- other conditions such as gastroparesis.

IV Insulin Infusion and Biochemical Monitoring of Patient with DKA

A fixed-rate intravenous insulin infusion should be administered (FRIII), calculated on 0.1 units per kilogram body weight per hour; for example, a 70 kg woman would receive 7 units of insulin per hour. The initial rate of insulin should not exceed 14 units per hour (Joint British Diabetes Society Inpatient Care Group, 2017).

Biochemical Monitoring

CBG, blood ketones, potassium and bicarbonate need to be monitored regularly to assess progress and adjust therapy in DKA (see Table 34.1). If these treatment targets are not achieved, then the FRIII rate should be increased. This is more likely to be necessary in insulin-resistant states such as pregnancy.

It is also often necessary to administer an intravenous infusion of 10% glucose in order to avoid hypoglycaemia and permit the continuation of a FRIII to suppress ketogenesis. Introduction of 10% glucose at 125 ml/h is recommended when the blood glucose falls below 14.0 mmol/l. It is important to continue normal saline fluid resuscitation to correct the circulatory volume. It may be necessary to infuse these solutions concurrently.

Hyperkalaemia and hypokalaemia are both common in DKA and need particular attention. Serum potassium is often high on admission (although total body potassium is low), but may fall precipitously upon treatment with insulin. Regular monitoring is mandatory. The patient may be severely dehydrated on presentation and is at risk of acute kidney injury; therefore, the British Joint Diabetes Societies' guidelines recommend that the initial resuscitative fluid is without potassium. Subsequent IV fluid replacement should then be with potassium-containing fluids: normal saline with potassium 40 mmol/l as long as the serum potassium level is below 5.5 mmol/l and the patient is passing urine.

Table 34.1 Biochemical monitoring and recommended treatment targets in DKA.

Biochemical parameter	Frequency of monitoring during DKA	Recommended treatment targets in DKA
CBG	Hourly	Reduction by 3.0 mmol per hour
Blood ketones	Hourly	Reduction by 0.5 mmol/l per hour
pH, bicarbonate, serum K+	At 1 hour, 2 hours and 4 hours	Increase in venous bicarbonate by 3.0 mmol/l per hour Maintain K+ at 4.0–5.5 mmol/l
Plasma electrolytes	4 hourly	

Resolution of DKA

The resolution of DKA depends upon the suppression of ketonaemia.

Resolution of DKA is defined as:

- pH > 7.3
- bicarbonate > 15.0 mmol/l
- blood ketone level < 0.6 mmol/l.

The fixed-rate infusion can be discontinued following DKA resolution and 30 min after the first dose of subcutaneous rapid-acting insulin is administered with a meal.

Continuation of subcutaneous long-acting basal insulin analogues during the initial management of DKA provides background insulin when the intravenous insulin is discontinued. This avoids rebound hyperglycaemia when intravenous insulin is stopped.

Normalisation of fetal heart tracing after correction of DKA may require 4–8 hours. There is no consensus on further fetal monitoring after complete resolution of DKA.

The specialist inpatient diabetes team must be involved in any patient presenting with DKA – UK guidance recommends by 24 hours after presentation, ideally even earlier. The diabetes specialist team will advise on management of the DKA episode and management of the patient's diabetes once the DKA episode has resolved. They will also counsel the patient regarding potential precipitating causes and early warning symptoms of DKA. They will also educate the patient on prevention of recurrence of DKA.

Bibliography

Joint British Diabetes Societies Inpatient Care Group. (2013). The Management of Diabetic Ketoacidosis in Adults; Second Edition; Update. Available from: www.diabetologists-abcd.org.uk/JBDS/JBDS.htm

(2017). Management of glycaemic control in pregnant women with diabetes on obstetric wards and delivery units. Available from: www.diabetologists-abcd.org.uk/JBDS/JBDS.htm

Kamalakannan, D., Baskar, V., Barton, D. M. and Abdu, T. A. M. (2003). Diabetic ketoacidosis in pregnancy. *Postgraduate Medical Journal*, 79, 454–457.

Mohan, M., Baagar, K. A. M. and Lindow, S. (2017). Management of diabetic ketoacidosis in pregnancy. *The Obstetrician & Gynaecologist*, 19, 55–62.

National Institute for Health and Clinical Excellence. (2015). Diabetes in pregnancy: management from preconception to the postnatal period.

Chapter

Subarachnoid Haemorrhage in the Postpartum Patient

Craig Carroll and Daniel Holsgrove

Scenario in a Nutshell

Postpartum headache and seizure from subarachnoid haemorrhage.

Stage 1: Fitting patient with prior history of headache immediately after delivery 3 days ago (negative septic screen/normal CT scan/negative lumbar puncture).

Stage 2: Fit stops with appropriate dose anti-convulsant therapy, proceeds to have respiratory compromise and no improvement in conscious level.

Stage 3: Sedation, intubation, ventilation, neuro-protective strategies and plan to transfer for CT scan.

Target Learner Groups

All members of the multidisciplinary obstetric team: anaesthetists, midwives, obstetricians, operating department practitioners/anaesthetic nurses and neurosurgical MDT.

Specific learning opportunities
Initial assessment and management of the acutely fitting patient
Differential diagnosis for postnatal seizure
Knowledge of neuroprotective strategies

Suggested learners (to represent their normal roles)	In the room from the start	Available when requested
Anaesthetic CT2/ST3+		√
Obstetric ST1–2/ST3+		√
Midwife Coordinator		√
Midwife responding to emergency	√	
Operating Department Practitioner (ODP)/ anaesthetic nurse		√
Neurosurgical registrar (if not available, a list of essential information will be provided)		√

Suggested learners (to represent their normal roles)	In the room from the start	Available when requested
Suggested facilitators		
Faculty member to play role of midwife who is performing the discharge of the patient when she starts fitting (facilitator must know all of the scenario summary information)	√	

Details for Facilitators

Patient Demographics

Name: Helen

Age: 34

Gestation: 3 days postpartum

Booking weight: 65 kg

Parity: P1

Scenario Summary for Facilitators

34-year-old, now P1 patient, who is 3 days post normal vaginal delivery following induction of labour for post dates (term +11 days).

Initial history relates to her delivery 3 days ago.

During labour, she had a lumbar epidural (uneventful insertion and provided good analgesia). There was no postpartum bleeding or ongoing obstetric concerns.

She commenced breastfeeding immediately after delivery, but developed a severe frontal headache in the hour after delivery. It was constant with no postural element or photophobia.

There were no neurological signs identified at this time, she had mildly raised blood pressure (140/80) with no proteinuria. Antenatal BP had been stable at 118/75 mmHg, with no proteinuria. All bloods, including PET bloods, were normal.

Due to the ongoing headache, she was discussed with the neurology team who suggested a septic screen

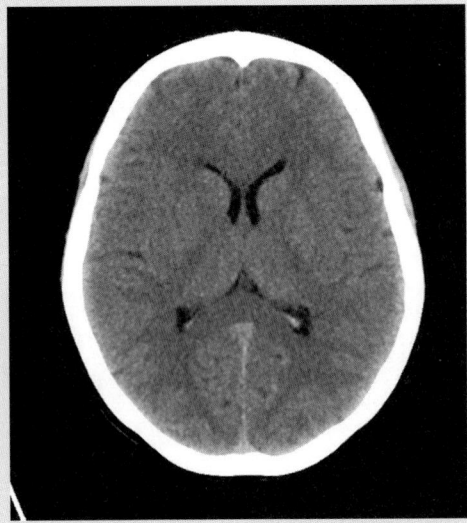

Figure 35.1 Normal CT head (image link https://radiopaedia .org/cases/normal-brain-ct).

(although CNS infection was felt to be unlikely). A CT brain was also performed two hours after onset, which showed no intracranial pathology (see Figure 35.1). The lumbar puncture was normal with no organisms on Gram stain, 5 red cells and no xanthochromia.

The headache improved significantly, she was mobilising well and she was due to be discharged later in the afternoon of day 3.

Current presenting complaint – on the afternoon of day 3, when the scenario starts.

The patient is being discharged from the ward by the midwife when she complains of headache and then collapses, becomes unresponsive then has a seizure.

The seizure terminates when appropriate anticonvulsant agents are administered. She remains unresponsive and becomes increasingly hypertensive and bradycardic with unequal pupils. She requires sedation, intubation, ventilation and institution of neuroprotective strategies while arranging for a CT scan and referral to neurosurgery. During the scenario differential diagnosis for the headache and seizure to be considered include:

1. eclampsia,
2. post dural puncture headache and acute subdural haematoma,
3. cerebral sinus thrombosis,
4. meningitis,
5. *de novo* epilepsy,
6. pituitary apoplexy,
7. acute intraparenchymal haemorrhage.

The actual pathology is a large subarachnoid haemorrhage resulting in acute interference with cerebral perfusion, seizure and loss of consciousness. She then develops acute hydrocephalus as a result of the blood load.

Her reduced GCS is a combination of:

1. acute disturbance of cerebral blood flow,
2. the resulting seizure,
3. the acute hydrocephalus causing potentially lethal rise in intracranial pressure (ICP), and
4. the mass effect generated by the intracranial blood load.

Set-up Overview for Facilitators

Clinical setting	Bed on postnatal ward
Patient position	Lying flat in bed having a generalised tonic clonic seizure
Initial monitoring in place	Nil monitoring
Other equipment	Any equipment normally available in postnatal ward
Useful manikin functions	Seizure Trismus Pupil dilatation Intubation

Medical Equipment

For core equipment checklist, see Chapter 9.

Additional equipment specific to scenario		
Arterial line	Pen torch	Tendon hammer
Midazolam	Magnesium (in case treat as PET)	Drugs for intubation
Lorazepam	Labetalol	
Mannitol	Hydralazine	

Information Given to the Learners

Emergency buzzer pulled and SBAR handover given by midwife in the postnatal bay (faculty)

Time: 11:00
SBAR handover given to the attending emergency team consisting of other responding midwives/obstetricians (anaesthetist not present until stage 2).
Situation: This patient is having a seizure.
Background: She is not known to suffer from epilepsy. 34 years old, P1 patient, who is 3 days post normal vaginal delivery following induction of labour for post maturity. No issues at delivery. Epidural during labour. She is a delayed discharge on account of headaches, but they had resolved and the patient was being discharged home. She became acutely distressed, clutched her head in pain and then collapsed.
Assessment: I performed observations just before she became symptomatic – SpO$_2$ 98%, RR 15 bpm, HR 80, BP 120/75. Since the seizure I have called for help immediately.
Recommendation: Can you help manage this patient?

Scenario Schedule

Stage 1: Fitting patient with prior history of headache immediately after delivery 3 days ago (negative septic screen / normal CT scan)	
Information given	**Expected actions**
Patient is having generalised tonic clonic seizure Lying supine on the postnatal bed	Commence ABCDE approach
	Call for senior midwifery, obstetric and anaesthetic help
	Keep patient safe Position in left lateral position
Jaw clenched A Guedel airway cannot be inserted at this time If a nasal airway is passed there is bleeding into the airway	Apply Oxygen via non-rebreathing mask at 15L/min, and support the airway as much as possible
	Apply monitoring
CBG 8mmol/L	Secure IV access Check all bloods including PET bloods, FBC, U+E, LFT, clotting, Magnesium, CBG (capillary blood glucose at bedside)
	Locate emergency resuscitation trolley
Further information given based on explored differential diagnosis: Eclampsia – pre seizure BP normal, normal PET bloods Hypoglycaemic – CBG 8mmol/L Epilepsy – not known to have Epidural complication – no evidence sepsis. Headache but no postural element, frontal in location with no photophobia CNS infection – mild temperature noted post-ictal, bloods NAD, no reported neck stiffness	Consider causes for seizure
Progress to stage 2 once initial assessment completed, blood sugar checked and differential diagnosis considered.	

Observations	
A	Jaw clench, no added noises
B	RR 40/min
	SpO$_2$ not recording
C	HR 130bpm
	BP 140/110
	CRT 1s
D	AVP**U**
E	Temp 37.4°C

Stage 2: Fit stops with appropriate dose anticonvulsant therapy, proceeds to have respiratory compromise and no improvement in conscious level

Information given	Expected Actions
Anaesthetist arrives	
The seizure will only terminate once the patient receives anticonvulsant medication (of the correct dose)	Acute seizure management ideally benzodiazepine, but depends upon what drugs are available (propofol, barbiturate are acceptable)
If magnesium is administered, this will have no effect on seizure activity	
Following appropriate anticonvulsant, patient stops fitting.	Once seizure free – reassess ABCDE
Breathing obstructed / noisy. Slow respiratory rate. Chest examination normal percussion, difficult to auscultate as transmitted upper airway noises but nil obvious added sounds	Airway / Breathing assessment Support ventilation with bag valve mask ventilation
Hypertensive. ECG monitor shows cardiovascular abnormality, periods of bradycardia and junctional rhythm	Circulation assessment
GCS 5: Eyes – closed to any stimulus 1, Motor score- extending to pain 2, Voice – incomprehensible groaning 2 Pupils dilated but reactive to light	GCS assessment Confirm patient not protecting airway, necessity to intubate and ventilate patient
	Consider causes of low GCS: Post ictal Anticonvulsant drugs Intracranial pathology
Although normoglycaemia confirmed in stage 1, a second blood sugar test is considered excellent practice (evidence exists of normoglycaemia recordings in hypoglycaemic patients owing to sugar on finger at time of testing)	Recheck blood sugar
Morning blood results Hb 102g/L WCC 12x10⁹/LNa 140 mmol/L K 4.3mmol/L Ur 4.5mmol/L Creatinine 50µmol/L Mg 0.8mmol/L	

Observations

A	Obstructed
B	RR 6/min
	SpO$_2$ 88% on air
	SpO$_2$ 97% with assisted ventilation and oxygen
C	HR 100bpm
	BP 210/110
	CRT 1s
D	AVP**U**
	GCS E1 M3 V2
E	Temp 37.0°C

Information given	Expected Actions
Team able to transfer to their chosen location eg theatres	Make arrangements to transfer to safe location with skilled assistance for sedation, intubation and ventilation
	Full monitoring with capnography, portable oxygen, assisted ventilation until intubated

Progress to stage 3 when seizures terminated and plans made for securing the airway and transfer

Stage 3: Sedation, intubation, ventilation, neuroprotective strategies and plan to transfer for CT scan

Information given	Expected actions
Theatre team present to receive patient	Arrive in safe location (eg theatres / recovery)
	Organise team (alert senior members if not already informed)
Grade 1 intubation	Safe sedation, paralysis and intubation It is essential to use induction agents and opiate to obtund cardiovascular response
	Insert arterial line
	Insert urinary catheter
	BP management to ensure appropriate Cerebral Perfusion Pressure (CPP= MAP-ICP)
Important the team do not attempt to achieve "normal BP" or to treat hypertension as for pre-eclamptic patients.	Measures to Reduce Cerebral Blood Volume Maintain normal $PaCO_2$ (pCO_2 4.5-5.0KPa) Head up with no venous constraints to reduce venous engorgement Reduction of Cerebral Metabolic Rate ($CMRO_2$) by avoiding seizure activity (which may not be seen on account of neuromuscular blockade) and ensuring appropriate levels of sedation Maintain normothermia Consider mannitol or hypertonic saline (Mannitol 0.5g/kg +/- Furosemide 0.5-1mg/kg to potentiate the effect of mannitol)
Signs of dangerously high ICP are now present; Dilated, unresponsive right pupil Severe hypertension Bradycardia	

Observations	
A	Intubated
B	RR as per ventilator setting
	SpO_2 98%
C	HR 50bpm
	BP 210/110
	CRT 2sec
D	Anaesthetised
E	Temp 37.0°C

291

Information given	Expected Actions
	Expect discussion of strategies to prevent secondary brain injury
	Organise urgent brain imaging The team need to identify the cause for deterioration with suitable imaging. An emergency plain CT Brain (CTB) is necessary (as delays with requesting CT angiogram or contrast CT and discussion with a neurosurgeon may introduce unacceptable delay)
ECG shows bradycardia with non-specific T wave changes (Figure 35.3)	ECG
	Organise rapid, safe transfer to radiology for CT Brain Full monitoring and trained transfer staff

ABG if requested

pH 7.30

pCO_2 6.1 kPa

pO_2 45 kPa

BE -5 mmol/L

Lactate 3 mmol/L

Hb 102 g/L

CBG 9 mmol/L

If the team elect to perform a lumbar puncture without having an up to date CTB, patient would be at risk of acute cerebellar tonsillar herniation through the foramen magnum

Main differential diagnosis to consider:

1. Subarachnoid haemorrhage
2. Intracerebral bleed
3. Cerebral venous thrombosis
4. Acute subdural haematoma
5. Pituitary apoplexy
6. de novo epilepsy
7. Intracranial infection
8. Hypoglycaemia
9. Eclampsia

Scenario ends once the patient is intubated, ventilated, neuroprotective strategies are in place and a decision has been made to transfer to CT scan.

The **CT Brain (CTB) (Figure 35.2)** shows extensive blood volume occupying the basal cisterns suggesting aneurysmal Subarachnoid haemorrhage with concomitant acute hydrocephalus.

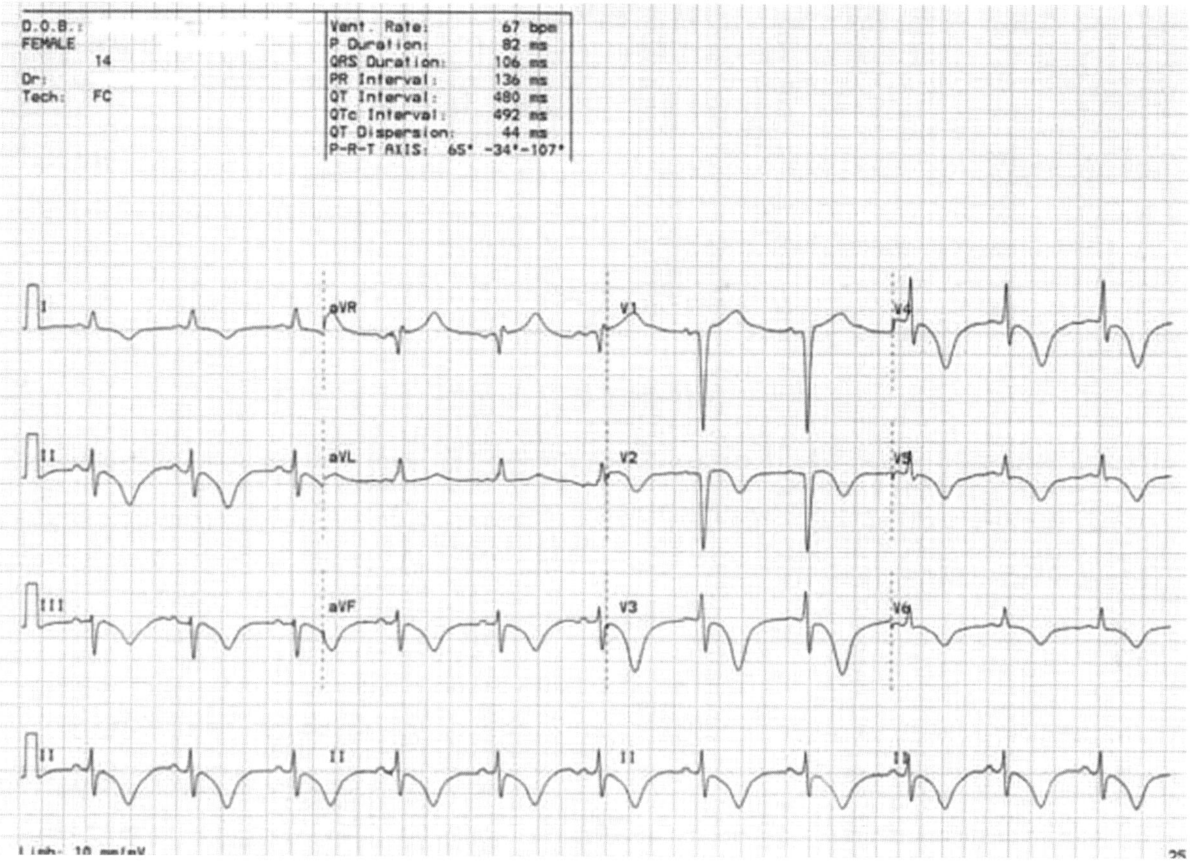

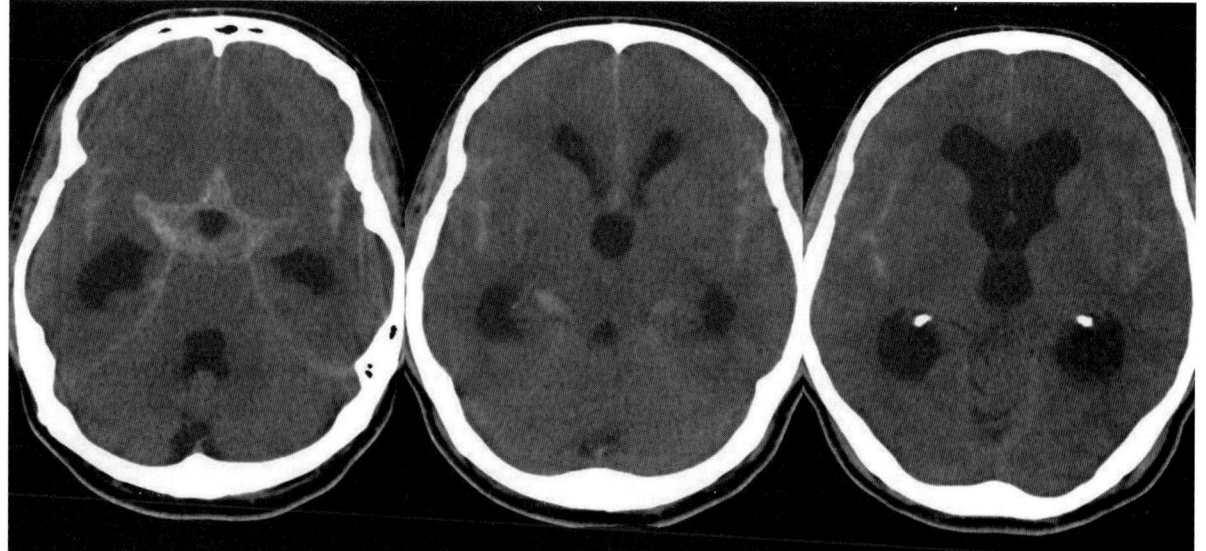

Figure 35.2 ECG. Non-specific T-wave changes associated with acute aneurysmal SAH.

Figure 35.3 CT head – series shows large blood load in the basal cisterns with blood in both Sylvian Fissures, with blood also overlying the tentorium cerebellae. The lateral ventricles are enlarged as are the temporal horns, the third and fourth ventricles. This is a classic appearance of extensive subarachoid bleeding with resultant acute hydrocephalus.

Suggested Topics for Debrief Discussion

- What causes for the seizure were going through your mind?
- How confident would you be managing prolonged seizure activity?
- What were your considerations for neuroprotective strategies?

Discussion

Aneurysmal subarachnoid haemorrhage (aSAH) can affect the obstetric population. The classical presentation of acute severe headache is not diagnostic; however, aSAH has to be seriously considered if a patient complains of a sudden-onset severe headache. Other presenting features of aSAH include vomiting, loss of consciousness or sudden death.

Cerebral aneurysms can be associated with other conditions: connective tissue diseases (Marfan's syndrome, Ehlers–Danlos syndrome, fibromuscular dysplasia), familiar polycystic kidney disease, coarctation of the aorta and intracranial arteriovenous malformations. A strong family history of aSAH should also alert the clinician to aSAH as a differential diagnosis.

The initial presentation depends upon the extent of the bleeding and how this impacts upon cerebral perfusion. Classic teaching states that a third of patients who suffer an acute subarachnoid bleed will die at the time of the bleed, a third will go on to suffer considerable complications and a final third will make a good recovery.

If the bleed is extensive, then intracranial pressure (ICP) may approximate mean arterial pressure (MAP) and hence arrest cerebral blood flow. (Cerebral perfusion pressure (CPP) = MAP – ICP.) This may account for the immediate loss of consciousness and high incidence of sudden death. Brain tissue that has been exposed to hypoxic or traumatic insult is at risk of swelling. The presence of any swelling or blood clot within the brain can add mass effect, increasing ICP and reducing CSF drainage. A reduction in conscious level and subsequent hypoventilation can lead to a rise in arterial CO_2, causing cerebral vasodilatation and further raise in ICP. The primary cerebral insult will also disrupt the normal protective autoregulatory mechanisms of cerebral perfusion and as such, cerebral blood flow will be dependent on MAP. Cardiac function can also be affected, with 30% of patients suffering

aSAH developing acute left ventricular dysfunction. Damage to brain homeostasis causes membrane instability which can precipitate seizures, further increasing cerebral metabolic demands.

Haemorrhage within the subarachnoid space can disrupt normal CSF physiology in the following ways:

1. inhibition of flow through the ventricular system,
2. inhibition of absorption of CSF in the arachnoid villae,
3. a combination of the two effects.

Following a primary bleed, there is high risk of rebleeding which is associated with high morbidity/mortality. It is therefore important to:

- recognise the urgency of the clinical situation,
- adopt neuroprotective strategies,
- seek expert opinion as to ongoing care.

Both aSAH and pre-eclampsia must be considered as differential diagnosis in patients with acute onset of headache in the obstetric population; it is vitally important to consider the differences in treatment that the two conditions require. In the acute setting of an intracranial bleed, immediate BP control to normality may be detrimental to cerebral blood flow and result in worsening of the acute brain injury.

Neuroprotective Strategies

1. *Reduce engorgement of the intracranial venous system.* It is important to facilitate venous drainage. Simple measures include: head-up tilt of 15–20° and avoidance of tight ligature effects of endotracheal tube ties. PEEP is unlikely to affect ICP significantly.
2. *Optimisation of cerebral perfusion.* Acknowledging that autoregulation is lost, the clinician should consider allowing permissive hypertension, as the reflex hypertension may reflect a requirement for such a pressure to overcome the effects of intracranial hypertension. The transducer for an arterial line should be at the level of the tragus.
3. *Reduce cerebral blood volume.* High $PaCO_2$ results in cerebral vasodilatation, causing increased intracranial blood volume and resultant increased ICP. Moderate hyperventilation will reduce the ICP. Be aware, however, that extreme hyperventilation ($PaCO_2 < 4$ kPa) will result in cerebral hypoperfusion and risk global cerebral hypoperfusion.
4. *Avoid cerebral vasodilatory medication*, e.g. GTN.

5. *Reduce brain volume* by the use of osmotic agents. Mannitol and hypertonic saline have been used as rescue agents when ICP is dangerously high – they may be indicated when there is a risk of 'coning' and on the advice of the Neurosurgical team when the patient is at particular risk of continued rise in ICP before emergency procedures can be performed.

6. *Reduce cerebral metabolic demands.* Anticonvulsant therapy is of great importance, and standard seizure management should be considered, including the use of benzodiazepines. Further seizure control can be achieved using valproate, levetiracetam or phenytoin. In the context of ongoing seizure, agents that are available in the obstetric setting (propofol, thiopentone) may be the appropriate ones to use. Drugs and doses used for seizure control: lorazepam (IV) 0.1 mg/kg, midazolam (IV) 0.2 mg/kg. The dose of thiopentone or propofol necessary to terminate seizures is likely to require the clinician to support the airway and possibly provide ventilator support.

Avoidance of hyperthermia is also important, as is glycaemic control.

The Emergency of the Situation

In this scenario, the patient is developing acute hydrocephalus and potentially lethal intracranial hypertension as a result.

Any of the neuroprotective strategies are only temporising measures and all effort must be made to minimise delay in diagnosing the cause of the initial deterioration and transfer to the neurosurgical theatre for immediate CSF drainage (with possible additional therapies of clot evacuation or decompressive craniectomy).

Effective communication between the care team, radiology and the receiving neurosurgical team (including receiving anaesthetic staff) is essential. 'Time is neurones' in this context! The team must work effectively, with delegation of specific roles to minimise time taken to perform tasks such as arterial cannulation and urinary catheterisation.

Arterial line insertion allows reliable $PaCO_2$ measurement (to guide ventilation) and real-time evaluation of MAP and hence an estimate of cerebral perfusion pressure. (In an unconscious patient with acute brain injury, estimate that ICP is in excess of 20 mmHg.) A urinary catheter may be appropriate (again if it incurs no delay), especially if administering osmotherapy (mannitol). There is very little to be gained (if anything) from central venous catheter insertion. Efforts should be made to expedite a safe transfer and avoid distraction from non-essential technical tasks that require skill, equipment and take valuable time. The staff facilitating transfer need to be aware of the time-dependent nature of the situation, and hence effective communication is paramount.

Cardiac Complications

Thirty per cent of patients suffering aSAH develop acute left ventricular dysfunction. This can present with acute respiratory and cardiovascular compromise, including acute pulmonary oedema. Negative pressure pulmonary oedema can also occur in this setting in the fitting patient who makes strong respiratory effort against a closed glottis or obstructed airway. Treatment by IPPV with additional PEEP should be considered.

ECG findings in aSAH commonly demonstrate diffuse T-wave changes that do not correspond to coronary vascular territory and may be as a result of high concentrations of catecholamines being secreted over the myocardium during the acute bleed period. Vascular territory changes are seen less frequently.

Conclusion

This scenario requires consideration of both obstetric and non-obstetric causes for headache, hypertension and reduction in conscious level. It requires a coordinated, goal-directed team approach to provide initial resuscitation, situation control, diagnosis and subsequent management, in order to efficiently prevent secondary complications. Treatment of this patient in a way designed to treat eclampsia would be very likely to result in a rapid decline in the patient's condition, with resultant coning and brain death.

Bibliography

MacLennan, K., O'Brien, K. and Macnab, W. R. (Eds.). (2015). *Core Topics in Obstetric Anaesthetics.* Cambridge: Cambridge University Press.

Nolan, J. and Soar, J. (Eds.). (2012). *Anaesthesia for Emergency Care.* Oxford Specialist Handbook. Oxford: Oxford University Press.

Obstetric Trauma

36

John Butler

Scenario in a Nutshell

Obstetric trauma with injury to chest, abdomen and pelvis.
    Stage 1: A front-seat passenger in a road traffic accident (RTA) arrives in A+E, haemodynamically compromised and in pain (left chest, left hip and abdomen).
    Stage 2: Haemodynamically compromised despite resuscitation secondary to splenic laceration and pelvic fracture.
    Stage 3: Maternal and fetal deterioration secondary to massive haemorrhage. Requires transfer to theatre for emergency laparotomy, pelvic fracture management and caesarean section.

Target Learner Groups

All members of the multidisciplinary obstetric team: anaesthetists, midwives, obstetricians. All members of the multidisciplinary A+E emergency team.

Specific learning opportunities
Recognise the importance of a structured handover in trauma
Understand the modifications of management in trauma for obstetric population
Consideration of teams to be called
Orientation to where obstetric emergency equipment is in your A+E department (delivery packs/drugs/checklists)
Specific skills able to be incorporated
• Manual uterine displacement • Chest drain insertion • Intubation with in-line stabilisation • FAST scan performance and interpretation

Suggested learners (to represent their normal roles)	In the room from the start	Available when requested
Anaesthetic ST3+	√	
Operating Department Practitioner (ODP)/ anaesthetic nurse	√	
Obstetric ST3+		√

Suggested learners (to represent their normal roles)	In the room from the start	Available when requested
Midwife		√
Surgical trauma team (as many as can attend)	√	
A+E trauma team (as many as can attend)	√	
Trauma team leader	√	
Neonatal team		√
Suggested facilitators		
Faculty to play role of lead paramedic	√	

Details for Facilitators

Patient Demographics

Name: Jessie

Age: 24

Gestation: 30

Booking weight: 58 kg

Parity: P0

Scenario Summary for Facilitators

Patient in RTA. Car vs. van. Patient front-seat passenger (not wearing seatbelt) in a car T-boned by a van at 50 mph. Impact to passenger side. Airbags deployed. Paramedics report significant intrusion into front-seat passenger side of car. Passenger was extricated from vehicle by Fire crew and Paramedics. Spinal immobilisation maintained during extrication. Patient conscious throughout.
The Paramedic crew send a pre-alert trauma call through control.
Scenario starts when patient arrives in A+E with AT-MIST-structured handover.
Haemodynamically compromised, with severe pain in left side of chest, abdomen and left hip.

Injuries sustained include simple left-sided pneumothorax, splenic laceration and pelvic fracture. Haemorrhagic shock, which initially responds to fluid resuscitation but then patient deteriorates.

Scenario ends with agreement for transfer to theatre for laparotomy, pelvic fracture management and caesarean section.

Other simulated blood components	O-negative blood	Chest drain kit	External pelvic binder
Drugs Tranexamic acid Anaesthetic drugs box	Arterial line	Pen torch	

Set-up Overview for Facilitators

Clinical setting	In A+E resuscitation bay
Patient position	Supine, on trolley, on spinal board with cervical collar and head straps
Initial monitoring in place	Pulse oximetry NIBP cuff ECG
Other equipment	Oxygen 15 l via non-rebreathe mask No IV access
Useful manikin features	Abnormal breath sounds (pneumothorax)

Medical Equipment

For core equipment checklist see Chapter 9.

Additional equipment specific to scenario			
Spinal board	Hard collar	Blocks/ tape	Rapid fluid infusor

Information Given to the Learners

Handover by lead paramedic to assembled emergency team

AT-MIST handover (see Chapter 8 for reference).

Age: 24-year-old, 30 weeks pregnant.

Time of injury: 17:10 (30 minutes ago).

Mechanism of injury: Car vs. van. Front-seat passenger (not wearing seatbelt) in a car T-boned by a van at 50 mph. Impact to passenger side. Airbags deployed.

Injuries sustained: Left-sided chest, abdomen and hip. Abdominal distension and tenderness.

Signs/symptoms: Airway patent, SpO$_2$ 93%, RR 35, HR 120 bpm, BP 80/40 mmHg, GCS 15, moving all 4 limbs, in pain.

Treatment: 15 l O$_2$, c-spine collar and spinal board.

Scenario Schedule

Stage 1: A front seat passenger in road traffic accident (RTA) arrives in A+E, haemodynamically compromised and in pain (left chest, left hip and abdomen)

Trauma team start assessment after AT MIST handover.

Observations		Information given	Expected actions
A	Clear		Commence ABCDE approach to patient
B	RR 35/min SpO$_2$ 90% on air (96% with O$_2$)	Patient shouting out with pain all down left side of abdomen and left hip, severe pain in groin on moving left leg	
C	HR 120bpm BP 80/40 CRT 4s		Team to apply full monitoring whilst assessment on going
		Airway clear	**A.** Perform airway assessment with spinal immobilisation
D	**A**VPU GCS 15/15		Apply 15L/min oxygen via non-rebreathing mask until stabilised then titrated oxygen to SpO$_2$ 94-98%
E	Temp 36.0°C		

Information given	Expected actions
	Maintain spinal alignment at all times (high risk of spinal injury). Alleviate aortocaval compression. Turn patient to left lateral position on spinal board. (If this is not possible, apply manual uterine displacement)
	Call for emergency obstetric and neonatal teams
Right side chest all normal. Left side chest, decreased chest expansion, decreased breath sounds, percussion note resonant. Trachea central	**B.** Assess breathing and ventilation
	Consider diagnosis of simple pneumothorax and discuss need and timing for intercostal chest drain (as stable likely confirm diagnosis on scan)
Heart sounds normal and clear Pregnant abdomen, no PV blood loss Left leg shortening Bruising on left side of chest and abdomen	**C.** Assess circulation with haemorrhage control Look for signs of haemorrhage. (Chest/ Abdo/Pelvis/ Long Bones/ per vaginal (PV))
	Diagnose shock - likely haemorrhagic
	Secure 2x large bore IV access Take blood for FBC, U+E, LFT, Coagulation including fibrinogen and X match, VBG.
VBG result pH 7.22 pO_2 4.4kPa pCO_2 4.6kPa BE -12mmol/L Lactate 6.3mmol/L Hb 87g/L Gluc 6.8mmol/L	
	Stop external haemorrhage. Consider pelvic binder in view of suspicion of pelvic fracture. Accept maybe difficult in pregnancy
	Activate major haemorrhage protocol
	Locate A+E obstetric emergency trolley (if unit has one)
	Commence 2 units 0-ve RBC, infused as per local policy

Observations at the end of stage 1	
A	Clear
B	RR 24/min-SpO$_2$ 96% on O$_2$
C	HR 110bpm BP 110/50 CRT 3s
D	**A**VPU
E	Temp 35.9°C

Information given	Expected actions
	Administer Tranexamic acid 1G IV (over 10 mins)
Pupils equal and reactive GCS 15 CBG 6.8mmol/L	**D.** Assess pupils, GCS, CBG
	Administer IV analgesia
	Keep patient warm
Bruising all down left side of chest and abdomen, nil obvious bleeding, no obvious injuries on back if log rolled	Expose patient and review all areas including back with log roll
	Repeat all observations

Progress to stage 2 once primary survey complete and initial resuscitation commenced.

Stage 2: Haemodynamically compromised despite resuscitation secondary to splenic laceration and pelvic fracture

Observations	
A	Clear
B	RR 29/min SpO$_2$ 96% on O$_2$
C	HR 130bpm BP 85/45 CRT 4s
D	A**V**PU
E	Temp 36.1°C (if patient warmed)

Information given	Expected actions
Obstetric, midwife and neonatal team arrive	
Patient initially responded to resuscitation but now becoming more drowsy, complaining of pain on left side of chest, abdomen and pelvis	Repeat ABCDE assessment following interventions made in stage 1
	Repeat all observations
Left upper abdomen very tender. Uterus feels normal for gestation. Not tender. No PV blood loss	Obstetrician to examine patient
Sonicaid fetal heart rate 160bpm. U/S fetal heart rate confirmed 160bpm, posterior placenta clear of os, no abnormalities seen	Fetal heart rate assessment. (U/S assessment if equipment available)
Physiological signs of ongoing haemorrhage. Patient clammy with cool shut down peripheries	
Massive haemorrhage Pack 1 arrives 4u RBC, 4U FFP	Continue to resuscitate patient with blood and blood products
	Send TEG/ROTEM
ABG result (if requested) pH 7.19 pCO$_2$ 4kPa pO$_2$ 18kPa BE -15mmol/L Lactate 8 mmol/L Hb 78g/l	Consider arterial line insertion Perform ABG

Information given	Expected actions
	Team to consider differential diagnosis for cause of haemorrhage: Intra-abdominal Long bone fracture Pelvic fracture Chest Uterine Consider best management for diagnosing – imaging vs surgery for suspected source of bleeding
	Consider initial FAST U/S scan v CT scan
	If not already present, inform obstetric and anaesthetic consultants

Progress to stage 3 once plans for imaging have been discussed

Observations	
A	Clear
B	RR 35/min SpO$_2$ 96% on O$_2$
C	HR 135bpm BP 78/35 CRT 5s
D	AV**V**PU
E	Temp 36.1°C (if patient warmed)

Stage 3: Maternal and fetal deterioration secondary to massive haemorrhage. Requires transfer to theatre for emergency laparotomy, pelvic fracture management and caesarean section.

Information given	Expected actions
Patient responding to voice – groaning in pain	Note deterioration in ABCDE assessment
Abdomen distending and greater swelling over pelvis.	Re-examine patient
	Repeat all observations
	Continue resuscitation with blood products
Emergency theatre is free and able to receive the case	Team discussion re need for urgent theatre, not scan, in view of deterioration Coordinate with theatre Team to arrange appropriate equipment and monitoring for transfer to theatre
	Liaise with blood bank for further blood components – guided by TEG/ROTEM
	Discuss plan to continue spinal immobilisation throughout transfer, anaesthesia, intubation and surgery
	Insertion of left sided chest drain if not already in place
	Surgical Plan: General surgeons for laparotomy Orthopaedics with radiology to image hip / pelvis in theatre Obstetricians for caesarean section with neonatologists for baby

301

Information given	Expected actions
	Discuss plan for further assessment including full body CT scan after haemostasis achieved in theatre.
	Need for full secondary survey
	Consideration of Maternal Blood group Rhesus status
	Insertion urinary catheter in theatre (if not already inserted)
Scenario ends when patient is ready for transfer to theatre with full monitoring in place	

Suggested Topics for Debrief Discussion

- How confident did you feel managing trauma in a pregnant patient?
- Was your environment appropriately equipped?
- Was the decision to transfer to scan or theatre easy?

Discussion

The worldwide incidence of injury is very significant, accounting for 12% of the world's burden of disease. According to the WHO, approximately 5.8 million people of all ages and economic groups die every year from unintentional injuries and violence. Road traffic injuries alone cause more than 1 million deaths annually and an estimated 20–50 million significant injuries. Injury-related deaths are expected to rise dramatically by 2020 when it is expected that 1 in 10 people will die from injuries.

Trauma in Pregnancy

Fortunately, the incidence of trauma in pregnancy is rare. Most mechanisms of injury are the same as for non-pregnant patients. However, there are important alterations in anatomy and physiology that can influence the evaluation of injured pregnant patients by altering the signs and symptoms of injury, the approach and response to resuscitation, and the interpretation of diagnostic tests. It is estimated that about 60% of blunt trauma in pregnancy is caused by RTCs (road traffic collisions), with 22% as a result of falls and 17% due to direct assaults (Shah and Kilcline, 2003). The abdominal wall, uterus and amniotic fluid act as a buffer to protect the fetus from injury; however,

fetal injury can still occur from direct impact to the abdominal wall from impact with a steering wheel or car dashboard. Indirect fetal trauma can be secondary to compression, deceleration or shearing forces, which can result in placental abruption. Unrestrained pregnant women in RTCs have a higher risk of premature delivery and fetal deaths compared with passengers wearing a seatbelt. The type of seatbelt worn appears to influence outcome. Lap belts alone allow flexion and uterine compression with the risk of uterine rupture and abruption. If the belt is too high then force may be applied directly to the uterus on impact. Evidence suggests that the traditional three-point seatbelts reduce the risk of injury to the greatest degree. Interestingly there appears to be no greater risk to the mother or fetus from airbag deployment in RTCs. As the pregnancy progresses the uterus increases in size, making it more likely to be injured during penetrating trauma. The uterine musculature, amniotic fluid and fetus can all act to slow any penetrating missiles and also reduce the incidence of injury to other organs in the mother. Consequently, this low incidence of extrauterine maternal organ injury generally leads to good maternal outcomes from penetrating trauma. Unfortunately, this is not the same for the developing fetus, where there is a high incidence of reported injury in these rare cases.

Adaptations in Pregnancy

Pregnancy results in significant changes both physiologically and anatomically. It is important to be aware of these adaptations when assessing a pregnant trauma patient.

For expected physiological changes in pregnancy, see Chapter 9.

Uterine adaptations: The uterus remains an intra-pelvic organ until 12 weeks of gestation. It is a thick-walled structure at this stage. By week 20 it is at the level of the umbilicus, with the small fetus protected by its own copious amniotic fluid. However, this fluid can give rise to amniotic fluid emboli if it enters the maternal circulation. The uterus reaches the costal margin by about 34 weeks. At this stage, the uterus is large and relatively thin-walled. As the fetal head engages the uterus drops slightly. With the head engaged in the pelvis the remainder of the body sits above the pelvic brim. Pelvic fractures in the third trimester can result in fetal skull fractures and intracranial injury. The placenta is a relatively inelastic structure and significant shear forces can lead to a placental abruption. In addition, the placenta is very sensitive to endogenous catecholamine stimulation. As a consequence, any catecholamine production in response to maternal haemorrhage can lead to increases in uterine vascular resistance and reductions in fetal oxygen delivery, even in the presence of normal maternal vital signs.

Approach to the Pregnant Trauma Patient

The initial approach to the pregnant trauma patient is the same as in a non-pregnant patient. However, the treating team need to remember that there are two patients (or maybe even more) to manage. It is the type and severity of the maternal injuries that determine outcome for both mother and child. Fortunately, the best treatment for the fetus is to resuscitate and optimise the treatment of the mother. It is prudent to consult with a senior obstetrician and anaesthetist at an early stage when these patients present to the ED.

Trauma teams should focus the initial assessment and resuscitation on the mother followed by an assessment of the fetus. During the primary survey and resuscitation, as with non-pregnant adult trauma, ensure a patent airway, adequate ventilation and effective circulatory volume. The initial ABCDE approach recommended by ATLS is:

A Airway maintenance with cervical spine protection
B Breathing with ventilation
C Circulation with haemorrhage control
D Disability: neurological status
E Exposure/environment.

Some points to remember when managing the pregnant trauma patient include the following.

- Oxygen consumption is increased 20% in pregnancy, so ensure good oxygenation.
- Delayed gastric emptying increases aspiration risk.
- Difficult intubation is more likely – call anaesthetic help early.
- In the supine position, uterine compression of the vena cava can reduce cardiac output by 30%, owing to a reduction in venous return. To avoid this, displace the uterus manually to the left side. If the patient is positioned on a spinal board, roll the board to the left (approx. 15°) and keep supported in this position. Spinal immobilisation should be maintained at all times, until the spine has been cleared clinically and, if necessary, radiologically.
- Pregnant patients demonstrate signs and symptoms of hypovolaemia LATE! Fetal circulation will be affected before maternal signs of compromise. The commonest cause of fetal death from trauma is maternal shock and maternal death. Do not delay maternal resuscitation.
- During maternal haemorrhage, early use of blood and blood products will be needed. Activation of, and adherence to, local major haemorrhage pathways will facilitate rapid resuscitation. Be aware, vasopressors can further reduce fetal blood flow.
- Dilatation of pelvic vessels can lead to significant retroperitoneal haemorrhage following a pelvic fracture.

Tranexamic Acid and Trauma

Many trauma centres in the UK are now using tranexamic acid (TXA) in the hospital phase of care as an adjunct to early haemorrhage control in order to improve trauma outcomes. At present, there is still only one large randomised clinical trial (Clinical Randomisation of an Antifibrinolytic in Significant Haemorrhage 2 (CRASH-2)) that examined the efficacy of in-hospital TXA in trauma and documented that all-cause mortality was reduced from 16.0% to 14.5% (1.5% absolute reduction, RR 0.91, 95% CI 0.91 (0.85 to 0.97), $p = 0.0035$, NNT 67) and risk of death caused by bleeding was reduced from 5.7% to 4.9% (0.8% reduction, NNT 121) (Shakur et al., 2010). Importantly, for bleeding deaths, early TXA treatment was better: TXA given ≤ 1 hour after injury was more protective than when given 1–3 hours after injury, and TXA given after 3 hours was associated with an increased risk of death. In the CRASH-2 subgroup analysis, the most significant mortality benefit for TXA was in the severe shock cohort, trauma patients with admission systolic blood pressure (SBP) ≤ 75 mmHg with 28-day all-cause mortality of 30.6% for TXA vs. 35.1% for placebo (RR 0.87, 99% CI 0.76 to 0.99). Administration doses of TXA should follow local policy.

Other Considerations

Placental abruption may be revealed, concealed (behind the placenta) or a mixture of both. It is associated with vaginal bleeding (70%), uterine tenderness, uterine contractions and irritability with a hard wooden consistency. Uterine ultrasound may be limited by pain and a normal ultrasound *cannot* exclude the diagnosis.

Uterine rupture is a rare injury associated with fetal compromise, abdominal tenderness, peritonism, abdominal fetal lie, or the palpation of fetal parts.

Feto-maternal haemorrhage can result in iso-immunisation if the mother is rhesus-negative. All Rh-negative mothers should be considered for Rh immunoglobulin therapy within 72 hours of injury.

Obstetric teams will guide the mode of fetal monitoring. Sonicaid/CTG/US may all be used and should be available; however, it should always be remembered that maternal resuscitation is the priority.

Appropriate imaging should be undertaken for the pregnant trauma patient, the benefits outweigh the risks to the fetus. Indications for CT, FAST scanning, are as for non-pregnant patients.

Perimortem caesarean section (PMCS) may be indicated in pregnant trauma patients who experience hypovolaemic cardiac arrest. It is more likely to be successful if performed within 4–5 minutes of the arrest. See Chapter 25 for further information on PMCS.

Bibliography

American College of Surgeons. (2012). *Advanced Trauma Life Support Course Manual, 9th edition*. Chicago, IL: American College of Surgeons.

Harris, T. (2012). Early fluid resuscitation in severe trauma. *British Medical Journal*, 345, e5752.

NICE. (2012). Evidence Summary: Significant haemorrhage following trauma: tranexamic acid.

(2016). Guidelines on Major Trauma: Assessment and Initial Management (NG39).

Shah, A. J. and Kilcline, B. A. (2003). Trauma in pregnancy. *Emergency Medicine Clinics of North America* 21, 615–629.

Shakur, H., Roberts, I., Bautista, R., et al. (2010). CRASH-2 trial collaborators. Effects of tranexamic acid on death, vascular occlusive events, and blood transfusion in trauma patients with significant haemorrhage (CRASH-2): a randomised, placebo-controlled trial. *Lancet*, 376, 23–32.

37

Newborn Life Support (Preterm Delivery)

Jonathan Hurst

Scenario in a Nutshell

This scenario focuses on the initial management and resuscitation of a preterm newborn infant and could be run simultaneously with some of the obstetric scenarios in other chapters.

Resuscitation and stabilisation of a significantly preterm infant prior to transfer to the neonatal intensive care unit (NICU) including newborn life support (NLS), consideration of thermoregulation, intubation and surfactant delivery.

Stage 1: Imminent delivery of preterm infant. Call to neonatal team and effective handover from maternity team. Checking of equipment and role allocation.

Stage 2: Delivery of the preterm infant, assessment regarding delayed cord clamping.

Stage 3a: Establishing thermoregulation and pulmonary gas exchange.

Stage 3b: (Only proceed to stage 3b if effective ventilation not achieved). Infant deteriorates, need to ensure effective inflation breaths.

Stage 4: Intubation, surfactant delivery and planning for transfer to NICU.

Target Learner Groups

Midwifery and neonatal teams.

Specific learning opportunities
Demonstrate knowledge of the Newborn Life Support (NLS) algorithm and effective NLS skills
Understand the special considerations for the preterm infant relating to thermoregulation and ventilatory support
Demonstrate effective team communication and handover of information

Suggested learners (to represent their normal roles)	In the room from the start	Available when requested
Midwife	√	
Midwife 2		√
Junior Neonatal Nurse		√
Senior Neonatal Nurse		√
Neonatal ST1–3/foundation doctor/junior trainee		√
Neonatal ST4+/registrar/senior trainee		√
Midwife Coordinator		√
Suggested facilitators		
Faculty to play role of baby's mother	√	
Faculty to play role of baby's father	√	
Faculty to play role of neonatal consultant if advice requested		√

Details for Facilitators

Patient Demographics

Details	Baby Smith
Age	25+5 weeks gestation (at time of delivery)
Weight	Estimated 510 g (2nd centile)
Sex	Female

Scenario Summary for Facilitators

Mother – Emma Smith, 28 years old, primiparous with uneventful pregnancy and normal antenatal scans. Emma has developed severe pre-eclampsia requiring delivery. Has had nifedipine and IV labetalol to control BP. Has had one complete course of dexamethasone, last dose 12 hours before delivery, and magnesium sulphate for neuroprotection (and severe pre-eclampsia). No perinatal risk factors for sepsis.

25-week gestation infant is born by vaginal delivery and is found to be in poor condition, requiring initial inflation and ventilation breaths, proceeding to intubation and administration of endotracheal surfactant for lung immaturity.

If effective airway and breathing support is given, the heart rate will respond and there will be no cardiovascular compromise (i.e. chest compressions and drugs will not be required).

The scenario also focuses on decision-making regarding transfer to the neonatal unit and awareness of needing to update the family.

Set-up Overview for Facilitators

Clinical setting	In a delivery room, baby about to be delivered
Mother's position	In lithotomy
Initial monitoring in place	None for baby
Other equipment	Resuscitaire in room
Useful manikin functions	The manikin used should ideally be an intubatable preterm manikin (e.g. Laerdal Premie Anne®, Life/form Micro-Preemie Simulator®, Gaumard Premie HAL®) which can be mask-ventilated and is intubatable with a size 2.5 mm endotracheal tube

Medical Equipment

Airway		
Oxygen supply with appropriate tubing (piped/cylinders)	Resuscitaire and power supply and overhead heater	Face masks – standard set of neonatal resuscitation masks (premature to infant) – may include Fisher Paykel 35 mm and 42mm for extreme preterm
Suction (portable/on resuscitaire/oxylitre suction regulator and tubing)	Yankauer	Suction catheter (5–10Fr; 2 of each)
T piece (compatible with resuscitaire)	Bag-valve mask (in case of power failure)	ETT Sizes (2), 2.5, 3, 3.5, (4) Size 2 and 4 tubes optional dependent on unit practices
Laryngoscopes Miller sizes 00, 0, 1	Paediatric stethoscope	Oropharyngeal airway(s) sizes ISO 3.5 (pink), 5 (blue), 5.5 (grey)
Saturation probe + posiwrap (to shield out excess light from around the probe)	CO_2 detector (for < 1 kg and > 1 kg)	ET tube fixation device
Transport incubator with ventilator and tubing	Spare AA batteries (for laryngoscope)	Surfactant drawing up and delivery apparatus (incl. appropriate syringe)
Cardiovascular		
ECG leads	UVC (4Fr) insertion kit	Cord clamp and tie
Exposure/Miscellaneous		
Thermometer	Towels (3) and hat (sizes to fit range of infants – preterm and term)	Polythene bag (food bag)
Drugs/infusion equipment		
Adrenaline 1:10,000	Sodium bicarbonate 4.2%	Dextrose 10% (500 ml bag)
0.9% sodium chloride (100 ml bag)	Surfactant (120 mg and 240 mg vials)	

Syringes 1, 3, 5, 10, 20, 50 ml (3 of each)	Needles for drawing up emergency drugs
Paperwork	
Copy of resuscitation record sheet with emergency drug doses	Drug chart

Information Given to the Learners

Handover given to midwife caring for the mother from facilitator:

G (Gestation) – This is Emma Smith. She is a para 0, gravida 1 and 25+5 weeks gestation.

A (Antenatal history) – The antenatal scans have been normal, with nothing to note on her booking bloods. She is O rhesus positive.

M (Maternal problems and medications) – Emma is pre-eclamptic, and we are struggling to control her blood pressure with labetalol and nifedipine. She has completed one full course of dexamethasone 12 hours ago and has been on a magnesium sulphate infusion for over 4 hours.

E (Examination) – The plan is for a vaginal delivery. She is fully dilated and pushing. There are no signs of sepsis in mum.

S (Suggestions) – The delivery of the baby is imminent, can you contact the neonatal team to be present at this delivery?

Scenario Schedule

Stage 1: Imminent delivery of preterm infant. Call to neonatal team and effective handover from maternity team. Checking of equipment and role allocation	
Information given	**Expected actions**
	The midwife should call for the neonatal team to be present urgently (given the imminent delivery)
	(This may involve an SBAR phone call initially then presenting the information given above to the neonatal team)
	The team (including the midwife) should check the resuscitaire / resuscitation equipment ensuring: • Temperature set at maximum, appropriate size hat, polythene bag available to deliver the baby into / put in as soon as possible after delivery • Inflation pressures should be reduced to 20cm H2O, with air/oxygen blender set to 21-30%, and saturation probe ready to place on right arm • Suction equipment should be checked (may replace Yankauer with 10Fr suction catheter (no smaller)) • Endotracheal tubes (sizes 2 and 2.5) may be prepared or sought, with appropriate fixation device
	Team roles should be discussed and allocated.
Progress to stage 2 now even if neonatal team have not been called or full preparation of equipment has not occurred in a timely fashion.	

Stage 2: Delivery of the preterm infant, assessment regarding delayed cord clamping

Information given	Expected Actions
Baby is just delivered, cord not clamped yet	If midwife hasn't called neonatal team in stage 1, midwife needs to activate emergency buzzer, commence newborn resuscitation and urgently call neonatal team
	If neonatal team called in stage 1, they will commence resuscitation
	Start the clock as soon as the whole baby is born
	The infant should be either born into a clear polythene bag, or placed in very soon after delivery
	Assess colour, tone, breathing effort and heart rate on delivery of the infant
If delay in recognising the need for resuscitation, the infant does not improve and the team will be prompted by the facilitator explaining that the infant has stopped breathing completely.	The team should realise quickly that this infant requires resuscitation
	Clamp and cut cord and take infant to the resuscitaire under the radiant heater (if no means of providing effective resuscitation at bedside, e.g. lifestart trolley)

Observations	
A	No crying, floppy infant
B	Irregular gasps seen, blue
C	Heart rate below 60bpm
D	Floppy, not responding to stimulation
E	Cold environment

Progress to stage 3a once cord cut and baby taken to resuscitaire or lifestart trolley in situ (if delayed cord clamping offered, the infant must receive effective airway and breathing support simultaneously. If not, then proceed directly to stage 3b).

Stage 3a: Establishing thermoregulation and pulmonary gas exchange

Information given	Expected actions
	Ensure that the clock has been started
	Dry infant's head and apply hat
	Infant (in the polythene bag) placed under the radiant heater on maximum setting / on transwarmer®
	The infant's head should be placed in the neutral position and appropriate size facemask sought

	Observations
A	Floppy, flexed (should put in neutral position)
B	Irregular gasps / no breaths, blue
C	Heart rate initially below 60bpm. If chest rise seen, heart rate will rise to above 100bpm.
D	Floppy, little response to stimulation
E	Cold environment unless put in polythene bag under heater with hat in place.

Information given	Expected actions
	The team may reassess colour, tone, breathing and heart rate
	Give 5 inflation breaths, with peak pressures of 20cmH$_2$O each lasting for 2-3 seconds, looking for chest movement with each breath (If PEEP is available it should be supplied at 5cmH$_2$O).
	A saturation probe should be placed on the right arm (preductal), though until a steady trace achieved, one team member should assess the apical heart rate with a stethoscope.

If facilitator sees effective chest movement, the heart rate will increase to above 100 (**progress to stage 4**). If no chest movement seen, heart rate remains below 60, with a poor saturation trace (**progress to stage 3b**).

Stage 3b: (only proceed to stage 3b if have not delivered effective inflation breaths in stage 3a) Infant deteriorates, need to ensure effective inflation breaths.

	Observations
A	Floppy, need to recheck and ensure **neutral** position
B	Not breathing, SpO2 not reading
C	HR slow (below 60bpm), blue
D	Floppy, no response to stimulation
E	Cold environment unless in polythene bag under heater with hat in place

Information given	Expected actions
Heart rate will not respond until chest movement has been seen. Once effective inflation breaths are provided, then heart rate increases to above 100bpm.	Re-establish a neutral head position and repeat the inflation breaths
Any attempt at cardiac compressions (ratio 3 compressions: 1 breath) or drugs before effective sustained chest movement is seen will be futile and the infant will continue to deteriorate.	
If the infant is not adequately covered with plastic bag / hat, i.e. thermoregulation has not been addressed, the heart rate will only increase slowly when chest movement is seen.	

Progress to stage 4 once ventilation effective and heart rate increases

Stage 4: Intubation, surfactant delivery and planning for transfer to neonatal intensive care unit (NICU)

Observations	
A	Neutral position, floppy (so needs to be maintained)
B	Irregular gasps seen, improving in frequency, SpO_2 (preductal) 50% in air-30% O_2 **at 3 minutes**
C	HR 120bpm on monitor and auscultation
D	Some active movement, floppy
E	Cold environment unless put in polythene bag under heater with hat in place.

Information given	Expected actions
	Give ventilation breaths (rate approximately 30/minute)
Require over 40% oxygen before saturations are acceptable	Increase oxygen in view of low saturations
If mention CPAP, highlight gasps still present, prompting need for intubation	Assess infant's respiratory effort and consider use of CPAP
	Intubation of infant (manikin spontaneous respiratory rate needs turning off for this procedure)
If intubation successful: • Chest movement should be seen and air entry equal (the ETT insertion distance varies; some manikins may not differentiate between an ETT in the trachea or bronchus – estimated oral insertion distance should be around 6cm at the lips (some manikins may require the ETT further in; facilitators should know this prior to the simulation)) • Oxygen saturations should increase to above 80% • Heart rate should increase (e.g. around 140-160bpm) • CO2 detector should change colour (blue / purple to yellow – depending on type of device used)	Assessment of endotracheal tube(ETT) position should include: • Observe chest movement • Auscultation for air entry • Assessment of heart rate and saturations • CO2 detector (not relying on this alone)
If intubation attempt unsuccessful: • Chest movement should not be seen • Heart rate should fall to below 60bpm • Oxygen saturations should fall to below 40% • No colour change on CO2 detector	Recognise intubation unsuccessful Remove the ETT Recommence mask ventilation and ensure adequate chest expansion prior to any further intubation attempt (consider need for senior help at the point if not done before, e.g. consultant)
If suggest giving surfactant on NICU, drop saturations slowly after successful intubation, so more oxygen is required and prompts its need prior to transfer	Gives surfactant (The whole 120mg vial should be given (normal convention))
	Liaise with NICU regarding setup of bedspace and ventilator, and also discuss how the team are going to get the baby to NICU and keep warm (may use pre-warmed transport incubator / transwarmer®).

Scenario ends with an update to parents (facilitator) with an explanation of what has happened and what is planned next

Suggested Topics for Debrief Discussion

- How was the handover from midwifery to neonatal team?
- How well prepared was the equipment for neonatal resuscitation and equipment for transfer to NICU of a preterm infant?
- Did the team follow the Newborn Life Support algorithm, with particular emphasis on managing a preterm infant?

Discussion

Teamwork and Effective Handover

Effective teamwork and communication are essential in ensuring that resuscitation or stabilisation, including thermoregulation, is instigated as early as possible in a significantly preterm infant.

This requires clear, structured conversations to occur between all members of the perinatal team throughout. Using structured tools such as SBAR (Situation, Background, Assessment, Recommendation) and GAMES (Gestation, Antenatal problems, Maternal problems and medication, Examination findings, Suggested actions) allows cohesive, succinct communication between teams, so that situations can be anticipated and dealt with in a timely, effective manner. In this scenario, it is imperative that the message gets from the maternal to the neonatal team in good time to allow planning and role allocation to take place before the infant is born, so that effective measures can be put in place early, increasing the chance of success.

When the neonatal resuscitation team is assembled, or ideally even beforehand, it is vital that appropriate equipment is available and checked, with adjustments made in line with the gestation of the infant to be delivered.

Teams need to be well prepared with a clear leader and roles assigned, especially in the setting of a preterm delivery. It is well known that planning prevents problems arising and an effective team leader needs to have overall situational awareness, be able to prioritise tasks and delegate appropriately, make clear decisions and communicate these succinctly to the team and anticipate problems that might arise. Teams are much more efficient when tasks are addressed simultaneously rather than in a linear fashion. This requires effective leadership and followership. Team members

need to know to whom feedback should be directed, using closed-loop communication. Depending on the skills of the team members, the leadership role may have to be passed on during the scenario, as it is well documented and appreciated that one cannot lead effectively while performing a task, e.g. intubation. The passage of this role needs to be clear to all members of the team.

Thermoregulation in the Preterm Infant

The preterm infant is particularly vulnerable to heat loss due to immature skin, large surface area to volume ratio, reduced subcutaneous fat and poor thermoregulatory mechanisms. There is a significantly increased mortality associated with hypothermia in infants of around 28% for every 1 °C below 36 °C. Not only this, but hypothermia has a significant effect on an infant's ability to produce surfactant to aid lung maturity, and is associated with hypoxia, pulmonary hypertension, hypoglycaemia and coagulation problems. Resuscitating a cold infant is much more difficult and prolonged than if thermoregulation was considered at the beginning and throughout the resuscitation process. This can be done by:

- ensuring an adequate environmental temperature, ideally at least 26 °C, and minimising drafts;
- the early application of a hat on the infant's head, where a large amount of the heat loss takes place;
- for the preterm infant, placing the infant in a polythene bag under a radiant heater, as soon as possible after birth.

These procedures to minimise heat loss should be maintained during the resuscitation/stabilisation process and continued during transfer to the neonatal unit. For infants born below 32 weeks' gestation, it is recommended that multiple methods of minimising temperature loss are employed. These can also include the use of a warming infant transport mattress, e.g. TransWarmer®, especially if the infant is still found to be cold during resuscitation.

Cord Clamping in Preterm Infants

Although there are significant benefits of delayed cord clamping for preterm infants (increased circulating blood volume and subsequent cardiovascular stability, decreased need for blood transfusions and decreased risk of intraventricular haemorrhages and necrotizing enterocolitis), these have only been seen in infants with evidence of an effective circulation. It is important to be able to make this clinical decision quickly and also paying attention to the infant's temperature. If there is doubt around the stability of the infant or thermoregulation is compromised, it is wise to clamp and cut the cord quickly and instigate any necessary resuscitation measures, unless these measures can be performed safely and effectively by the bedside while ensuring adequate thermoregulation.

Airway and Ventilation Management in the Preterm Infant

The fragility of the preterm lung needs to be considered. For the term infant, peak inspiratory pressures are usually preset at 30 cmH_2O, but using these pressures initially on a preterm would cause huge tidal volume delivery and significantly increase the risk of air leaks, as well as later chronic lung disease. Studies have shown that even using sustained peak pressures of 20–25 cmH_2O can produce tidal volumes in excess of 10 ml/kg, and that a more gentle approach may be beneficial. This means commencing the inflation breaths, to replace the pulmonary fluid with air, using initial peak pressures of 20–25 cmH_2O, ideally in the presence of PEEP (positive end-expiratory pressure), set at 5 cmH_2O. Studies have also shown that the unnecessary use of high oxygen concentrations, especially in the preterm infant, can be harmful to the developing organs, and hence resuscitation is commenced in room air 30%-O_2, with early use of a saturation monitor in place to assess the need for additional oxygen.

During mask inflation and ventilation breaths, attention needs to be focused on creating an effective mask seal, ensuring correct size of mask (covering the nose and mouth, without encroaching over the eyes or chin) and that its position, pressure placed through the mask and providing a chin support are maintained. Practitioners need to be aware of the distribution of the pressure they are exerting through the mask, so as not to create a leak and avoid excessive pressure being passed through the infant's head, causing unnecessary bruising. To aid assessment of efficacy, the early placement of a saturation probe not only assists the team with whether additional oxygen is required to avoid hypoxia (or hyperoxia, which can have significant adverse longer-term effects), but also assessment of the heart rate (for which a rise signifies sufficient chest inflation has occurred). The quoted acceptable saturations (see Figure 37.1) are based on a study of over 450 infants, although only 39 were under 32 weeks' gestation. However, when the data was subanalysed, the readings for this preterm group were only very slightly less than their term counterparts and hence the published acceptable right arm saturations hold for preterm infants also.

Although a large majority of more mature preterm infants require stabilisation using CPAP (continuous positive airway pressure) in the spontaneously breathing infant, it is important to anticipate in the more immature infant that ventilator support may be required and endotracheal intubation performed in the delivery room. This involves prior preparation of a range of endotracheal tubes, based on the infant's weight and gestation, and appropriate suction device. A Yankauer device may be difficult to use in the extreme preterm infant, so a large bore (10 Fr) flexible suction catheter should be available and checked.

Intubation should ideally only be considered when the infant is stable, after successful mask inflation and rise in heart rate. It is important that when performed, it is done with the least disruption to the transitional physiology as possible. Human factors are of huge importance in this process and should be explored in any debrief. The practitioner should also be aware of the need for the correct size tube and position (as a rule of thumb, the distance inserted at the lips should equal 6 + weight (in kilograms) (if above 1 kg)). Multiple methods should be used to check for its correct insertion into the trachea, not merely relying on the CO_2 detector changing colour (false negative with very small tidal volumes, low cardiac output; false positive after contact with surfactant). Once intubated, and especially if surfactant is given, the infant should ideally be connected to a ventilator where tidal volume delivery can be measured and excessive tidal volumes avoided. The peak inspiratory pressure usually requires decreasing after intubation and surfactant delivery to prevent the delivery of excessive tidal volumes.

Communication with Families

Communication with families following any kind of resuscitation is of utmost importance and great care is required to provide clear, honest and open messages. It is important to establish what is already known and their understanding of the situation, ideally at least referring to the infant's gender, or name (if given). Admission to a neonatal unit usually involves prolonged separation between families and the newborn infant, which in turn increases anxiety, which can be reduced by timely updates with the family and allowing

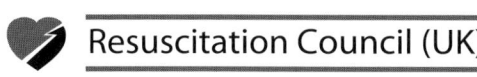 **Resuscitation Council (UK)** GUIDELINES 2015 **Newborn Life Support**

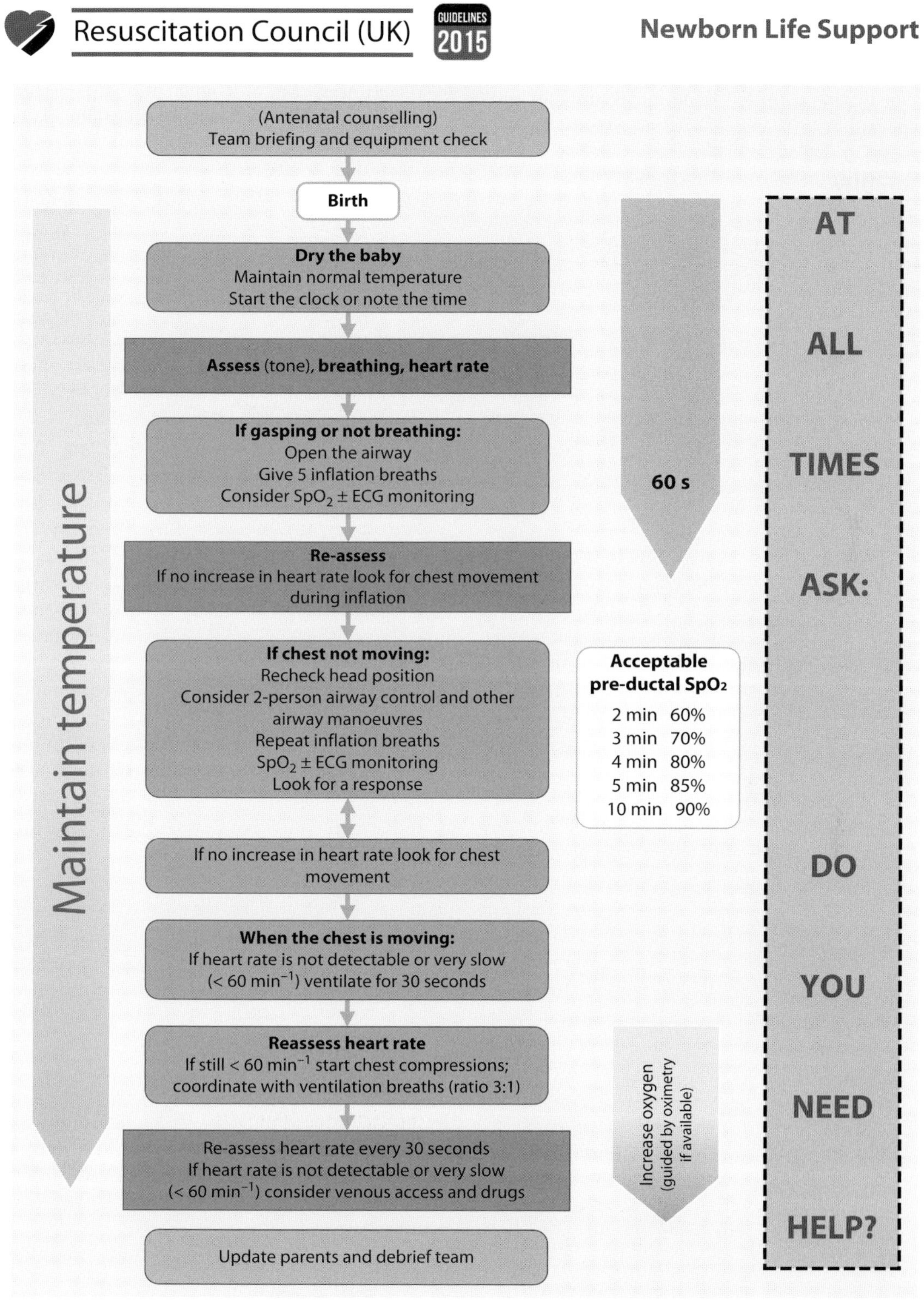

Maintain temperature

(Antenatal counselling)
Team briefing and equipment check

Birth

Dry the baby
Maintain normal temperature
Start the clock or note the time

Assess (tone), **breathing, heart rate**

If gasping or not breathing:
Open the airway
Give 5 inflation breaths
Consider SpO_2 ± ECG monitoring

Re-assess
If no increase in heart rate look for chest movement
during inflation

If chest not moving:
Recheck head position
Consider 2-person airway control and other
airway manoeuvres
Repeat inflation breaths
SpO_2 ± ECG monitoring
Look for a response

If no increase in heart rate look for chest
movement

When the chest is moving:
If heart rate is not detectable or very slow
(< 60 min^{-1}) ventilate for 30 seconds

Reassess heart rate
If still < 60 min^{-1} start chest compressions;
coordinate with ventilation breaths (ratio 3:1)

Re-assess heart rate every 30 seconds
If heart rate is not detectable or very slow
(< 60 min^{-1}) consider venous access and drugs

Update parents and debrief team

60 s

**Acceptable
pre-ductal SpO_2**

2 min   60%
3 min   70%
4 min   80%
5 min   85%
10 min 90%

Increase oxygen
(guided by oximetry
if available)

AT

ALL

TIMES

ASK:

DO

YOU

NEED

HELP?

Figure 37.1 NLS 2015 Algorithm. Reproduced with the kind permission of the Resuscitation Council (UK).

access to see their child. These conversations are the beginning of building trusting relationships between the healthcare team and the family, which are paramount for infants admitted to neonatal units for prolonged periods.

Bibliography

BLISS. (2011). Making critical care decisions for your baby. Available from: www.bliss.org.uk (accessed March 27, 2017).

Fawke, J. and Cusack, J. (2014). *Advanced Resuscitation of the Newborn Infant*, 1st edition. London: Resuscitation Council UK.

Wyllie, J., Ainsworth, S., Tinnion, R. and Hampshire, S. (2016). *Newborn Life Support*, 4th edition. London: Resuscitation Council UK.

Index